CONTENTS

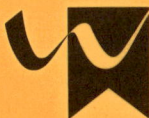

UNDERSTANDING AND CHANGING HEALTH BEHAVIOUR

UNDERSTANDING AND CHANGING HEALTH BEHAVIOUR

From Health Beliefs to Self-Regulation

Edited by

Paul NORMAN
University of Sheffield, UK

Charles ABRAHAM
University of Sussex, UK

and

Mark CONNER
University of Leeds, UK

harwood academic publishers
Australia • Canada • France • Germany • India
Japan • Luxembourg • Malaysia • The Netherlands
Russia • Singapore • Switzerland

Amsteldijk 166
1st Floor
1079 LH Amsterdam
The Netherlands

British Library Cataloguing in Publication Data.

A catalogue record for this book is available from the British Library.

ISBN: 90-5823-073-2 (hard cover)

LIST OF FIGURES

LIST OF TABLES

PREFACE

The identification of the factors predicting health behaviours has become a major focus of research in health psychology and related disciplines. The identification of such factors not only increases our understanding of health behaviour but also identifies cognitive targets for interventions designed to change health behaviour and recommends potentially effective approaches to health promotion. This book focuses on a range of social cognitive factors, from health beliefs to self-regulation processes, that have been highlighted as the proximal determinants of health behaviour. The book brings together work from two recent special issues of *Psychology & Health* on 'Social Cognition Models in Health Psychology' (Guest Editors: Mark Conner and   Paul Norman) and 'Self-Regulation and Health' (Guest Editors: Charles Abraham and Marie Johnston). A selection of papers from these two special issues, as well as two new papers, have been included to (i) outline the contribution that a social cognitive approach can make to our understanding of the determinants of health behaviour, (ii) highlight current conceptual and methological issues in this field, (iii) explore the way in which cognitive change is link to behaviour change, (iv) indicate cognitive targets for interventions designed to promote change, (v) link cognitive models of change to techniques designed to promote change, and finally, (vi) suggest promising directions for future research.

The book is split into six sections. Section 1 consists of an introductory chapter that provides an overview and integration of the social cognitive approaches presented in this book. In this chapter Abraham and Sheeran consider the key social cognitive antecedents of health behaviour. Drawing upon models such as the Theory of Planned Behaviour and Social Cognitive Theory they outline a core model of 'motivation' (i.e. intention formation). They then consider how intentions may be translated into action through volitional or 'action control' process, highlighting the importance of preparatory acts, planning and rehearsal. Finally, they discuss the way in which particular goals may or may not be prioritised, acknowledging the multi-goal context in which everyday action control occurs.

Section 2 presents a number of applications of social cognition models (i.e. Protection Motivation Theory, the Health Belief Model, and the Theories of Reasoned and Planned Behaviour) to the prediction of health behaviour (i.e. condom use, breast self-examination, and cycle helmet use). In Chapter 2 Morrison, Baker and Gillmore report the results of a longitudinal study examining the predictive utility of the Theory of Reasoned Action in relation to condom use among high-risk heterosexual teens over a three month period. The Theory of Reasoned Action provided strong predictions of intentions to use condoms with both steady and casual partners, but was less predictive of actual condom use. Milne and Orbell (Chapter 3) consider another popular model of health behaviour, Protection Motivation Theory, to examine the predictors of beast self-examination (BSE). This study represents one of the few longitudinal studies of Protection Motivation Theory. The results of the study highlighted self-efficacy as the key predictor of women's intentions to perform BSE over the next month which, in turn, were predictive of subsequent BSE behaviour. However, further analyses revealed that the Protection Motivation Theory variables were unable to mediate the influence of previous BSE behaviour, suggesting that the model is not sufficient. In Chapter 4, Quine, Rutter and Arnold present a comparison of two social cognition models of the attitude-behaviour relationship – the Health Belief Model and the Theory of Planned Behaviour. In a longitudinal study of cycle helmet use among schoolboy cyclists, they found the Theory of Planned Behaviour to provide a more powerful prediction of behaviour than the Health Belief Model. Quine, Rutter and Arnold proceed to outline a number of reasons for the better predictive utility of the Theory of Planned Behaviour.

Section 3 considers some extensions to social cognition models of health behaviour. Two of the chapters in this section focus on the common distinction made between attitudinal and normative influences on health behaviour. In Chapter 4 Trafimow evaluates a number of arguments that question the validity of the attitude-normative distinction before presenting a range of evidence to support the distinction. Empirical support for this distinction has important implications for models that seek to understand, predict and change health behaviour, for example, in relation to the separate measurement and targeting of normative beliefs. Given the validity of this distinction, Agnew (Chapter 6) considers various methods for assessing behavioural beliefs (which constitute attitudes) and normative beliefs as outlined in the Theories of Reasoned Action and Planned Behaviour. Studies using these theories will typically conduct a pilot study to identify the 'model salient' behavioural and normative beliefs. These beliefs are taken to be representative of important beliefs relevant to the specified behaviour among the studied population and are measured in the main study. However, a number of researchers have suggested that asking respondents to generate and rate their own personal beliefs might provide a better method for assessing behavioural and normative beliefs. Agnew reports a study comparing these two methods of belief elicitation and concludes that the slight gains in predictive and ecological validity provided by self-generated beliefs need to be weighted against practical considerations of the extra effort involved in collecting these data. In Chapter 7 Gibbons, Gerrard, Ouellette and Burzette question the utility of 'rational' models of health behaviour to explain potentially health-compromising behaviours such as smoking, drinking, driving and unprotected sex. They argue for a distinction between two 'pathways' to risk behaviour – a 'reasoned' path which proceeds through behavioural intention (or behavioural expectation), and a 'social reaction' path which proceeds through behavioural willingness (i.e. one's willingness to engage in the behaviour given certain opportunities to do so). Thus, for example, while a person might not intend to have unprotected sex, he or she might be willing to do so given certain circumstances. Gibbons *et al.* present results from two studies that confirm the additional predictive utility of behavioural willingness in relation to adolescent smoking behaviour and drink driving. In addition, their results suggest that behavioural willingness to engage in a risk behaviour may be associated with a denial of the risks involved.

Section 4 examines the utility of stage models of health behaviour. Recent work has suggested that there may be qualitatively different stages in the initiation and maintenance of health behaviour and that different cognitions may be important at different stages. Two of the studies presented here examine one of the most widely used stage models – the Transtheoretical Model of Change. According to the most widely applied version of the Transtheoretical Model of Change, there are five stages of change: precontemplation, contemplation, preparation, action and maintenance. Individuals are seen to progress through each stage to achieve successful maintenance of a new behaviour. DeVries and Mudde (Chapter 8) present results from a prospective study with individuals attempting to quit smoking. Those in different stages in relation to smoking cessation were found to differ on several social cognition variables and, more importantly, different cognitions were predictive of stage progression for those at different stages. However, while Courneya, Nigg and Estabrooks (Chapter 9) found Theory of Planned Behaviour constructs to be predictive of exercise stage over a three-year period, their data do not support the addition of Transtheoretical Model, stage-of-change, measures to predictive models. Courneya and colleagues criticise the distinctions between stages in the Transtheoretical Model of Change and this point is elaborated on by Sutton in Chapter 10. Sutton reviews the empirical evidence from recent studies on smoking cessation for the existence of different stages, stage transitions and the efficacy of stage matched-mismatched interventions. He concludes that the results of these studies question the validity and utility of the Transtheoretical Model of Change.

Section 5 focuses on the development and application of self-regulation models of health behaviour. These models seek to identify cognitive processes involved in setting, prioritising and implementing goals. In doing so they extend cognition models beyond attitudes and behaviour and provide health psychologists with new intervention targets. Gollwitzer and Oettingen (Chapter 11) explain how advances in self-regulation modelling illuminate the process of goal setting and allow us to distinguish between intentions which are and are not translated into action. They outline a model of action phases and related mindsets and illustrate the importance of developing specific context-related plans to implement action (i.e. 'implementation intentions'). They also consider how positive fantasies may inhibit action but can also be employed to motivate health behaviour change when contrasted with negative realities. In Chapter 12 Bagozzi and Edwards report a longitudinal study of weight loss demonstrating how self-regulatory resources can be measured and used to predict attainment of a health-related goal. Drawing upon a similar theoretical background to that developed by Gollwitzer and Oettingen, they investigate the links between psychological antecedents of intention formation (including self-efficacy, subjective norms, attitudes and desire), intention formation, efforts to control one's behaviour, preparatory actions (or instrumental acts) and actual goal achievement. They also report a second study which introduces a new approach to the exploration of goal hierarchies within which health-related intentions may be embedded. Bandura (Chapter 13) describes social cognitive theory and compares its health promotion application to those of similar models such as the Theory of Planned Behaviour. He shows how an understanding of self-regulation processes can provide the basis for effective health promotion and illustrates this by describing a computer-based system capable of giving patients personalised feedback on their self-regulatory progress. Bandura also makes a convincing case for the importance of developing 'collective self-efficacy' by raising public awareness and developing local-level action plans aimed at achieving changes of everyday relevance to participants. In doing so he reminds us that health psychology has always had a community-development agenda and points to the role of health psychologists as community psychologists.

Finally, in Section 6, Abraham, Norman and Conner focus on the implications of work described in the book for the development of a psychology of behaviour change which could inform health promotion practice. They discuss the utility of defining stages of cognitive change and explore relationships between cognition tendencies, personality and health-related behaviour. This discussion has implications for how interventions should be developed and targeted for particular audiences. They then consider the more practical question of what kind of cognitive change techniques can be employed to promote health-related behaviour, that is, how can we change cognition and behaviour? Finally, they outline the potential implications of some advances in social cognitive and self-regulation theory, including the diffusion of successful interventions and the design of interventions focusing on responsibility for action as well as the links between health-related behaviour and underlying motivators, such as looking and feeling good.

We would like to finish by taking the opportunity to thank all the authors who have contributed their work to this book. This collection of work illustrates the importance of a social cognitive approach for furthering our understanding of health behaviour and informing the development of interventions designed to change health behaviour.

Paul NORMAN, Charles ABRAHAM and Mark CONNER

LIST OF CONTRIBUTORS

Charles Abraham
School of Social Sciences, University of Sussex, Brighton, UK

Christopher R. Agnew
Department of Psychological Sciences, Purdue University, West Lafayette, USA

Laurence Arnold
Department of Psychology, University of Kent at Canterbury, UK

Richard P. Bagozzi
Michigan Business School, University of Michigan, Ann Arbor, USA

Sharon A. Baker
Department of Psychology, University of Washington, Seattle, USA

Albert Bandura
Department of Psychology, Stanford University, California, USA

Rebecca Burzette
Department of Psychology, Iowa State University, Ames, USA

Mark Conner
School of Psychology, University of Leeds, UK

Kerry S. Courneya
Faculty of Physical Education, University of Alberta, Edmonton, Canada

Hein De Vries
Department of Health Education, University of Limburg, Maastricht, The Netherlands

Arie Dijkstra
Department of Clinical and Health Psychology, University of Leiden, The Netherlands

Elizabeth A. Edwards
College of Business, Eastern Michigan University, Ypsilanti, USA

Paul A. Estabrooks
Faculty of Kinesiology, University of Western Ontario, London, Canada

Meg Gerrard
Department of Psychology, Iowa State University, Ames, USA

Frederick X. Gibbons
Department of Psychology, Iowa State University, Ames, USA

Mary Rogers Gillmore
Department of Psychology, University of Washington, Seattle, USA

Peter M. Gollwitzer
Department of Psychology, New York University, USA

Sarah E. Milne
Department of Psychology, University of Bath, UK

Diane M. Morrison
Department of Psychology, University of Washington, Seattle, USA

Aart N. Mudde
Department of Health Education, University of Limburg, Maastricht, The Netherlands

Claudio R. Nigg
Department of Experimental Psychology, University of Rhode Island, Kingston, USA

Paul Norman
Department of Psychology, University of Sheffield, UK

Gabriele Oettingen
Department of Psychology, New York University, USA

Sheina Orbell
Department of Psychology, University of Sheffield, UK

Judith A. Ouellette
Department of Psychology, Iowa State University, Ames, USA

Lyn Quine
Department of Psychology, University of Kent at Canterbury, UK

Derek R. Rutter
Department of Psychology, University of Kent at Canterbury, UK

Paschal Sheeran
Department of Psychology, University of Sheffield, UK

Stephen Sutton
Health Behaviour Unit, University College London, UK

David Trafimow
Department of Psychology, New Mexico State University, Las Cruces, USA

Section 1 –
Introduction

CHAPTER ONE

Understanding and Changing Health Behaviour: From Health Beliefs to Self-Regulation

Charles ABRAHAM & Paschal SHEERAN

A series of 'social cognition' models which specify modifiable cognitive antecedents of action have been proposed (Conner & Norman, 1996; Eagly & Chaiken, 1993). In this introductory chapter we review the development of these models and identify core constructs representing correspondences between them. We also discuss recent theorising which, looking beyond motivation, has focused on action control and self-regulation processes. In doing so we map progress from early attempts to model health-related beliefs (Hochbaum, 1958) to recent explorations of the cognitive underpinnings goal-related action initiation and maintenance (Gollwitzer & Bargh, 1996).

Social cognition models have been tested by using differences in self-reported cognitions to predict health-related behaviour. For example, differences in reported health beliefs have been used to predict reported preventive action such as condom use (Abraham, Sheeran, Spears & Abrams, 1992) and recorded attendance at screening appointments (King, 1982). Reviews suggest that self-report measures based on these models do reliably distinguish between those who do and do not undertake a range of health behaviours (e.g., Bandura, 1992; Godin & Kok, 1996; Sheppard, Hartwick & Warshaw, 1988). On this basis it has been argued that interventions targeting cognitions specified by these models could effectively promote health-enhancing behaviour and/or improve the outcomes of healthcare services. In general the evidence has been supportive. Since the earliest tests of the health belief model, interventions designed to change theory-specified cognition have been shown to promote health-related behaviour (Haefner & Kirscht, 1970). Moreover, in some areas, interventions based on social cognition models have been shown to be more effective than interventions without such theoretical foundations. For example, the rapid development of interventions designed to promote HIV-preventive behaviour resulted in few theoretically-based programmes or campaigns and almost none of these were found to influence sexual behaviour (Fisher & Fisher, 1992; Oakley et al., 1995). By contrast, more recent HIV-preventive interventions based on social cognition models have proved to be effective in controlled trials (Bryan, Aiken & West, 1996; Fisher et al., 1996; Kalichman, Carey & Johnson, 1996; Schaalma et al., 1996).

3

Thus these models appear to offer a theoretical, evidence-based foundation for health promotion activities. Moreover, the relationship between social cognition theorists and health promoters may be symbiotic because evaluative studies of theory-based interventions can provide validity tests of the models themselves. There are also promising indications that recent theorising concerning control processes, such as action initiation and maintenance, may facilitate the development of even more effective behaviour-change interventions (see e.g., Chapters 11–13 by Gollwitzer & Oettingen, Bagozzi & Edwards, and Bandura, respectively).

DEVELOPMENT OF A MODEL OF REASONED MOTIVATION

The availability of many overlapping social cognition models may itself discourage consistent application to intervention design. Bandura (Chapter 13 & Bandura, 1998) is critical of the proliferation of such models and, in our view, the identification of a summary model which is both 'content-free' and 'parsimonious' (Ajzen, 1998) would be useful to those involved in intervention design. Such a model would highlight common theoretical understandings of the cognitive antecedents of motivation but could be extended to incorporate behaviour-specific antecedents in a problem-based manner (see Ajzen, 1998; Kok & Schaalma, 1998). Four key advances in this area provide a basis for such a summary model.

First, the development of the health belief model (HBM) (Rosenstock, 1974). The HBM specifies a series of subjectively rational beliefs that could account for individual differences in motivation and action. The model highlights threat perceptions as a central component of motivation and conceptualises such appraisals in terms of beliefs about the extent of perceived *susceptibility* to and *severity* of a health problem (e.g., 'It is unlikely that I will contract lung cancer' and 'I would die soon after contracting lung cancer', respectively). Susceptibility and severity beliefs are outcome expectancies, that is, beliefs about what will happen if the person does or does not perform a particular action or sequence of actions. Both have been shown to correlate with measures of health-related behaviour. However – and perhaps surprisingly – such correlations tend to be small (Janz & Becker, 1984; Sheeran & Abraham, 1996). Harrison, Mullen and Green (1992), for example, found that these measures accounted for 1–2% of the variance in behaviour across studies.

A number of explanations for these weak relationships have been considered. Perceived severity may correlate poorly with behaviour (Maddux & Rogers, 1983; Schwarzer, 1992; Schwarzer & Fuchs, 1996; Wurtele & Maddux, 1987) because perceptions of severity only influence motivation when severity exceeds a certain threshold, and, once this threshold is reached, perceived susceptibility may be a more important component (Sheeran & Abraham, 1996; Weinstein, 1988). There has also been some debate about the meaning of correlations between perceived susceptibility to a health hazard and preventive action and about the most appropriate measures of susceptibility beliefs (see e.g., Gerrard, Gibbons & Bushman, 1996; Weinstein, 1988; Weinstein & Nicolich, 1993). Two points are worth highlighting here. First, there is a difference between simple awareness of a risk ('Have you heard of X?') and estimates of the magnitude of the risk to oneself ('How likely is X to happen to you over the next five years?') (Weinstein, 1988; Weinstein & Sandman, 1992). Secondly, when previous behaviour is not controlled for, correlations may reflect the impact of behaviour on perceived susceptibility, rather than vice versa, so that those who take more precautions perceive less risk (Weinstein & Nicolich, 1993). This latter problem may be addressed by controlling for reported health behaviours and measuring anticipated personal susceptibility in the absence of taking precautions (Sheeran & Abraham, 1996; Van der Pligt, 1998). For example, Van der Velde, Hooykaas and Van der Pligt (1996) found that 'conditional' measures of perceived susceptibility (which specified taking no precautions) were more likely to be related to intention than 'unconditional' assessments. Overall then, perceived severity may be less important than perceived susceptibility and the latter may be less central to health-related motivation than is suggested by the HBM. Nevertheless, there is little doubt that ensuring people are aware of a health threat and persuading them that they are susceptible to it unless they act (i.e., reducing defensive optimism, Schwarzer, 1998) is likely to be prerequisite to the promotion of health-related action (Weinstein, 1988; Wurtele, 1988).

Perceived barriers to action and perceived effectiveness of health-related actions (i.e., '*response efficacy*') are also included in the health belief model. The former may be a component of self-efficacy (see below) (e.g., 'It is difficult for me to get through the day without a cigarette.') and both refer to relationships between outcome expectancies and individual goals (e.g., 'I will not be able to concentrate at work without cigarettes.' and 'Cutting down on cigarettes reduces the chances of contracting lung cancer.'). However, the specification of 'barriers' and 'response efficacy' may underestimate the importance of other outcome expectancies. For example, the perceived likelihood of negatively evaluated emotional or social consequences of health-protective actions may be more important than health-protective outcomes (e.g., Abraham, et al., 1992; Richard, van der Pligt & de Vries 1995, see below).

A second crucial advance was made by Fishbein and Ajzen who demonstrated that behavioural prediction depended upon the use of cognition measures which describe the action/s concerned at the same level of specificity as the behaviour measure (Ajzen & Fishbein, 1977; Fishbein & Ajzen, 1975; Ajzen, 1988). For example, when identifying the cognitive antecedents of a particular action, such as destroying all your remaining cigarettes when you get home, statements used to assess individual beliefs, or cognitions should refer to this *particular action* towards this *target* in this *context* at this *time*. Similarly, when measuring cognitions relevant to the achievement of a behavioural goal which involves a sequences of actions over time, such as not smoking over the next week, cognition measures should specify that particular goal e.g., not smoking over the next week.

A third important advance was made when Fishbein and Ajzen proposed that *intention* formation provides a mechanism by which action-relevant beliefs and outcome expectancies affect behaviour (e.g., Fishbein & Ajzen, 1975). The theory of reasoned action (TRA) specifies attitudes and subjective norms (see below) as antecedents of intention formation and has been extensively tested over a twenty year period (e.g., Fishbein & Ajzen, 1975; Van den Putte, 1991). For example, the TRA has been employed to identify beliefs correlated with safer sex intentions which, in turn, have been shown to predict reports of subsequent safer sexual behaviour amongst a variety of samples (Fisher, Fisher & Rye, 1995; Sheeran, Abraham & Orbell, 1999).

There is considerable variability in the strength of the intention-behaviour relationship across different health behaviours but reported intentions are reliably and moderately correlated with a range of health actions (Armitage & Conner, in press; Godin & Kok, 1996; Randall & Wolff, 1994; Sheppard, Hartwick & Warshaw, 1988). For example, in a review of studies of health behaviours, Godin and Kok (1996) report intention-behaviour correlations of 0.35 across six studies of screening attendance, 0.52 across eight applications to exercise behaviour, 0.56 across five applications to addictive behaviour and an overall correlation of .46 (across twenty six applications). Comparisons of intention-behaviour correlations using self-report and observational behavioural measures suggest that correlations are somewhat lower when observational behavioural measures are employed (Armitage & Conner, in press). However, across studies, we can expect intention measures to account for 20%–25% of the variance in health behaviour measures. This indicates that other cognitive antecedents of health behaviour need to be considered but, nonetheless, establishes reported intention strength as a key indicator of cognitive preparedness for action. This is underlined by Sutton (1998) who identifies nine reasons, including inherent methodological limitations, why better behavioural prediction has not been achieved. In addition Sutton points out that percentage of variance explained is a 'pessimistic' effect size measure. He shows, for example, that, even when only 16% of the variance in behaviour is explained, this can correspond to a 40% success rate difference between an intervention and control group and an odds ratio of 5.4.

A fourth key advance is described by Ajzen (1998) as follows: 'If one had to point to one profound insight produced by work on self-regulation, it is probably the tremendous importance of self-efficacy beliefs or perceived behavioural control' (p. 738). The addition of perceived behavioural control to the theory of reasoned action, created the theory of planned behaviour (Ajzen, 1991; Ajzen & Madden, 1986).

There is some debate about of the definition of perceived behavioural control and its relationship to self-efficacy beliefs (see e.g., Sparks, Guthrie & Shepherd, 1997; Terry & O'Leary, 1995). Self-efficacy has been typically defined in terms of perceived personal competence or confidence (e.g., 'I believe I can do X successfully.') while perceived behavioural control also includes measures of perceived barriers and difficulties (e.g., 'Doing X would be difficult.'). Conner and Sparks (1996) note that some studies have found low reliabilities for multi-item scales designed to incorporate both these aspects of perceived control and Sparks et al., (1997) present evidence from two studies showing that perceived control and perceived difficulty have different relationships to intentions to change eating behaviours. By contrast, it has been argued (e.g., Schwarzer, 1992) that self-efficacy is related to a variety of perceptions of the self, social context and task demands and that multi-item measures which assess personal confidence in relation to perceived barriers can take account of these various components (e.g., 'I believe I can successfully do X even when difficulty Y is present.') This alternative view suggests that self-efficacy and perceived behavioural control can be regarded as synonyms (see Ajzen, 1998; Bandura, 1998) and, in the interests of conceptual simplification, we shall use the term '*self-efficacy*' to mean an overall sense of control taking account of both personal resources and perceived barriers (in the HBM sense).

Bandura and others have demonstrated that self-efficacy to successfully perform an action is predictive of actual success (e.g., Bandura, 1992; Bandura, 1997; Schwarzer & Fuchs, 1996). Those who believe they will succeed are, in general, more likely to: formulate intentions to act (e.g., De Vries & Backbier, 1994), set themselves higher goals, exert greater effort, regard errors as learning experiences and persevere for longer. They are also less likely to be distracted by anxiety and self-doubt during performance (Bandura, 1992). The TPB suggests that self-efficacy promotes action primarily through bolstering strength of intention and this view is supported by evidence showing that that, while self-efficacy is correlated with behaviour, it does not necessarily add to the prediction of behaviour achieved by intention measures (Godin & Kok, 1996). This is illustrated in Chapter 2 by Morrison, Baker and Gillmore (see also Morrison, Baker & Gillmore, 1998). In a longitudinal study of study of high-risk heterosexual teenagers Morrison and colleagues found that self-efficacy did not add to the variance explained in condom use once strength of intention had been taken into account. Note, however, that in their study of safety helmet use amongst schoolboy cyclists, Quine, Rutter and Arnold report (in Chapter 4) that self-efficacy did add to the model's capacity to predict helmet use, although this ceased to be the case once previous behaviour was included (see also, Quine, Rutter & Arnold, 1998). Self-efficacy may be most likely to enhance prediction when the action/s concerned are perceived as being generally less controllable (Madden, Ellen & Ajzen, 1992). For example, Godin & Kok (1996) found that self-efficacy measures explained most behavioural variance (in addition to that explained by intention measures) in the case of addictive behaviours.

Figure 1.1 maps out core cognitive constructs which have been used to predict a variety of health behaviours. The dotted line between self-efficacy beliefs and behaviour is derived from the theory of planned behaviour (TPB) (e.g., Ajzen, 1991) and represents variability in the additional variance explained by self-efficacy after the association between intention and behaviour has been considered.

The TPB presents intentions and self-efficacy beliefs as the immediate predictors of behaviour. Other cognitions are throught to promote action through their effects on intention formation or perceived self-efficacy (Fishbein & Ajzen, 1975; Bandura, 1992). Health-related intentions may develop from a variety of values, perceptions and understandings which are inadequately represented by the HBM. This is illustrated by Milne and Orbell in Chapter 3 (see also Hodgkins & Orbell, 1998) who test protection motivation theory, a model derived from the health belief model, and observe that only self-efficacy predicted strength of intention. They also point out that past behaviour, rather than the specified cognition measures, was the most powerful predictor of

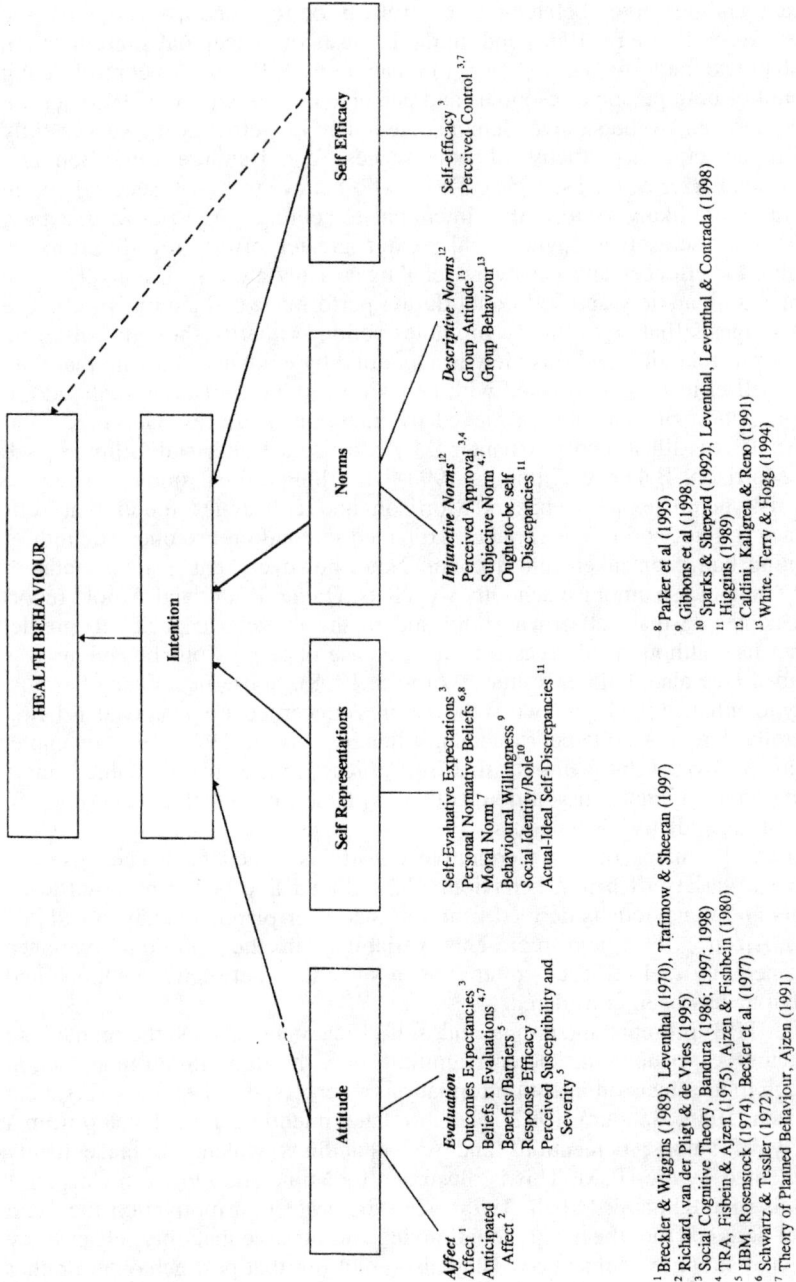

Figure 1.1   Core cognitive antecedents of health behaviours

future behaviour, suggesting that the model does not adequately describe the cognitive antecedents of either intention or behaviour. Of course, this does not mean that strength of intention is unrelated to such health beliefs. In Chapter 4, Quine, Rutter and Arnold report that the health belief model accounted for 22% of the variance in strength of intentions to wear helmets. However, TPB measures, including self-efficacy, accounted for 34% of the variance in the same intention. Similarly, in Hodgkins and Orbell's study, self-efficacy alone accounted for 20% of the variance in intention.

Bagozzi (1992) proposed that *desires* (e.g., 'I want to do X.') and self-efficacy are key precursors of intention formation. Desires may in turn be based on *attitudes* or *outcome expectancies* (see Bagozzi & Edwards, Chapter 12). Outcome expectancies (Bandura, 1992, 1998) overlap with 'attitude' measures specified by the TRA/TPB framework (e.g., 'For me, using a condom would be good/bad.') (see Ajzen, 1998). According to the TRA, beliefs concerning the likelihood of various outcomes (e.g., 'A condom is likely to protect me against HIV/AIDS.') multiplied by the individual's evaluations of those outcomes (e.g., 'Protecting myself against HIV/AIDS is important to me.') index a person's attitude towards a behaviour. Studies have shown that people who do or do not engage in specified behaviours may differ both in relation to anticipated outcomes (e.g., of taking medication) and in relation to how positively or negatively they evaluate those potential consequences (e.g., Werner & Middlestadt, 1979). Thus it is important not to make assumptions about respondents' goals, outcome expectancies or evaluations. For example, young pregnant women may justify smoking in relation to the (positively evaluated) outcome of having a small baby (Lawson, 1994). In that case changing the evaluation of this outcome should precede attempts to discourage smoking on the basis of the increased likelihood of this outcome.

This underlines the need to pilot questionnaires with particular client groups in order to accurately represent the range of potentially important outcome expectancies and evaluations (Fishbein & Ajzen, 1975; Fisher & Fisher, 1992; Godin & Kok, 1996). Such piloting need not be complex. In Chapter 6, Agnew describes a pilot study used to identify 'modal beliefs' specified by the TRA in relation to students' condom use (see also Agnew, 1998). He shows that questions based on this pilot corresponded closely to individual condom-relevant beliefs generated in a free-response questionnaire and also demonstrates that the modal beliefs provided as good a predictive model of condom use intentions as individual beliefs. Note, however, that this suggests that direct attitude measures which ask respondents to rate how good/bad, pleasant/unpleasant, wise/foolish etc. a health-related action is, may not adequately identify differences between people's underlying beliefs about the consequences of that behaviour (Ajzen & Fishbein, 1980; Conner & Sparks, 1996). Studies employing such measures may not be able to specify the kind of educational intervention likely to promote more positive evaluations of a recommended action.

Breckler and Wiggins (1989) have argued that there is evidence to support a separation between cognitive/evaluative (e.g., how good or bad performing this behaviour would be) and affective (e.g., how good or bad would I feel about performing/having performed this behaviour) components of attitudes. This distinction is supported by Ajzen's (1991) observation that evaluative beliefs explain only 10% to 36% of the variance in attitude measures across studies – even after optimal re-scaling. Affective beliefs may be based upon direct experience (e.g., greater familiarity produces more positive or negative feelings about a behaviour; cf. Zajonc, 1968). Evaluative beliefs, on the other hand, are likely to be derived from social communication concerning the likelihood of particular outcomes. Trafimow and Sheeran (1998) used factor analytic and clustering in free recall paradigms to demonstrate that people distinguish between evaluation and affect in their attitudes towards health behaviours and showed that both components influence intentions. Other studies have also presented evidence indicating that *'anticipated affect'* may be a powerful motivator (Richard et al., 1995; Parker, Manstead & Stradling, 1995). For example, Richard et al., (1995) found that respondents who anticipated that they would feel regret or worry if they did not use a condom were more likely to intend to use one.

Many health promotion campaigns have assumed that *fear* arousing communications which persuade people of the likelihood of threatening outcomes following health risk behaviour will motivate behaviour change because of individuals' desire to reduce their fear. Leventhal (1970) noted that efforts to reduce fear could involve strategies other than adoption of a recommended health behaviour (e.g., denial of the threat). However, Leventhal (1970) and Sutton (1982) both concluded that the greater the fear aroused by communications the greater their impact on intention formation and behaviour, especially when specific instructions on how to avoid the feared outcome were included (see below).

Beliefs about other people's approval for one's behaviour (i.e., *normative beliefs*) are also outcome expectations and, in Chapter 13, Bandura categorises them as 'social outcome expectations'. However, there is evidence indicating that people distinguish between normative beliefs and other outcome expectancies (Fishbein, Middlestadt & Trafimow, 1993; Trafimow & Fishbein, 1995). In general, normative beliefs have been found to be less strongly associated with intentions than attitude (and other outcome expectancy) measures (e.g., Armitage & Conner, in press). However, there is also evidence suggesting that normative beliefs are especially influential in relation to a particular set of behaviours and/or for particular people (Trafimow & Finlay, 1996). In Chapter 5 Trafimow argues that normative beliefs should be regarded as separate cognitive antecedents of intention formation and action control and that interventions should be primarily directed towards either general outcome expectancies or normative beliefs depending on the relative strength of their relationship to target intentions (see also Trafimow, 1998).

The TRA specifies that people's motivation may relate to the approval of a *range* of specified others, implying that the variety of people whose approval is important for a particular behaviour must be assessed (see e.g., Agnew's pilot study in Chapter 6). Ratings of perceived approval are multiplied by ratings of the desire to comply with their wishes (i.e., 'motivation to comply') to form a *'subjective norm'* measure (Ajzen & Fishbein, 1980). However, beliefs about what others are thinking and doing (i.e., *'descriptive norms'*) can be as important as beliefs about others' approval/disapproval of one's performance of the action/s in question (i.e., '*injunctive norms*') (Cialdini, Kallgren, & Reno, 1991). For example, in the case of condom use Sheeran et al. (1999) report stronger correlations between condom use and descriptive norms than between use and subjective norm. Descriptive norms include beliefs about others' attitude towards the action in question ('group attitude') and perceptions of their behaviour ('group behaviour') (White, Terry & Hogg, 1994).

The TRA implies that personal behavioural standards or morality are inseparable from normative beliefs (as represented by subjective norm measures) (Fishbein & Ajzen, 1975). However, a number of researchers have suggested that separate measurement of personal standards may help clarify individual differences in behaviour. Triandis (1977) suggested that *personal normative beliefs* (e.g., 'I feel I should do X.') influenced action and, in Chapter 13, Bandura refers to the role of self-sanctions in regulating behaviour. Schwartz and Tessler (1972) found that such personal normative beliefs were strong predictors of intention and Parker et al. (1995) demonstrated that they explained additional variance in intentions after measures specified by the theory of planned behaviour had been accounted for. This corresponds to Ajzen's (1991) finding that, for certain behaviours, a measure of *moral obligation* enhanced the prediction of intentions achieved by the theory of planned behaviour.

In Chapter 7, Gibbons, Gerrard, Oullette and Burzette make a distinction between intentions and *behavioural willingness*, where the latter indicates a tendency to engage in situation-prompted but unpremeditated health risks (see also Gibbons et al., 1998). The willing (but not intending) respondent is indicating a personal latitude of acceptance for specified behaviours that may make him or her more likely to undertake health risk behaviours in the context of unanticipated situational opportunities (than someone reporting less willingness). Behavioural willingness, moral obligation and personal normative beliefs all appear to measure personal behavioural standards and future research may clarify relationships between these measures and their relevance to particular behaviours.

It has been argued that measures of *self-identity* can enhance models of the cognitive antecedents of behaviour (Eagley & Chaiken, 1993). For example, Charng, Piliavin and Callero (1988) observed that a role identity measure explained variance in blood donation in addition to that accounted for by attitude measures and that role identity was stronger amongst those who had donated blood more often. Similarly, Sparks and Shepherd (1992) showed that a self-identity measure added to the explained variance in intentions (to eat organic vegetables) after theory of planned behaviour measures had been considered. Kelly and Breinlinger (1995) suggest that such measures may reveal differences between the intention formation processes of those with stronger versus weaker self-identification. Drawing upon the work of Charng et al., (1988) and on self-categorisation theory (Turner et al., 1987), they suggest that when a behaviour is thought to represent or expresses a salient social identity, normative expectations regarding how people sharing that identity should act will be more important than individual assessments of potential outcomes (i.e., outcome expectancies). This view was supported by the observation that a single-item measure of identity relevance ("Would you describe yourself as someone who is actively involved in promoting women's issues?") moderated the effect of attitudes on intentions (to participate in women's meetings and campaigns) so that attitudes were only significantly associated with intentions for weak identifiers (Kelly & Breinlinger, 1995). Similar findings by Terry and Hogg (1996) showing that perceived norms are more strongly related to strength of intention amongst strong identifiers are discussed by Trafimow in Chapter 5.

Such findings suggest that different types of self-representations may result in different intention formation processes. Higgins's (1987) self-discrepancy theory suggests that perceived differences between our ideal and actual selves and between the selves we feel we ought to be and our actual selves shape both our emotions and motivation. Carver (1996) has related this to the TRA, noting a potential correspondence between the proposed motivational effects of personal attitudes (including outcome expectancies) and subjective norm by the TRA and the directive influence of *ideal-actual self-discrepancies*, on the one hand, and *ought-to-be-actual self-discrepancies*, on the other. Carver suggests that intentions based primarily on normative or 'ought-to' influences may be quite different in their emotional or affective components to intentions based on attitudes, personal behavioural standards or goals associated with an ideal-self. This is based on Higgins's proposal that discrepancies between perceived self and the self we feel we ought to be are likely to give rise to fear and anxiety while discrepancies between the ideal and actual self lead to emotions of dejection such as disappointment, sadness and depression. These ideas are related to Trafimow's proposal, in Chapter 5, that some people are largely under 'attitude control' while others are under 'normative control'. However, consideration of self-representations suggests that this could change depending on how strongly one's social identity was related to the goal in question, i.e., strong social identification could promote greater normative control. It seems clear that further research on self-representations and the normative and attitudinal bases of intention formation could have important implications for health-related interventions (see Trafimow's discussion of this issue in Chapter 5). Not least because Sheeran, Norman and Orbell (1999) have demonstrated that intentions based on attitudes better predict behaviour than intentions based on norms.

In conclusion, it appears that a summary model of motivation could be based on Bandura's social cognitive theory (Bandura, 1997; 1998) or on the theory of planned behaviour (Ajzen, 1991) and should include: intention and self-efficacy (including perceived barriers to action) as the most proximal cognitive antecedents of behaviour. Population-relevant outcome expectancies, that is, anticipated consequences (including affective outcomes and personal suscept-ibility to negative outcomes – currently and in the absence of precautions) and evaluations of these consequences are likely to be prerequisites of intention formation. Similarly, descriptive and subjective norms (including perceptions of others' attitudes towards the behaviour, others' behaviour, their potential approval of the behaviour and respondents' motivation to comply with their wishes) are also likely to prompt intention formation. Finally, self-representa-tions, including personal normative beliefs and self-identification are likely to affect intention formation and action control. Although not all of these constructs (and associated measures) will be relevant to any particular health-related behaviour they provide a generic or content-free framework which is likely to include the core cognitive antecedents of many health behaviours. Figure 1 summarises relationships between these constructs and lists some relevant references. Previously tested items, or multi-item scales, are available for all these cognitive measures and in many cases assessments of the extent to which they relate to a variety of health-related behaviours have also been published (e.g., Ajzen & Fishbein, 1980; Bandura, 1992; 1997; Conner & Sparks, 1996; Godin & Kok, 1996; Parker et al., 1995; Richard, van der Pligt & de Vries, 1995; Schwarzer & Fuchs, 1996; Sheppard et al., 1988; Sheeran & Abraham, 1996; Sparks & Shepherd, 1992).

ACTION CONTROL: FROM INTENTION FORMATION TO VOLITIONAL PROCESSES

The preceding discussion has focused mainly on modelling the cognitive antecedents of strength of intention. The exception being direct effects of self-efficacy reports on behavioural prediction (i.e., variance in behaviour explained, over and above that accounted for intention). We have noted that such effects are not always evident but, when they are, they indicate a cognitive readiness to act that is distinct from strength of intention. Social cognition models have shed little light on such post-intentional action readiness. Yet it seems likely that interventions designed to facilitate action amongst those who intend to act could have important implications for health promotion. As Gollwitzer and Oettingen point out in Chapter 11, it may be that problems with getting started or maintaining action, rather than formulating intentions, prevent people from engaging in recommended action.

Theoretical work on self-regulation has increasingly encompassed voitional processes involved in the initiation and maintenance of specified action which may lead to goal achievement. Bagozzi (1992) has highlighted the importance of 'instrumental acts', that is, specific *preparatory behaviours*, involved in goal achievement (such as resisting buying cigarettes before meeting a friend or explicitly asking friends not to share their cigarettes when trying to give up smoking). Relatedly, Schwarzer (1992; Schwarzer and Fuchs, 1996) has noted that 'action phase' cognitive processes include the formulation of specific plans, specific action-control perceptions (i.e., self-efficacy) and appraisals of contextual factors which may constrain or facilitate action.

This focus on specific preparatory behaviours is an extension of Fishbein and Ajzen's (1975) recommendations regarding the specificity of attitude and intention measures (see Fishbein, 1993). Bagozzi's model reminds us that many health goals involve complex sequences of action across time (see also Bandura, 1998). For example, in Chapter 12, Bagozzi and Edwards demonstrate how dieting and exercise behaviours both contribute to the overall goal of losing weight (see also Bagozzi & Edwards, 1998). Similarly, prior to condom use a person may have to acquire condoms, carry or store them, suggest their use to a sexual partner, negotiate their use if their partner is reluctant and resist invitations to have unprotected sex. Each of these preparatory behaviours may be preceded and determined by behaviour-specific attitudes, self-representations, normative beliefs, self-efficacy beliefs and intentions. Moreover, the importance of different cognitive antecedents may vary across different preparatory behaviours and an individual's cognitive preparedness may be greater for one preparatory behaviour than another. For example, an individual's self-efficacy may be high in relation to using a condom but low in relation to suggesting condom use to a partner. Analysis of this kind can specify preparatory behaviours which particular individuals have greatest difficulty enacting en route to the overall goal. This, in turn suggests particular cognitive interventions for particular people (see e.g., Bandura in Chapter 13). Some individuals may, for example, lack self-efficacy in relation to condom acquisition while others may feel strong normative pressures which militate against suggesting condom use to a sexual partner. Thus cognitive modelling is likely to be most effective when it addresses the cognitive antecedents of *specific behaviours* rather than *goal-related* cognitions (see e.g., Conner & Norman, 1996b).

The importance of sub-goal planning and attainment has long been recognised in behaviour modification and cognitive behaviour therapy (Gambrill, 1977; Clark & Fairburn, 1996) and is supported by research into the cognitive effects of sub-goal achievement. For example, Stock and Cervone (1990) have shown that sub-dividing a complex task into a series of sub-goals leads to higher self-efficacy at task outset, heightened self-efficacy and satisfaction at the point of sub-task completion and greater overall goal persistence.

In Chapter 11, Gollwitzer and Oettingen (see also Gollwitzer & Oettingen, 1998) provide further insights into action initiation. They propose that intentions are more likely to be enacted if they are translated into '*implementation intentions*' specifying when and where a particular act is to be undertaken. This focus on specific plans is reminiscent of earlier research which demonstrated that fear appeals were most likely to influence behaviour when they were accompanied by instructions on how to act (e.g., where and when to go for a check-up) (Leventhal, 1970). The approach also emphasises Bagozzi's (1992) discussion of action-specific cognitions and underlines Schwarzer's (1992) suggestion that cognitive representations of the action context are important. Gollwitzer (1993) has shown that those who have formed implementation intentions are better able to recall presented descriptions of the means to carry out an action, more likely to identify environmental cues relevant to their planned action and faster to initiate action in response to situational prompts. He suggests that the elaboration of intentions into implementation intentions facilitates the identification of action-relevant context cues and that these, in turn, lead to action initiation in an automatic fashion.

This reference to automaticity or unconscious control is useful because critics of social cognition models have pointed out that people do not experience action as involving a process of checking through outcome expectancies and beliefs concerning others' potential approval. Most of the time we experience action as an automatic response to situational demands. This suggests that we have access to ready-made sets of instructions capable of directing action in a context-appropriate manner with minimal conscious monitoring. Bargh's 'auto-motive' model (Bargh 1990; Bargh & Barndollar, 1996) describes how this might operate. Bargh proposes that when we repeatedly perform a behaviour in a particular context, the motive and its implementation instructions become integrated into our representation of that situation. Consequently, once we perceive the situation, the overall motive or goal and the means to implement it (through specific actions) are automatically triggered in memory. This process facilitates action without deliberation or conscious decision-making. In other words, implementation intentions are prompted by the perception of previously represented context cues and are immediately given regulatory priority. Where the necessary skills have also been learnt, the individual can produce an immediate and competent performance without hesitation or deliberation. Similar contextual prompting and unconscious action control may also operate when strongly held attitudes or attitudes based on prior personal experience are cued by a particular context (Fazio, 1990), resulting in action that is apparently not preceded by conscious intention formation.

This account of the inclusion of action regulation instructions in situational representations sketches a cognitive explanation of 'stimulus-response behaviour'. Previous learning enables environmental stimuli to prompt ready-made context-relevant intentions which, when combined with implementation instructions, can be executed automatically. As Gollwitzer (1993) notes, the individual can pass control of a behaviour to a self-chosen environmental (and discriminative) stimulus. Similarly, Bargh's auto-motive model provides a psychological account of 'habit' and 'past-behaviour' effects. Practice results in the pairing of a behaviour and the context of performance in memory such that encountering the context prompts the behaviour (e.g., Orbell, Hodgkins & Sheeran, 1997). In the case of health-enhancing behaviours this suggests that context-specific practice will result in increasingly effortless enactment. However, in the case of health-risk behaviours, it suggests that repeated relegation of intention-act sequences to unconscious control in a particular situation will make change more difficult. Behaviour change, in these circumstances will require conscious dismantling of these unconsciously activated routines (see Gollwitzer & Oettingen in Chapter 11). For example, a smoker who has regularly smoked with friends while drinking alcohol may find that, although successfully resisting smoking during the day, s/he experiences very strong desires for a cigarette while drinking and, seemingly without thinking, asks friends for cigarettes. A clear understanding of why this happens, self-monitoring of such automatic desires, and conscious initiation of alternative, cognitively-rehearsed implementation intentions (e.g., declaring craving and asking for social support as soon as the desire is felt) may, through practice, disrupt this automatic, context-prompted behaviour. Cognitive behavioural approaches to behaviour change can facilitate such disruption. For example, a 'desire for a cigarette' scale taped onto a cigarette packet may serve as the context cue for smoking cessation implementation intentions.

The most optimistic aspect of the Gollwitzer/Bargh account is the suggestion that cognitive rehearsal of intentions and the context of their enactment can mimic the practice effects inherent in habit formation. For example, Gollwitzer (1993) notes that the differences in speed of response between those who have and have not formed implementation intentions is similar, in some respects, to observed differences between people who have had direct experience of the behaviour in question and those who have not. This suggests that we can 'programme' health-enhancing behaviours to become automatic. By imagining the situation in which we intend to act and planning what we will do, we make it more likely that our future thoughts in that situation will turn to this intention and that the intended action will gain cognitive priority. Orbell et al., (1997), for example, have demonstrated that questions which prompt context-specific planning (i.e., implementation intention formation) can increase the likelihood of preventive health action and reduce the impact of past behaviour on future action. These findings support health education methods focusing on cognitive rehearsal of action and script-based action planning (e.g., Miller, Bettencourt, DeBro, & Hoffman, 1993; Schinke & Gordon, 1992). They also suggest that self-report measures of the extent to which people have planned action may usefully assess intenders' readiness to act on their intentions (see e.g., Abraham, Sheeran, Norman, Conner, de Vries, & Otten, 1999).

GOAL PRIORITISATION: FROM ACTION CONTROL TO SELF-REGULATION

Karoly (1998) identified the 'twin demons' of self-regulation as 'goal imprecision' and 'intergoal conflict'. We have noted that planning (e.g., implementation intention formation) can enhance action control through the generation of context-specific action instructions, but even a precisely defined action sequence may be abandoned if it conflicts with a more important personal agenda. Weinstein's (1988) views everyday intergoal conflict as analogous to an executive's management of a 'messy desk' that directs her attention to a series of competing priorities. Thus understanding why some people undertake health-related behaviour while others do not is likely to require clarification of the cognitive processes involved in prioritising health-related goals in the face of competing distractions.

Goal prioritisation may be especially difficult when the completion of preparatory actions is experienced as difficult. In Chapter 11 Gollwitzer and Oettingen illustrate how self-efficacy in relation to overcoming obstacles and, consequently, action control, can be enhanced by cognitive preparation to ignore anticipated distractions. Similar rehearsal techniques, involving verbal description and imagery, have been employed by cognitive behaviour therapists to develop action-maintaining, cognitive resources (Clark & Fairburn, 1996). For example, Meichenbaum's (1977) self-instruction therapy involves practising self-talk that can highlight sub-tasks and positive outcome expectancies during performance. Scheier and Carver (1988) have also noted that contextual self-focus cues (such as the presence of a mirror) can reduce discrepancies between attitudes and behaviour, on the one hand, and behavioural standards and actual performance, on the other. Collectively, these findings suggest that rehearsal and positive, action-orientated self-talk may be important to maintaining goal priority in the face of difficulties.

This may be especially true when skill levels are low. Kanfer (1996) argues that skill development relies on conscious control and requires substantial attentional resources. Activities which invite self-evaluation during this development process can be detrimental because they divert attention away from the task. Trying tasks without evaluation is, therefore, recommended in the early stages of skill acquisition. Moreover, for those who find skill acquisition challenging, cognitive strategies that enhance affective/emotional control (e.g., self instruction to ignore feelings of worry or disappointment) have been found to be more helpful than motivation control strategies (such as focusing on maximising effort) (Kanfer, 1996). Thus Karoly (1998) recommends health promotion programmes which provide external monitoring, feedback on cognitive and behaviour change and action instructions over time (see, for example, the self-regulatory computer-based programmes described by Bandura in Chapter 13).

Measures which assess individual differences in goal prioritisation resources are likely to add to our understanding of health-related behaviour and the operation of health promotion interventions (see Karoly, 1993 for a review). For example, Klinger's Concerns Dimensions Questionnaires measure a variety of cognitions in relation to a range of goals in order to identify the characteristics of frequently thought-about goals (Klinger, Barta and Maxeiner, 1980). Cognitions include: positive value, importance and desire (all of which appear to be related to Bagozzi and Edwards's measure of 'desire'), previous investment (which could include preparatory actions), anticipated affect, perceived likelihood of success, perceived barriers to achievement and, finally, commitment.

Measures of the *relative* importance of competing intentions may also improve behavioural prediction over measures of goal intention. Sheppard et al., (1988) found that the theory of reasoned action predicted behaviour more accurately when a choice between alternatives was specified (with weighted average intention-behaviour correlations rising from $r = .49$ when no choice was specified to $r = .77$ for choice behaviours). Sheppard et al., suggest that specification of alternatives may allow respondents to assess their intentions more precisely. Related experimental work has indicated that the importance of intentions affects their retrieval in memory (Kvavilashvili, 1987) implying that intenders who act may be differentiated from those who do not by the importance they attach to competing intentions in choice situations. This is supported by Abraham et al. (1999) who found that intenders who reported using a condom in a specified encounter rated the importance of condom use more highly than the importance of having sexual intercourse while intending non-users indicated that having intercourse was more important than condom use. In this study the relative importance measure was the strongest discriminator between intenders who reported use and non-use (see also Davidson & Morrison, 1983, within-subjects analysis of intentions to use different types of contraception). Such measures help clarify 'how health goals relate to contra-health intentions' (Karoly, 1998, p. 743) and point to the need for extended cognitive models of self-regulation. Theories such as the theory of planned behaviour, while taking account of a variety of influences on intention formation, do not adequately conceptualise the goal conflict at the heart of self-regulation.

Scheier and Carver (1988) have highlighted the way in which goals are embedded in complex hierarchies and Bagozzi and Edwards demonstrate how such hierarchies can be revealed. Action identification theory (Vallacher & Wegner, 1987) suggests that action representations may reflect higher or lower order goals in a goal hierarchy. For example, an implementation intention such as 'I shall go swimming on Thursday afternoon at the local pool' is a lower order (and more precisely defined) goal, than 'I intend to exercise three times a week' (since the former can be derived from the latter). We have noted the importance of precision above. However, Vallacher and Wegner (1987) point out that higher order goal formulations are important to motivational stability. Intentions with higher level identifications are more likely to be implemented in the face of contextual variation (e.g., if something comes up on Thursday afternoon then a suitably re-scheduled exercise intention can be implemented in the gym that evening). Higher order intentions are also more likely to be attributed to dispositional rather than situational factors (e.g., I exercise because it's important to me rather than because the local pool is convenient). Higher order goals may, therefore, facilitate prioritisation in the face of situational constraints and may be more easily linked to valued identities or self-representations. Dispositional attributions may help to embed goals in valued identities and simultaneously increase goal-related self-efficacy following successful performances. Cognitive links between higher-order goals and valued identities may influence the allocation of cognitive resources to prioritise a particular intention. Thus the place of an intention within higher order goal hierarchies may determine the likelihood of its enactment (i.e., the intention-behaviour correlation).

Fuhrmann and Kuhl (1998) emphasise the importance of linking goals to the self and argue that the inability to discriminate between self-chosen and recommended goals deprives the individual of important self-regulatory resources, leaving action control dependent on negative, failure-avoiding motivation which may lead to long-term mood-regulation and action control deficits. The importance of the identity to which health goals are anchored may also limit the extent to which these goals are likely to be re-evaluated when competing social identities becoming salient in situations where the planned action can be implemented (see e.g., Levine & Reicher, 1996). For example, if 'being fit' becomes a central identity then awareness of competing goals (such as maintaining one's reputation as a productive worker) is less likely to result in exercising being devalued or postponed (e.g., in order to meet work deadlines). Such identity relevance may also mean that perceived discrepancies between ideal selves and actual behaviour (Higgins, 1987) or between fantasy and reality (Gollwitzer & Oettingen, Chapter 13) are especially motivating. We have noted that repeated behaviours may become integrated into identities and that the self-relevance of a behaviour may be more important to intention formation than outcome expectancies (Kelly & Breinlinger, 1995). Future research may clarify relationships between self-representation measures and the measures of planning and rehearsal.

SUMMARY

We have discussed cognitive resources which may be assessed to predict whether an individual is more or less likely to undertake a particular course of action. We have summarised research into the reasoned basis of intention formation and highlighted the importance of context-specific planning and rehearsal. Finally, we have noted the need to develop measures which relate intentions and plans to goal hierarchies and identities. As more sophisticated measures of these cognitive resources are developed, they are likely to enhance our understanding of health-related behaviour and the operation of health promotion interventions. This in turn should provide a framework for (i) the identification of cognitive changes likely to result in health-related behaviour (at individual and group levels), (ii) defining intervention targets in cognitive terms and (iii) the measurement of behavioural change resulting from health-related interventions that target cognitive change.

REFERENCES

Abraham, C., Sheeran, P., Norman, N., Conner, P., de Vries, N., & Otten, W. (1999). When good intentions are not enough: Modeling post-intention cognitive correlates of condom use. *Journal of Applied Social Psychology*, 12, 2591–2612.

Abraham, C., Sheeran, P., Spears, R. & Abrams, D. (1992). Health beliefs and the promotion of HIV-preventive intentions amongst teenagers: A Scottish perspective. *Health Psychology*, 11, 363–370.

Agnew, C. R. (1998). Modal versus individually-derived beliefs about condom use: Measuring the cognitive underpinnings of the theory of reasoned action. *Psychology and Health*, 13, 271–287.

Ajzen, I. (1988). *Attitudes, Personality and Behavior*. Milton Keynes, UK: Open University Press.

Ajzen, I. (1991). The theory of planned behavior. *Organizational Behavior and Human Decision Processes*, 50, 179–211.

Ajzen, I. (1998). Models of human social behaviour and their application to health psychology. *Psychology and Health*, 13, 735–739.

Ajzen, I. & Fishbein, M. (1977). Attitude-behavior relations: A theoretical analysis and review of empirical research. *Psychological Bulletin*, 84, 888–918.

Ajzen, I. & Fishbein, M. (1980). *Understanding Attitudes and Predicting Social Behavior*. Englewood Cliffs, NJ: Prentice-Hall.

Ajzen, I. & Madden, T. J. (1986). Prediction of goal-directed behavior: Attitudes, intentions and perceived behavioral control. *Journal of Experimental Social Psychology*, 22, 453–474.

Armitage, C. J. & Conner, M. (in press). Efficacy of the theory of planned behaviour: A meta-analytic review. *British Journal of Social Psychology*.

Bagozzi, R. P. (1992). The self-regulation of attitudes, intentions and behaviour. *Social Psychology Quarterly*, 55, 178–204.

Bagozzi, R. P., & Edwards, E. A. (1998). Goal setting and goal pursuit in the regulation of body weight. *Psychology and Health*, 13, 593–621.

Bandura, A. (1992). Exercise of personal agency through the self-efficacy mechanism. In R. Schwarzer (ed.) *Self-Efficacy: Thought Control of Action*, (pp. 3–38). Washington: Hemisphere Publishing Corporation.

Bandura, A. (1986). *Social Foundations of Thought and Action: A Congnitive Social Theory*. Englewood Cliffs, NJ: Prentice-Hall.

Bandura, A. (1997). *Self-Efficacy: The Exercise of Control*. New York: Freeman.

Bandura, A. (1998). Health promotion from the perspective of social cognitive theory. *Psychology and Health, 13*, 623–649.

Bargh, J. A. (1990). Auto-motives: Preconscious determinants of thought and behavior. In E. T. Higgins & R. M. Sorrentino (eds.) *Handbook of Motivation and Cognition: Foundations of Social Behavior*, (Vol. 2, pp. 93–130). New York: The Guildford Press.

Bargh, J. A. & Barndollar, K. (1996). Automaticity in action: The unconscious as repository of chronic goals and motives. In P. M. Gollwitzer & J. A. Bargh (Eds.) *The Psychology of Action: Linking Cognition and Motivation to Behaviour*, (pp. 457–481). New York: The Guildford Press.

Becker, H. M., Heafner, D. P., Kals, S. V., Kirscht, J. P., Maiman, L. A. & Rosenstock, I. M. (1977). Selected psychosocial models and correlates of individual health-related behaviours. *Medical Care, 15* (5, supplement), 27–46.

Breckler, S. J. & Wiggins, E. C. (1989). Affect versus evaluation in the structure of attitudes. *Journal of Experimental Social Psychology, 25*, 253–271.

Bryan, A. D., Aiken, L. S. & West, S. G. (1996). Increasing condom use: Evaluation of a theory-based intervention to prevent sexually transmitted diseases in young women. *Health Psychology, 15*, 371–382.

Carver, C. S. (1996). Some ways in which goals differ and some implications of those differences. In P. M. Gollwitzer & J. A. Bargh (eds.) *The Psychology of Action: Linking Cognition and Motivation to Behaviour*, (pp. 645–672). New York: The Guildford Press.

Charng, H., Piliavan, J. A., & Callero, P. L. (1988). Role identity and reasoned action in the prediction of repeated behaviour. *Social Psychology Quarterly, 51*, 303–317.

Cialdini, R. B., Kallgren, C. A., & Reno, R. R. (1991). A focus theory of normative conduct: A theoretical refinement and re-evaluation of the role of norms in human behavior. *Advances in Experimental Social Psychology, 24*, 201–234.

Clark, D. M, & Fairburn, C. G. (1996). *Science and Practice of Cognitive Behavioural Therapy*. Oxford: Open University Press.

Conner, M. & Norman, P. (1996). *Predicting Health Behaviour: Research and Practice with Social Cognition Models*, Buckingham, UK: Open University Press.

Conner, M. & Norman, P. (1996b). Body weight and shape control: Examining component behaviours. *Appetite, 27*, 135–150.

Conner, M. & Sparks, P. (1996). The theory of planned behaviour and health behaviours. In M. Conner & P. Norman (eds.) *Predicting Health Behaviour: Research and Practice with Social Cognition Models*, (pp. 121–162), Buckingham, UK: Open University Press.

Davidson, A. R. & Morrison, D. M. (1983). Predicting contraceptive behavior from attitudes: A comparison of within- versus across-subjects procedures. *Journal of Personality and Social Psychology, 45*, 997–1009.

De Vries, H. & Backbier, E. (1994). Self-efficacy as an important determinant of quitting amongst pregnant women who smoke: the ø-pattern. *Preventive Medicine, 23*, 167–174.

Eagly, A. H. & Chaiken, S. (1993). *The Psychology of Attitudes*. Fort Worth: Harcourt, Brace Jovanovich.

Fazio, R. H. (1990). Multiple processes by which attitudes guide behavior: The MODE model as an integrative framework. In M. P. Zana (ed.) *Advances in Experimental Social Psychology, 23*, (pp. 75–109). San Diego: Academic Press.

Fishbein, M. (1993). Introduction. In D. J. Terry, C. Gallois & M. McCamish (eds.) *The Theory of Reasoned Action: Its Application to AIDS-Preventive Behaviour*, (pp. xv–xxv). Oxford: Pergamon.

Fishbein, M. & Ajzen, I. (1975). *Belief, Attitude, Intention and Behavior: An Introduction to Theory and Research.* Reading, MA: Addison-Wesley.

Fishbein, M., Middlestadt, S. E., & Trafimow, D. (1993). Social norms for condom use: Implications for HIV prevention interventions of a KABP survey with heterosexuals in the eastern Caribbean. *Advances in Consumer Research, 20,* 292–296.

Fisher, J. D. & Fisher W. A. (1992). Changing AIDS risk behavior. *Psychological Bulletin, 111,* 455–474.

Fisher, J. D., Fisher W. A., Misovich, S. J., Kimble, D. L. & Malloy, T. E. (1996). Changing AIDS risk behaviour: Effects of an intervention emphasizing AIDS risk reduction information, motivation and behavioral skills in a college student population. *Health Psychology, 15,* 114–123.

Fisher W. A., Fisher, J. D. & Rye B. J. (1995). Understanding and promoting AIDS-preventive behavior: Insights from the theory of reasoned action, *Health Psychology, 14,* 255–264.

Fuhrmann, A. & Kuhl, J. (1998). Maintaining a healthy diet: Effects of personality and self-reward versus self-punishment on commitment to and enactment of self-chosen and assigned goals. *Psychology and Health, 13,* 651–686.

Gambrill, E. D. (1977) *Behavior Modification: Handbook of Assessment, Intervention, and Evaluation.* San Francisco: Jossey Bass.

Gerrard, M., Gibbons, F. X., & Bushman, B. J. (1996). The relation between perceived susceptibility and precautionary sexual behavior. *Psychological Bulletin, 119,* 390–409.

Gibbons, F. X., Gerrard, M., Oullette, J. A. & Burzette, R. (1998). Cognitive antecedents to adolescent health risk: Discriminating between behavioral intention and behavioral willingness. *Psychology and Health, 13,* 319–339.

Godin, G. & Kok, G. (1996). The theory of planned behavior: A review of its applications to health-related behaviors. *American Journal of Health Promotion, 11,* 87–97.

Gollwitzer, P. M. (1993). Goal achievement: The role of intentions. *European Review of Social Psychology, 4,* 142–185.

Gollwitzer, P. M. & Bargh, J. A. (eds.) (1996). *The Psychology of Action: Linking Cognition and Motivation to Behaviour.* New York: The Guildford Press.

Gollwitzer, P. M. & Oettingen, G. (1998). The emergence and implementation of health goals. *Psychology and Health, 13,* 687–715.

Haefner, D. P. & Kirscht, J. P. (1970). Motivational and behavioural effects of modifying health beliefs. *Public Health Reports, 85,* 478–484.

Harrison, J.A., Mullen, P.D. & Green, L.W. (1992). A meta-analysis of studies of the health belief model with adults. *Health Education Research, 7,* 107–116.

Higgins, E. T. (1987). Self-discrepancy: A theory relating self to affect. *Psychological Review, 94,* 319–340.

Hochbaum, G. M. (1958). Public participation in medical screening programs: A sociopsychological study. *Public Health Service Publication No 572,* Washington, United States Government Printing Office.

Hodgkins, S. & Orbell, S. (1998). Can protection motivation theory predict behaviour? A longitudinal test exploring the role of previous behaviour. *Psychology and Health, 13,* 237–250.

Janz, N. & Becker, M. H. (1984). The health belief model: A decade later. *Health Education Quarterly, 11,* 1–47.

Kalichman, S. C., Carey, M. P. & Johnson, B. T. (1996). Prevention of sexually transmitted HIV infection: A meta-analytic review of the behavioral outcome literature. *American Behavioural Medicine, 18,* 6–15.

Kanfer, R. (1996). Self-regulatory and other non-ability determinants of skill acquisition. In P. M. Gollwitzer & J. A. Bargh (eds.) *The Psychology of Action: Linking Cognition and Motivation to Behaviour.* New York: The Guildford Press.

Karoly, P. (1993). Mechanisms of self-regulation: A systems view. *Annual Review of Psychology, 44,* 23–52.

Karoly, P. (1998). Expanding the conceptual range of health self-regulation research: A commentary. *Psychology and Health, 13,* 741–746.

Kelly, C. & Breinlinger, S. (1995). Attitudes, intentions and behavior: A study of women's participation in collective action. *Journal of Applied Social Psychology, 25,* 1430–1445.

King, J. B. (1982). The impact of patients' perceptions of high blood pressure on attendance at screening. *Social Science Medicine, 26,* 1079–1091.

Klinger, E., Barta, S. G., & Maxeiner, M. E. (1980). Motivational correlates of thought content frequency and commitment. *Journal of Personality and Social Psychology, 39,* 1222–1237.

Kok, G. & Schaalma, H. (1998). Theory-based and data-based health education programmes. *Psychology and Health, 13,* 747–751.

Kvavilashvili, L. (1987). Remembering intention as a distinct form of memory. *British Journal of Psychology, 78,* 507–518.

Lawson, E. J. (1994). The role of smoking in the lives of low-income adolescents: A field study. *Adolescence, 29,* 61–79.

Leventhal, H. (1970). Findings and theory in the study of fear communications. In L. Berkowitz (ed.) *Advances in Experimental Social Psychology, 5,* (pp. 119–186). San Diego: Academic Press.

Leventhal, H., Leventhal, E., A. & Contrada, R. J. (1988) Self-regulation, health and behaviour: A perceptual-congnitive approach. *Psychology and Health, 13,* 171–133.

Levine R. M. & Reicher S. D. (1996). Making sense of symptoms: Self-categorization and the meaning of illness and injury. *British Journal of Social Psychology, 35,* 245–256.

Madden, T. J., Ellen, P. & Ajzen, I. (1992). A comparison of the theory of planned behavior and the theory of reasoned action. *Personality and Social Psychology Bulletin, 18,* 3–9.

Maddux, J. E. & Rogers, R. W. (1983). Protection motivation and self-efficacy: A revised theory of fear appeals and attitude change. *Journal of Experimental Social Psychology, 19,* 469–479.

Meichenbaum, D. (1977). *Cognitive Behaviour Modification: An Integrative Approach.* New York: Plenum Press.

Miller, L. C., Bettencourt, B. A., DeBro, S. C. & Hoffman, V. (1993). Negotiating safer sex: Interpersonal dynamics. In J. B. Pryor & G. D. Reeder (eds.) *The Social Psychology of HIV Infection,* (pp. 85–123). Hillsdale, New Jersey: Lawrence Erlbaum.

Morrison, D. M., Baker, S. A. & Gillmore, M. R. (1998). Condom use among high-risk heterosexual teens: A longitudinal analysis using the theory of reasoned action. *Psychology and Health, 13,* 207–222.

Oakley, A., Fullerton, D., Holland, J., Arnold, S., France-Dawson, M., Kelley, P. & McGrellis. S. (1995). Sexual health education interventions for young people: A methodological review. *British Medical Journal, 310,* 158–162.

Orbell, S., Hodgkins, S., & Sheeran, P. (1997). Implementation intentions and the theory of planned behaviour. *Personality and Social Psychology Bulletin, 23,* 945–954.

Parker, D., Manstead, A. S. & Stradling, S. G. (1995). Extending the theory of planned behaviour: The role of personal norm. *British Journal of Social Psychology, 34,* 127–137.

Quine, L. Rutter, D. R. & Arnold, L. (1998). Predicting and undestanding safety helment use among schoolboy cyclists: A comparison of the theory of planned behaviour and the health belief model. *Psychology and Health, 13,* 251–269.

Randall, D. M. & Wolff, J. A. (1994). The time interval in the intention-behaviour relationship: Meta-analysis. *British Journal of Social Psychology, 33,* 405–418.

Richard, R., van der Pligt, J. & de Vries, N. K. (1995). The impact of anticipated regret on (risky) sexual behaviour. *British Journal of Social Psychology, 34*, 9–21.

Rosenstock, I. M. (1974). Historical origins of the health belief model. *Health Education Monographs, 2*, 1–8.

Schaalma, H. P., Kok, G., Bosker, R. J., Parcel, G. S., Peters, L., Poelman, J., & Reinders, J. (1996). Planned development and evaluation of AIDS/STD education for secondary-school students in the Netherlands: Short-term effects. *Health Education Quarterly, 23*, 469–487.

Scheier, M. F. & Carver, C. S. (1988): A model of behavioral self-regulation: Translating intention into action. In L. Berkowitz (ed.) *Advances in Experimental Social Psychology, 21*, (pp. 303–346). New York: Academic Press.

Schinke, S. P. & Gordon, A. N. (1992). Innovative approaches to interpersonal skills training for minority adolescents. In R. J. DiClemente (ed.) *Adolescents and AIDS: A Generation in Jeopardy*, (pp. 181–193). Newbury Park, California: Sage.

Schwartz, S. H. & Tessler, R. C. (1972). A test of a model for reducing measured attitude behavior discrepancies. *Journal of Personality and Social Psychology, 24*, 225–236.

Schwarzer, R. (1992). Self-efficacy in the adoption and maintenance of health behaviors: Theoretical approaches and a new model. In R. Schwarzer (ed.) *Self-Efficacy: Thought Control of Action*, (pp. 217–243). Washington: Hemisphere.

Schwarzer, R. (1998). Optimism, goals and threats: How to conceptualize self-regulatory processes in the adoption and maintenance of health behaviours. *Psychology and Health, 13*, 759–766.

Schwarzer, R. & Fuchs, R. (1996). Self-efficacy and health behaviours. In M. Conner & P. Norman (eds.) *Predicting Health Behaviour: Research and Practice with Social Cognition Models*, (pp. 163–196). Buckingham, UK: Open University Press.

Sheeran, P. & Abraham C. (1996). The health belief model. In M. Conner & P. Norman (eds.) *Predicting Health Behaviour: Research and Practice with Social Cognition Models* (pp. 23–61). Buckingham, UK: Open University Press.

Sheeran, P., Abraham, C., & Orbell, S. (1999). Psychosocial correlates of condom use: A meta-analysis. *Psychological Bulletin, 125*, 90–132.

Sheeran, P., Norman, P. & Orbell, S. (1999). Evidence that intentions based on attitudes better predict behaviour than intentions based on subjective norms. *European Journal of Social Psychology, 29*, 403–406.

Sheppard, B. H., Hartwick, J. & Warshaw, P. R. (1988). The theory of reasoned action: A meta-analysis of past research with recommendations for modifications and future research. *Journal of Consumer Research, 15*, 325–343.

Sparks, P., Guthrie, C. A. & Shepherd, R. (1997). The dimensional structure of the perceived behavioral control construct. *Journal of Applied Social Psychology, 27*, 418–438.

Sparks, P. & Shepherd, R. (1992). Self-identity and the theory of planned behavior: Assessing the role of identification with 'Green consumerism'. *Social Psychology Quarterly, 55*, 388–399.

Stock, J. & Cervone, D. (1990). Proximal goal setting and self-regulatory processes. *Cognitive Therapy and Research, 14*, 483–498.

Sutton, S. R. (1982). Fear arousing communications: A critical examination of theory and research. In J. R. Eiser (ed.) *Social Psychology and Behavioural Medicine*, (pp. 303–337). New York: Wiley.

Sutton, S. (1998). Predicting and explaining intentions and behavior: How well are we doing?. *Journal of Applied Social Psychology, 28*, 1317–1338.

Terry, D. J. & Hogg, M. A. (1996). Group norms and the attitude-behavior relationship: A role for group identification. *Personality and Social Psychology Bulletin, 22*, 776–793.

Terry, D. J. & O'Leary, J. E. (1995). The theory of planned behavior: The effects of perceived behavioural control and self-efficacy. *British Journal of Social Psychology*, *34*, 199–220.

Trafimow, D. (1998). Attitudinal and normative processes in health behavior. *Psychology and Health*, *13*, 307–317.

Trafimow, D. & Finlay, K. A. (1996). The importance of subjective norms for a minority of people: Between subjects and within-subjects analysis. *Personality and Social Psychology Bulletin*, *22*, 820–828.

Trafimow, D. & Fishbein, M. (1995). Do people really distinguish between behavioural and normative beliefs? *British Journal of Social Psychology*, *34*, 257–266.

Trafimow, D. & Sheeran, P. (1998). Some tests of the distinction between cognitive and affective beliefs. *Journal of Experimental Social Psychology*, *34*, 378–397.

Triandis, H. C. (1977). *Interpersonal Behavior*. Monterey, CA: Brooks/Cole.

Turner, J. C., Hogg, M. A., Oakes, P. J. Reicher, S. D. & Wetherell, M. (1987). *Rediscovering the Social Group: A Self-Categorization Theory*. Oxford, UK: Blackwell.

Vallacher, R. R. & Wegner, D. M. (1987). What do people think they're doing? Action identification and human behavior. *Psychological Review*, *94*, 3–15.

Van den Putte, B. (1991). *20 years of the theory of reasoned action of Fishbein and Ajzen: A meta-analysis*. Unpublished manuscript, University of Amsterdam, Amsterdam.

Van der Pligt, J. (1998). Perceived risk and vulnerability as predictors of precautionary behaviour. *British Journal of Health Psychology*, *3*, 1–14.

Van der Velde, F. W. Hooykaas, C. & Van der Pligt, J. (1996). Conditional versus unconditional risk estimates in models of AIDS-related risk behaviour. *Psychology and Health*, *12*, 87–100.

Weinstein, N. D. (1988). The precaution adoption process. *Health Psychology*, *7*, 355–386.

Weinstein, N. D. & Nicolich, M. (1993). Correct and incorrect interpretations of correlations between risk perceptions and risk behaviors. *Health Psychology*, *12*, 235–245.

Weinstein, N. D. & Sandman, P. M. (1992). A model of the precaution adoption process: Evidence from home radon testing, *Health Psychology*, *11*, 170–180.

Werner, P. D. & Middlestadt, S. E. (1979). Factors in the use of oral contraceptives by young women. *Journal of Applied Social Psychology*, *9*, 537–47.

White, K. M., Terry D. J. & Hogg, M. A. (1994). Safer sex behaviour: The role of attitudes, norms and control factors. *Journal of Applied Social Psychology*, *24*, 2164–2192.

Wurtele, S. K. (1988). Increasing women's calcium intake: The role of health beliefs, intentions and health value. *Journal of Applied Social Psychology*, *18*, 627–639.

Wurtele, S. K. & Maddux, J. E. (1987). Relative contributions of protection motivation theory components in predicting exercise intentions and behavior. *Health Psychology*, *6*, 453–466.

Zajonc, R. B. (1968). Attitudinal effects of mere exposure. *Journal of Personality and Social Psychology*, *9*, 1–27.

Section 2 –
Applications of Social Cognition Models

CHAPTER TWO

Using The Theory of Reasoned Action to Predict Condom Use Among High-Risk Heterosexual Teens

Diane M. MORRISON, Sharon A. BAKER, and Mary Rogers GILLMORE

The advent of AIDS, as well as high rates of STDs among teenagers, has focused attention on the need for sexually-active teenagers to use condoms for disease prevention (Brooks-Gunn, Boyer & Hein, 1988; Holmes, Karon & Kreiss, 1990; Stiffman & Earls, 1990). Although most adults would prefer that teens protect themselves from pregnancy and disease by remaining sexually abstinent until adulthood, a substantial proportion of teens engage in intercourse during their high school years (Hayes, 1987; Wattleton, 1987). Consistent use of latex condoms for penetrative sex is widely regarded as the most effective method to prevent acquisition of disease (Carey et al., 1992; Centers for Disease Control, 1988).

Few sexually-active teenagers use protection consistently, however, leaving themselves at risk for disease at least some of the time (Mosher & Pratt, 1990). Teens are thus apt targets for interventions to increase condom use, for this and other reasons. There is growing recognition that interventions, to be effective, need to be grounded in the beliefs of the population of interest (cf., Fisher, Fisher & Rye, 1995). According to behavioural decision theories, intentions to engage in a behaviour are based on expected consequences of the behaviour. Intentions can change when beliefs about the expected consequences change. An important step, therefore, in designing a behaviour change intervention, should be to determine what beliefs underlie the behaviour. Intervention efforts can then be addressed to changing or discrediting negative beliefs, adding new positive beliefs, or enhancing existing positive beliefs. To this end, the study presented here is an investigation of the beliefs about condoms of teenagers who are at high risk for AIDS and STDs.

The Theory of Reasoned Action

This study is based on the Theory of Reasoned Action (TRA), an influential expectancy-value model that has been widely used to model a variety of health-related behaviours (cf., Carter, 1990). The TRA is a cognitive model that describes a process of combining information to direct a decision about a behaviour. It assumes that individuals who are making decisions about a behaviour (whom we will call "actors") hold certain expectations and beliefs about the consequences of the behaviour and about social norms regarding the behaviour, and base their decisions on those expectations and beliefs. The theory states that the best predictor of a behaviour like condom use is the actor's intention to perform the behaviour (in this case, use condoms).

Intention is posited to be a function of both the attitude toward performing the behaviour and subjective norm about the behaviour. Attitude is an evaluative dimension, reflecting an overall feeling of favourableness or unfavourableness toward the behaviour. It is based on a set of beliefs about the consequences of the behaviour, each of which is the product of (1) how likely the outcome is and (2) how good or bad it is. An example an outcome belief about condom use might be that it will prevent pregnancy. An actor may evaluate preventing positively or negatively, depending on whether a pregnancy is desired at this time (evaluation), and may perceive that condoms are very likely or very unlikely to effectively prevent pregnancy (likelihood).

Subjective norm reflects the actor's perception of what others want the actor to do. It is based on a set of beliefs about the norms of salient others and motivation to comply with them. For example, a normative referent for condom use might be one's health care provider. The normative belief is composed of the actor's judgements of (1) whether the provider is supportive of, or opposed to, the actor's use of condoms, and (2) how motivated the actor is to comply with the provider.

The TRA as a Model of Condom Use

A number of empirical studies have been undertaken to test the ability of the TRA, or some of its constructs, to account for condom use and other sexual behaviours that influence a person's risk of contracting HIV. With rare exceptions, intentions to use condoms consistently have been found to be positively associated with condom use. Sheeran and Orbell (1998) recently published the results of a meta-analysis of 28 tests of the association between condom use and intentions reported in both published and unpublished studies. They found a 'medium to strong sample-weighted average correlation between intentions and condom use ($r = .44$)' (p. 231). Other studies suggest that the relationship is quite generalisable, in that it has been demonstrated in both straight (St. Lawrence et al., 1998) and gay samples (Fisher, Fisher, & Rye, 1995; but only for insertive, not receptive, oral or anal sex; Ross, 1990; Wulfert, Wan, & Backus, 1996); among adolescents (Reinicke, Schmit, & Ajzen, 1996) as well as adults (Heckman et al,. 1996); among persons of colour (St. Lawrence et al., 1998) as well as whites in the U.S.; and, cross-nationally, in samples of German adolescents (Reinecke et al., 1996), adolescents and young adults in St. Vincent and the Grenadines (Albarracin, Fishbein, & Middlestadt, 1998;), Australian gay men (Ross & McLaws, 1992) and Australian university students (White, Terry, & Hogg, 1994). Only rarely have intentions been found to be unrelated to condom use, such as in one convenience sample of high school U.S. adolescents (Fisher et al., 1995), and a sample of U.S. contraceptive clinic users (Valdiserri, Arena, Proctor, & Bonati, 1989).

The relationship between attitudes toward, and subjective norms about, condom use with intentions to use condoms has been examined in many more studies than has the intention-behaviour relationship. Studies of adolescents' intentions to use condoms consistently have found both attitude and subjective norms related to intentions, in Canada (Godin, Fortin, Michaud, Bradet & Kok, 1997), Germany (Reinecke et al., 1996; Krahe & Reiss, 1995), Norway (Rise, 1992), the Netherlands (Schaalma, Kok & Peters, 1993), and the U.S. (Jemmott, Jemmott & Hacker, 1992), suggesting that these results are quite generalisable. Exceptions include a study of Malawian adolescents (Bandawe & Foster, 1996) in which attitude, but not norm, predicted intentions, and a study of U.S. high school students (Fisher et al., 1995) in which both attitude and norm were related to intentions among females, but only attitude predicted the intentions of males.

Among adults, the picture is somewhat more complicated. Among gay and bisexual men, for example, some studies have found both attitude and norm associated with intentions (Fishbein et al., 1992; Fisher et al., 1995); others have found only norm related to intentions (Ross & McLaws, 1992), and still others find only attitude related to intentions (Wulfert et al., 1996). Among heterosexuals, both attitude and norm seem to predict intentions (White, Terry, & Hogg, 1994; Kashima, Gallois, & McCamish, 1993; Chan & Fishbein, 1993) when partner type is not taken into account. However, when partner type (main or steady vs. non-main or casual) is taken into account, the relationship is less clear. Catania, Coates, and Kegeles (1994) found, in a probability sample of adults, that norm, but not attitude, predicted intentions with casual partners. In Baker, Morrison, Carter and Verdon's (1996) study of STD clinic clients, they report similar findings, but only for women. For men, only attitude, but not norm, predicted intention to use condoms with casual partners, and both attitude and norm predicted intentions with steady partners. The reasons for these inconsistencies is not clear. Taking the literature as a whole, the TRA seems to have utility in explaining decisions to use condoms, and the formation of condom-use intentions. Relationships between attitude, norm, and intentions to use condoms have been demonstrated cross culturally, both among adolescents, as described above, and across distinct ethnic groups of adults (Godin et al., 1994).

The Addition of Self-efficacy or Perceived Behavioural Control

One limitation of the TRA as a model of condom use is that the TRA models volitional behaviour, and makes no provision for the effects of factors outside of the actor's control; these are seen in the TRA either as distal variables that shape the initial outcome and normative beliefs, or as post-decision factors, which intervene between intention and behaviour, but do not influence intention *per se*. In forming an intention to use condoms, however, the actor may well take his or her partner's anticipated cooperation into account. That is, an individual might have a positive attitude toward using condoms and might perceive generally positive norms toward using condoms, but believe that his or her partner would flatly refuse. If we predicted such a person's intention from attitude and norm alone we would predict a positive intention to use condoms, but the belief that an attempt would be unsuccessful might change the actor's intention to negative: Why bother to try if you are sure that you will fail? This reasoning suggests that the addition of a measure of the actor's perception that he or she can carry out the behaviour – what Bandura (1977) calls self-efficacy – should increase prediction of intention for non-volitional behaviour, over and above prediction attained from attitude and norm alone.

Insofar as perceived self-efficacy is an accurate reflection of the actor's influence, it may also influence the link between intention and behaviour: Individuals who have positive attitudes and subjective norms toward condom use but are not effectively persuasive may try to convince their partners, but fail. Self-efficacy may also affect the actor's persistence in the face of initial failure (Bandura, 1989). Individuals who are higher in self-efficacy may be more likely to attempt condom use, more likely to successfully implement condom use, and more likely to persist in attempts than those who are lower in self-efficacy.

We should note here that there is controversy about the operationalisation of self-efficacy and how it is similar to, or different from, what Ajzen and others have called perceived behavioural control (Ajzen, 1985). Our measure of self-efficacy is based on judgements of whether or not one *could* perform the behaviour, rated as a likelihood. This is similar to the way Bandura and others have measured self-efficacy (cf., Ozer & Bandura, 1990), and to confidence ratings sometimes used (cf., Galavotti et al., 1995). Others have conceptualised self-efficacy as the actor's rating of the ease or difficulty with which the behaviour could be implemented (cf., Terry & O'Leary, 1995), and Ajzen's conceptualisation of perceived behavioural control includes measures of both ease or difficulty and degree of control (cf., Ajzen & Madden, 1986).

Recent TRA studies of condom use that have included self-efficacy as an additional predictor have operationalised self-efficacy variously as certainty (Basen-Engquist & Parcel, 1992), degree of control (Boyd & Wandersman, 1991), likelihood one could use condoms (Morrison, Gillmore & Baker, 1995), likelihood one would not be used (Richard & van der Pligt, 1991), and difficulty of getting one's partner to use them (White, Terry & Hogg, 1994). Chan and Fishbein (1993) used a multi-item measure incorporating both expected ease or difficulty and degree of control. In general, the studies that supported the role of self-efficacy in prediction of intention or behaviour were those using a certainty or likelihood rating (Basen-Engquist & Parcel, 1992; Morrison et al., 1995; Richard & van der Pligt, 1991). In those studies in which self-efficacy was operationalised as perceived difficulty in performing the behaviour or degree of control (Boyd & Wandersman, 1991; Chan & Fishbein, 1993; White et al., 1994), there was no significant increase in prediction.

Additional Factors Considered Here

We also model the decision to use condoms separately for two types of partners: steady partners (those with whom the actor has an ongoing relationship) and casual partners (new partners or partners with whom the actor has occasional sex but no romantic relationship). Type of partner has proved an essential distinction in our previous research with high-risk heterosexuals (Baker et al., 1996; Gillmore, Morrison, Lowery & Baker, 1994; Morrison et al., 1995), as well as work by others (Richard and van der Plight, 1991; Weisman, Plichta, Nathanson, Ensminger & Robinson, 1991). In analyses of intention to use condoms among high-risk heterosexual adults, for example, we found attitudes to be more important than norms in predicting intention to use condoms with steady partners, but norms more important than attitudes for casual partners (Morrison et al., 1995). Baker et al. (1996) also found that the TRA predicted condom use intentions differentially for persons who had steady partners and for those who had casual partners, with stronger prediction of intention to use condoms with steady partners than with casual partners. Richard and van der Pligt (1991) demonstrated differences in the relative weights of attitude and subjective norm by partner type in their adolescent sample, with attitudes predictive of condom use only for respondents who have only steady partners. In this study, we expect to find better prediction for steady than for casual partners, because the characteristics of casual partners are less well known to the actor, leading to greater ambiguity in the formation of, and follow-through on, intentions to use condoms.

We have also included gender, and the interactions of each of the model variables (attitude, norm, and self-efficacy) with gender, as predictors of intention to use condoms. Gender may moderate the effects of attitudes and norms on intentions to use condoms insofar as condom use involves different behaviours for men and women. Women are more dependent on their male partners' cooperation, and this may be reflected in greater weight on perceived norms, particularly partner norms. Conversely, attitude may be more important for men than for women because they can act directly on their attitudes, rather than having to negotiate condom use with their partners.

The two studies that we are aware of that have directly examined sex differences in the relative weights of attitude and norm about condom use draw different conclusions. In our own research on adults' condom use (Morrison et al., 1995), we found interactions of gender with both attitude and norm for condom use with steady partners, such that attitude and norm had equal weight for women, but only attitude was predictive for men. For casual partners, norms carried a larger weight than attitudes for women, and attitudes a larger weight than norms for men. Adler and her colleagues (Adler, Kegeles, Irwin, & Wibbelsman, 1990), however, had quite contrary results: Attitude, but not norm, was significantly associated with condom use intentions for women. In contrast, subjective norm, but not attitude, was significantly associated with condom use intentions for men. Examination of these interactions in this third sample, which resembles Adler et al.'s sample in age, and resembles our adult sample in other characteristics (such as high-risk status), should help to clarify these contrasting results.

A final addition to the model is the interaction of attitude and norm. The TRA does not predict such an interaction, but it has been observed in some previous research. Baker et al. (1996) found that only those who had both positive attitudes and positive subjective norms intended to use condoms. Given that using a condom is a dyadic behaviour, it seems reasonable to expect that only when both norms and attitudes are positive will intentions be positive. If the actor's attitude is negative, she or he is unlikely to intend to use condoms, irrespective of subjective norm. If attitude is positive but subjective norm is negative (such as might be the case when the actor expects that his or her partner, a very salient referent, does not want us to use condoms), the actor may be dissuaded from even suggesting condom use. This may be particularly true of teens, insofar as teens are although to be greatly concerned about how they are perceived by their peers.

In summary, the present research is a test of an expansion of Fishbein and Ajzen's TRA model for predicting high risk heterosexual teens' decisions to use condoms. We test not only whether attitude and norm independently predict intentions to use condoms, as posited by the TRA, but also (a) whether intentions predict subsequent condom use, (b) whether attitude and norm interact to predict intention, (c) whether condom use self-efficacy adds to the prediction of intention or behaviour, net of the TRA variables, and (d) whether gender interacts with attitude, norm, or self-efficacy in the prediction of condom use intentions. Finally, we examine the relationship of attitude and norm to specific outcome and normative beliefs, which are important to consider in designing interventions.

METHOD

Overview of Research Design

The study is a longitudinal survey designed to assess decision making with regard to condom use. Predictor variables measured at Time 1 included all TRA variables: intention to use condoms in the next three months; attitudes toward condom use; subjective norms about using condoms; perceived likelihood and evaluation of salient outcomes of using condoms; perceived norms of salient referents and motivation to comply with those referents with regard to condom use. Perceived condom use self-efficacy was also measured. Specific outcome beliefs, normative referents, and self-efficacy situations were developed based on open-ended interviews with 83 male and female, white and African-American clients in the STD clinic and correctional facilities. The Time 2 target behaviour was self-report of condom use in the previous three months.

Subjects

Teenage respondents (ages 14–19) were recruited from two sources: (1) clients registering for services at a large, urban public health department STD clinic located in the northwest, and (2) teens incarcerated in the county juvenile detention facility who were referred by clinicians based on the teen's requests for sexual health care and/or other indications that the teenager was sexually active.

Table 2.1 presents data describing the demographic characteristics of the sample. The sample was stratified by race and gender, and eligibility was restricted to whites and African-Americans, the ethnic groups represented in the largest numbers in the clinics. The sample of 467 includes 135 African-

Table 2.1   Subject Characteristics

Subject Characteristics	
Mean age	16.91
Race	*n (%)*
White	218 (47%)
African American	249 (53%)
Education	
Less than high school	219 (47%)
High school or GED	198 (42%)
Some post high school	50 (11%)
Live with	
Parents or guardian	282 (60%)
Alone	34 (7%)
Other	151 (32%)
Marital Status	
Never married	457 (98%)
Mother's education	
Less than high school	52 (11%)
High school or GED	132 (28%)
Some post high school	157 (34%)
College graduate	82 (18%)
Don't know/doesn't apply	42 (9%)
Missing	2 (<1%)
Total Family Income	
Under $5000	64 (14%)
$5001–$10,000	28 (6%)
$10,001–$20,000	39 (8%)
$20,001–$30,000	31 (7%)
$30,001 or more	72 (16%)
Don't know	228 (49%)
Missing	5 (1%)
Mean age at first intercourse	13.05
Median number of lifetime partners	5–10

Note. Total n = 467

American young women, 114 African-American young men, 130 white young women and 88 white young men. At Time 1, the majority of the respondents (84%) had steady partners, and almost half (49%) had casual partners; some had both types (33%). Follow-up questionnaires (Time 2) were obtained from 352 (75%) of the original 467 subjects. There were no differences between the longitudinal sample and the Time 1 sample on demographic characteristics or sexual history variables.

Procedure

All individuals registering for services at the STD clinic were given a written description of the study, with a form to return if they wished to participate. In detention, potential respondents were referred by staff clinicians. At both sites, potential respondents were then screened to ensure that they met our age, gender and race criteria and our stratification goals, and that they had engaged in heterosexual intercourse in the previous three months.

After giving informed consent, participants completed structured questionnaires in a private room with an interviewer present. To ensure inclusion of respondents with low reading levels, the interviewer offered to read the questionnaire to respondents. Most respondents preferred to self-administer the questionnaire and had no apparent difficulty with it. Completing the questionnaire typically took 30 to 45 minutes, slightly longer for those who had the questionnaire read to them. Respondents were paid $10 for completing the survey.

Extensive locator information was collected from respondents, with the understanding that we would contact them again in three months. The Time 2 survey, which was similar to, and slightly shorter than, the initial survey, was mailed to each respondent. If mailed surveys were not returned within a month, multiple efforts were made to locate the respondents and encourage them to return the questionnaire. Most of these respondents were contacted by phone and subsequently mailed their questionnaires; in some cases interviewers met respondents at their homes, our offices, or in the STD clinic. Respondents were paid $15 for completing the second survey.

Measures

All of the variables used in this analysis, with the exception of condom use behaviour, were asked with respect to using condoms in the *next* 3 months with either a steady or casual partner, and were measured at the Time 1 questionnaire administration. Condom use behaviour was also assessed separately for steady and casual partners, but was assessed at the Time 2 survey, and referred to the preceding three months (i.e., the interval between Time 1 and Time 2). Except where noted, all items used seven point Likert-type response scales. The wording and anchors of the items are listed below. Where items were worded differently for women and men, the female version is presented first and the male version is shown in brackets.

Intention to Use Condoms

'How likely are you to use condoms with your steady/casual partner(s) over the next three months?' The response scale anchors were 'very unlikely' and 'very likely', and the mid-point was labelled '50/50 chance.' Higher scores indicate greater likelihood. For steady partners, the mean was 4.30 (s.d. = 2.31); for casual partners, the mean was 5.78 (s.d. = 1.61).

Attitudes Toward Using Condoms

'Using condoms with my steady/casual partner(s) in the next three months would be...' Four semantic differential response scales were used for each type of partner. Anchors for the four scales were: bad/good, helpful/harmful, foolish/wise, and pleasant/unpleasant. Higher scores were assigned to the positive anchor. The average of the four items for that partner type was used as the respondent's overall attitude toward using condoms with that partner type. The reliabilities (Cronbach's alpha) for the scales were .84 for steady partners and .79 for casual partners. Mean attitudes toward using condoms were positive for both steady partners (mean = 5.44, s.d. = 1.41) and casual partners (mean = 5.99, s.d. = 1.15).

Subjective Norm Toward Using Condoms

Subjective norm was measured as the average of three items. 'Most people who are important to me think that with my steady/casual partner(s) I...,' and 'People whose opinion I respect think that with my steady/casual partner(s) I...' were used with a response scale anchored with 'definitely should not use condoms' and 'definitely should use condoms.' The third item, 'Thinking about my steady/casual partner(s), most people who are important to me...' used anchors 'strongly oppose our use of condoms' and 'strongly support our use of condoms.' Higher scores indicate more positive perceived norms. Reliabilities for the scales were .74 for steady partners and .77 for casual partners. Mean subjective norms were positive for both steady partners (mean = 5.51, s.d. = 1.39) and causal partners (mean = 6.10, s.d. = 1.28).

Outcome Beliefs

Twelve beliefs about the outcomes of using condoms were measured. These were: 'Protecting myself from getting VD;' 'Not getting [her] pregnant;' 'Less physical pleasure from sex for me;' 'Less physical pleasure from sex for my partner;' 'Having sex seem unnatural or artificial;' 'Making sex last longer;' 'Making sex less intimate and romantic;' 'My partner losing his [Losing my] erection and not being able to ejaculate ('cum');' 'Feeling he [she] doesn't trust me;' 'Getting [Having her get] dry and sore;' 'Interrupting sex;' and 'Causing a fight or argument.' Two items were constructed for each belief; the first was the individual's estimate of the likelihood of the outcome ['very unlikely' (coded 0) to 'very likely' (6)]; the second was the individual's evaluation of that outcome ['very bad' (−3) to 'very good' (+3)]. Following Ajzen and Fishbein (1980), the computed value of each belief item is the product of the likelihood and evaluation ratings. These product terms are then summed to form the overall value of the outcome beliefs.

Normative Beliefs

Norms of five referents were measured, under the general question, 'What do you think other people who are important to you think about you using condoms with your steady/casual partner(s)?'. The referents were: 'My sexual partner;' 'Most of my close friends;' 'My doctor or health care provider;' 'My mother;' and 'Most of my other family members.' Two items were constructed for each referent. We assessed the respondent's perception of each referent's norm: '[Referent] thinks that with my steady/casual partner(s) I...'. Response anchors were 'definitely should not use condoms' (−3) and 'definitely should use condoms' (+3). For each referent, respondents also rated the statement, 'Generally speaking, I want to do what [referent] think(s) I should do.' Response anchors were 'very little' (1) and 'very much' (7). Again, following Ajzen and Fishbein (1980), the computed value for each normative belief is the product of the perceived referent norm and motivation to comply with the referent. These product terms are then summed.

Self-efficacy

Self-efficacy was assessed separately for steady and casual partners. The self-efficacy items began with the stem, 'I could get my steady/casual partner to use condoms. . . ' and responses were on 7-point likelihood scales, with higher scores indicating greater likelihoods. For each partner type, respondents rated their likelihood of being able to use condoms in 10 specific situations: 'if condoms were handy when we had sex,' 'if I was worried about catching VD from him [her],' 'if I was worried about *giving* him [her] VD,' 'if I was worried about getting pregnant by him [getting her pregnant],' 'if he [she] objected to using them,' 'if I felt comfortable talking with him [her] about it,' 'if I was drunk or high,' 'if I thought he [she] was using needles,' 'if sex was unexpected or spur of the moment,' and 'if we were very 'turned on' sexually.' The 10 situational factors were those mentioned most frequently in the initial elicitation interviews, described earlier. The mean of these 10 ratings for each partner type formed the self-efficacy scale for that partner type. Means were 4.68 (s.d. = 1.51) for steady partners and 5.22 (s.d. = 1.25) for casual partners. Reliabilities for the scales were .85 for steady partners and .82 for casual partners.

Condom Use

'How often have you used condoms for vaginal sex with your steady/a casual partner in the past three months?' Five responses were: 'Never,' 'Less than half the time,' 'About half the time,' 'Over half the time,' and 'Every time we had vaginal sex in the last three months.' Those respondents who had only non-vaginal sex with that partner type in the last three months were excluded from the analysis.

Analysis Strategy

Partner types

We examined condom use separately for two types of sexual partners: steady partners ('someone you have sex with and also have an ongoing relationship with') and casual partners ('someone you have sex with and do not have an ongoing relationship with'). The casual partner definition specifically excluded sex for payment of money, drugs, gifts, or payment of rent. (Condom use with such partners was assessed for women who had paying partners, but is not reported here.) At each interview, subjects completed questions about steady partners only if they had a current steady partner; they completed casual partner questions only if they had had at least one casual partner in the past three months. Partners were those with whom the respondent had oral, vaginal, or anal sex in the prior three months. The subjects for the two analyses are therefore overlapping, but not identical. Those who have had both steady partners and casual partners in the past 3 months are in both analyses; those who have only steady or only casual partners are in only one analysis. These samples best mirror the population of individuals with that type of partner, avoiding the potential bias created by restricting analyses to those with only one type of partner, or to only those with both types of partners. Note that, for longitudinal analyses, only respondents who had that type of partner at *both* interviews can be included.

RESULTS

Analysis Strategy

Intention was regressed onto other model variables in steps. We first entered the standard TRA variables of attitude and norm, which tests the traditional TRA. At the second step, we entered the attitude/norm interaction, which both our own experience (Baker et al., 1996) and the experience of others (e.g., Shimp & Kavas, 1984; Smetana & Adler, 1980) suggest may increase prediction of intention. This interaction term must follow the main effects to be interpretable. At the third step, we entered self-efficacy, to test whether it adds to prediction of intention, over and above prediction from attitude, norm, and their interaction. At the fourth step we added a dummy variable for gender, to set the stage for testing gender interactions. Finally, on the fifth and final step, we entered the interactions of gender with attitude, norm, and self-efficacy, to test for gender differences in the relationship of these predictors to intention. Where interaction terms were used, the component variables were first 'centred' (i.e., transformed to deviation from the mean scores), as suggested by Cronbach (1987) and by Jaccard, Turrisi and Wan (1990), to alleviate problems of interpretation in the presence of multicollinearity among predictors.

Condom use at the second interview was regressed onto intention and self-efficacy at the initial interview, separately for each partner type. Intention was entered on the first step. Self-efficacy was entered on the second step, to determine its influence net of intention. These analyses use the longitudinal cohort.

Test of the Expanded TRA

Steady Partners

Table 2.2 summarises the steady partner regression results, showing the regression coefficients and multiple regression coefficients for each variable at each step. The initial regression of intention to use condoms with a steady partner onto attitude and norm yielded a significant R of .727. The regression weights for both attitude and norm were significant. The addition of the attitude-norm interaction in the second step did not produce a significant change in R. The additions of self-efficacy, in the third step, and gender, in the fourth step, both significantly increased R, but the final addition of the three gender interaction terms on the fifth step did not.

Table 2.3 summarises the results of regressions onto condom use with steady partners. The correlation between intention to use condoms at Time 1 and

Table 2.2   Regression of intention to use condoms with steady partners onto attitude, norm, self-efficacy, and gender

	Standardized Regression Coefficients				
	Step 1	*Step 2*	*Step 3*	*Step 4*	*Step 5*
Attitude	.638*	.642*	.606*	.622*	.621*
Norm	.165*	.167*	.147*	.148*	.163*
Attitude*Norm		.040(ns)	.041(ns)	.039(ns)	.043(ns)
Self-Efficacy			.169*	.163*	.160*
Gender				.153*	.152*
Gender*Attitude					.020(ns)
Gender*Norm					.000(ns)
Gender*Self-Efficacy					.055(ns)
R	.727	.728	.746	.761	.764
Adjusted R^2	.524	.523	.548	.569	.568
F of change in R^2	124.23*	0.72(ns)	12.96*	11.96*	0.71(ns)

Note: N = 225

 * p < .05

Table 2.3   Regression of condom use with steady partners onto intention, self-efficacy, and gender

	Standardized Regression Coefficients			
	Step 1	*Step 2*	*Step 3*	*Step 4*
Intention	.483*	.492*	.480*	.480*
Self-efficacy		-.026(ns)	-.225*(ns	−.211(ns))
Gender			.105(ns)	.104(ns)
Gender*Self-Efficacy				.007(ns)
R	.483	.484	.495	.496
Adjusted R^2	.230	.227	.234	.231
F of change in R^2	65.53*	0.68(ns)	0.82(ns)	0.90(ns)

Note: N = 217

 * p < .05

 (ns) not significant

condom use at Time 2 was .483. There was no significant relationship between self-efficacy and subsequent condom use, net of intention, although there was a small but significant univariate relationship (r = .15; p < .05). Neither gender nor the gender by self-efficacy interaction added significantly to the explained variation in condom use at Time 2, net of the effects of intention.

Casual Partners

Table 2.4 summarises the casual partner regression results, showing the regression coefficients and multiple regression coefficients for each variable at

Table 2.4 Regression of intention to use condoms with casual partners onto attitude, norm, self-efficacy, and gender

	Standardized Regression Coefficients				
	Step 1	*Step 2*	*Step 3*	*Step 4*	*Step 5*
Attitude	.520*	.542*	.574*	.574*	.583*
Norm	.326*	.338*	.339*	.341*	.386*
Attitude*Norm		.044(ns)	.058(ns)	.060(ns)	.114(ns)
Self-Efficacy			-.057(ns)	-.056(ns)	−.028(ns)
Gender				.007(ns)	.024(ns)
Gender*Attitude					.117(ns)
Gender*Norm					−.098(ns)
Gender*Self-Efficacy					−.019(ns)
R	.759	.760	.761	.761	.766
Adjusted R^2	.564	.560	.556	.550	.538
F of change in R^2	50.24*	0.18(ns)	0.44(ns)	0.01(ns)	0.37(ns)

Note: N = 77
    * p < .05
    (ns) not significant

each step. The initial regression of intention to use condoms with casual partners onto attitude and norm yielded a significant R of .759. As with the steady partners, the regression weights for both attitude and norm were significant. The additions of the attitude-norm interaction, self-efficacy, gender, and the interactions of gender with self-efficacy, attitude, and norm did not increase R.

Table 2.5 summarises the results of regressions onto condom use with casual partners. The correlation between intention to use condoms at Time 1 and condom use at Time 2 was .22, which was not significant. As with steady partners, there was no significant relationship between self-efficacy and subsequent condom use, net of intention. In this case, however, there was also no significant univariate relationship (r = .04; n.s.) and the partial coefficient for intentions to use condoms was reduced to marginal significance (p < .07). Neither the main effect of gender nor the gender by self-efficacy interaction added significantly to prediction of condom use net of the effect of intentions.

Analysis of Specific Outcome and Normative Beliefs

The correlations between the sum of the outcome belief cross-products and overall attitude were computed separately for both steady and casual partners, as were correlations between the sums of the normative beliefs product terms and overall subjective norm. These correlations assess the adequacy of the sets of beliefs to predict overall attitude or norm. Correlations between overall attitude and each outcome belief, and between overall subjective norms and each normative belief were also computed. These correlations assess the relationship of each specific belief or referent to overall attitude or subjective norm.

Table 2.5   Regression of condom use with casual partners onto intention, self-efficacy, and gender

| | *Standardized Regression Coefficients* | | | |
	Step 1	*Step 2*	*Step 3*	*Step 4*
Intention	.221*	.226(ns)	.230(ns)	.260*
Self-efficacy		−.019(ns)	−.024(ns)	−.031(ns)
Gender			−.066(ns)	−.058(ns)
Gender*Self-Efficacy				.091(ns)
R	.221	.222	.231	.247
Adjusted R^2	.036	.022	.013	.006
F of change in R^2	3.058#	0.26(ns)	0.32(ns)	0.54(ns)

Note: N = 74
  # .05 < p < .06
  * p < .05
  (ns) not significant

Table 2.6 shows the correlations of each outcome belief product term with overall attitude, and the correlation of attitude with the sum of the 12 outcome belief product terms, for both steady partners and casual partners. For steady partners, all but one (condoms makes sex last longer) of the specific outcome beliefs are significantly correlated with attitude toward using condoms. The

Table 2.6   Correlations of outcome belief product terms with overall attitude, by partner type

| | *Correlation with overall attitude toward condom use:* | | | |
| *Outcome belief* | *Steady partner* | | *Casual partner* | |
	r	*n*	*r*	*n*
Protecting myself from getting VD	.29***	225	.19(ns)	77
Not getting [her] pregnant	.34***	224	.35**	77
Less physical pleasure from sex for me	.35***	217	.14(ns)	74
Less physical pleasure from sex for my partner	.32***	219	.16(ns)	77
Having sex seem unnatural or artificial	.29***	224	.27*	77
Making sex last longer	-.05(ns)	223	.41***	77
Making sex less intimate and romantic	.35***	223	.21(ns)	75
My partner losing his [Losing my] erection and not being able to ejaculate ("cum")	.24***	224	.25*	77
Feeling he [she] doesn't trust me	.35***	222	.29**	77
Getting [Having her get] dry and sore	.15*	223	.15(ns)	73
Interrupting sex	.22***	219	.16(ns)	73
Causing a fight or argument	.18**	219	.40***	76
r, attitude with the sum of outcome beliefs	.49***	217	.42***	76

Note: *p < .05, 2-tailed; **p < .01; ***p<.001, 2-tailed; ns = not significant

Table 2.7 **Correlations of normative belief product terms with overall subjective norm, by partner type**

| Normative belief | Correlation with overall subjective norm toward condom use: | | | |
| | Steady partner | | Casual partner | |
	r	n	r	n
My sexual partner	.36**	226	.32*	78
Most of my close friends	.52**	224	.41**	78
My doctor or health care provider	.52**	224	.52**	77
My mother	.48**	221	.39**	74
Most of my other family members	.46**	223	.40**	76
r, subjective norm with the sum of normative beliefs	.69***	223	.60***	77

Note: *p<.01; **p < .001; 2-tailed; ***p<.001, 2-tailed

correlation of attitude with the sum of the outcome beliefs is positive and significant.

For casual partners, fewer outcome beliefs are significantly correlated with attitude, and the correlation of the sum of the outcome beliefs with attitude is lower. In contrast to the findings for steady partners, the beliefs that using condoms protects against STDs, result in less physical pleasure from sex for the respondent or partner, make sex less intimate and romantic, make the woman sore and dry, and interrupt sex were not significantly correlated with attitude.

Table 2.7 shows the correlations of the normative belief product terms with overall subjective norm, and the correlations of norms with the sum of the normative belief product terms, for both steady partners and casual partners. For both partner types, all of the specific normative beliefs are significantly correlated with subjective norm toward using condoms, and virtually all of the correlations are larger than the attitude/outcome belief correlations. The correlations of subjective norm with the sums of the normative beliefs are also significant for both partner types.

DISCUSSION

In these analyses, we tested the traditional TRA's ability to predict intention to use condoms, and subsequent condom use behaviour, in a sample of sexually active heterosexual teenagers at high risk for STDs, including HIV. We also tested an augmented TRA model, which examined the interaction of attitude and norm, self efficacy for condom use, gender, and the interaction of gender with model variables as predictors of intention to use condoms. We then examined the relationship between intention and subsequent behaviour, as well as the effect of self-efficacy on behaviour, net of the influence of intention. Finally, we examined the relationship between outcome beliefs and overall attitude, and of normative beliefs and overall subjective norm.

Predicting Condom-use Intentions

Traditional TRA

Consistent with previous findings, both attitudes and subjective norms for condom use were significantly related to intention to use condoms with both steady and casual partners. This finding contrasts with several other studies with teenagers which did not consistent relationships between subjective norm and intention (Adler et al., 1990; Basen-Engquist & Parcel, 1992; Richard & van der Pligt, 1991). This may reflect differences in our sample: Adler et al.'s sample was drawn from a primary care setting; and Basen-Engquist et al.'s and Richard et al.'s samples were drawn from school settings. These samples include both higher- and lower-risk teens. Our sample, recruited from teens receiving STD-related health services, was exclusively higher risk. Heightened awareness of STDs and of their own risk may have increased the salience of subjective norms. However, consistent with these studies and others based on both adult and teenager samples, attitude was a stronger predictor of intention than subjective norm (Adler et al., 1990; Basen-Engquist & Parcel, 1992; Chan & Fishbein, 1993; Morrison et al., 1995; Richard & van der Pligt, 1991; White et al., 1994).

Most studies using the TRA to understand the decision to use condoms have not distinguished between steady partners and casual partners (Boyd & Wandersman, 1991; Basen-Engquist & Parcel, 1992, Jemmott & Jemmott, 1991), but this is potentially a crucial distinction. Kelly and Kalichman (1995) have pointed out that the level of risk and the dynamics of risk reduction may be very different in an ongoing affectionate relationship, as opposed to a casual relationship. In our own research with adults (Morrison et al., 1995) prediction was consistently higher for steady partners than for casual partners. Yet, in the current study, which parallels the adult study in measurement and design, we find little difference in the proportion of variance accounted for by attitude and norm with steady partners ($R^2 = .53$) as opposed to casual partners ($R^2 = .58$). Richard and van der Pligt (1991) also found that the proportion of variance accounted for did not vary systematically by whether or not teens were in an exclusive relationship with a partner. Why would type of relationship predict differentially for teens and adults? Perhaps teens don't know *any* of their partners well, resulting in little difference between steady and casual partners. To test this, we compared the length of relationship with steady partners reported by adults and teenagers in our adult and teenage samples. We found, as expected, that teenagers' relationships with their steady partners were significantly shorter than adults, (t = 17.45, df = 380, p < .001). For the teens, the mean length of relationship with the steady partner was 12 months (mode = 2 months) and for adults the mean was 20 months (mode = 6 months). For the teens, steady partners may not be that much better known than are casual partners.

Augmented Theory

The dyadic nature of condom use behaviour suggests that attitude and subjective norm might be closely related and might interact in the decision making process. In this population, however, the interaction between attitude and subjective norm did not improve prediction of intention with steady or casual partners. This is consistent with our recent adult findings, but contrasts with an earlier finding, based on research in the same clinic, conducted several years earlier (Baker et al., 1996). One possible explanation for this difference may be historical; that social norms about condoms have changed, such that they are now more likely to be positively correlated with attitudes.

We also tested the addition of self-efficacy, and found that, with steady partners, the addition of self efficacy for the behaviour improved prediction of intention to use condoms, but only slightly. With casual partners, however, self-efficacy did not enter the equation; attitude and subjective norm were the only significant predictors of intention to use condoms. This is consistent with our study with high risk adults (Morrison et al., 1995), in which self-efficacy improved prediction of intention with steady partners, but not with casual partners. Why is self-efficacy for condom use apparently more important in steady than in casual relationships? In both studies, reported use of condoms and mean self-efficacy scores were higher with casual than with steady partners. Perhaps, because steady relationships carry an expectation of monogamy and of sexual safety, introducing the idea of using condoms into a steady relationship is much more challenging than it is with a casual partner.

Because the goal of condom use requires different behaviours for males, who use condoms, and females, who must request and persuade their partners to use condoms, we entered gender, and the interaction of gender with other model variables, into the regression predicting intention. With steady partners, we found a small effect for gender: Males had more positive intentions to use condoms than did females. With casual partners, there were no significant gender differences, and there were no interactions of gender with other model variables for either partner type, contrary to our expectations.

Although the introduction of variables extraneous to the TRA does enrich our understanding of adolescents' decision making with regard to condom use with steady partners, attitude and subjective norm remain the major predictors of intention to use condoms with both partner types, despite the fact that the goal of using condoms is not completely under the control of the individual. These results are similar to those we found with adults (Morrison et al., 1995).

Predicting Condom Use Behaviour

The TRA suggests that intention is the best predictor of a person's future behaviour. In these data, intention to use condoms with a steady partner was predictive of condom use ($r = .48$), but intention to use with a casual partner was only marginally associated with subsequent use ($r = .22$). We found a similar, though less dramatic difference in the adult study, with correlations of .38 and .27 for steady and casual partners, respectively. The strong difference in the predictive power of intention between partner types may reflect the unplanned character of teens' sexual encounters with casual partners, or the influence of situational factors (such as the availability of a condom at the time of intercourse) in determining whether or not condoms are used with a casual partner. Teens might benefit from frank discussion of the importance of being prepared for sex even when it is not explicitly planned: to carry condoms with them all the time, to have a prepared and rehearsed script for raising the issue with a new partner, to presume that any new partner is infectious until proven otherwise, rather than vice versa.

Although self-efficacy has shown direct effects on behaviour in some studies (e.g., Richard & van der Pligt, 1991; but note that this study did not control for the effects of intention), in this study, as in two previous studies of condom use (Morrison et al., 1995; White et al., 1994), self-efficacy was not related to condom use behaviour, net of the influence of intention. This should not be taken to mean that self-efficacy has no role; beliefs about one's ability to perform the behaviours necessary to successfully use condoms may be important components of attitude or intention.

Predicting Overall Attitude

As suggested by the TRA, the sum of outcome beliefs was significantly correlated with mean attitude toward using condoms, for both steady and casual partners. With steady partners, most of the outcome beliefs were significantly correlated with attitude at the bivariate level. Teenagers may be at particular risk in their relationships with steady partners, given the romantic expectations that make suggesting condom use more difficult and the short duration of those relationships. Attitude is the strongest predictor of intention to use condoms, and adolescents' attitudes toward condom use with their steady partners are related to a broad range of beliefs, all of which could and should be taken into account in intervention design.

The magnitude of the correlation between the sum of the outcome beliefs and attitude is slightly lower for casual than for steady partners, and fewer beliefs were significantly related to attitude for casual partners. Beliefs about the outcomes of using condoms may be less predictive for casual partners because casual partners are less well-known to the respondent. Physical pleasure and comfort were less salient with casual partners, while concerns about pregnancy, making sex last longer, and causing a fight or argument were more salient.

Predicting Overall Subjective Norm

The sum of normative beliefs is significantly correlated with the overall subjective norm for both steady and casual partners, as were each of the individual normative beliefs. The sex partner's norm is the least highly correlated, and health care providers' and peers' most highly correlated, with subjective norm for both steady and casual partners. Increasing adolescents' perceptions that their doctors and friends approve of condoms is likely to have a favourable influence on teens' attitudes toward using condoms.

Practical Implications

The findings of this study have implications for the design of interventions with high risk adolescents, as well as for the development of theory to understand adolescent decision making about that complex, emotionally charged, dyadic behaviour of condom use. The framework of the TRA provides a model for understanding the antecedents of behaviour. Insofar as the specific beliefs about the outcomes of condom use influence condom use, knowledge of which outcome beliefs underlie overall attitude is an essential step in designing interventions to change attitude, because attitude will change as a function of changes in those beliefs. In the same way, it is essential to understand which normative beliefs underlie subjective norm, and the relative weight of attitude and norm as predictors of intention.

The addition of self-efficacy permits the theory to begin to be applied to behaviours that are not fully under the volitional control of the actor, in that self-efficacy reflects the actor's assessment of whether or not he or she has the necessary situational control or skills that are required to successfully implement his or her preference. Our measure of self-efficacy was based on a set of specific efficacy beliefs, in a fashion parallel to outcome beliefs as components of overall attitude, and normative beliefs as components of overall subjective norm. This reflects our belief that changing an individual's perceived self-efficacy can be accomplished through changes in these underlying beliefs, in the same way attitude and perceived norm are changed through changes in those underlying beliefs.

A strength and a hindrance of the TRA model is that beliefs are specific to the population from which they are sampled. We identified the beliefs – outcome, normative and efficacy beliefs – that are salient for the high-risk teens we studied; whether these results can be generalised to lower-risk teens or to high-risk teens in other settings is an empirical question. An intervention for these teens could profitably focus on both norms and, in particular, on attitudes, based on the finding that both are significantly related to intention, with attitude carrying greater weight. To change attitudes toward using condoms with both casual and steady partners, one might focus on beliefs that are important components of attitudes toward condom use with both types of partners: protection from pregnancy, making sex seem less natural, preventing the male's ejaculation, raising issues of mutual trust, and causing a fight. Some of these could be addressed though education and dispelling of misinformation (such as about the efficacy of condoms in preventing pregnancy) and others with skills training (in making condom use a positive part of lovemaking, or raising concerns in socially skilled ways that do not engender feeling of distrust). All of the normative beliefs were positively related to subjective norm. Changing community norms is a large undertaking; however, a fairly easy and straightforward intervention might be to remind health care providers to remind teens of the efficacy of condoms and express approval of condom use for teens who are sexually active. The finding that self-efficacy is related to intention for use only with steady partners suggests teaching skills for successfully initiating condom use within an ongoing relationship.

Summary

The TRA was originally proposed to understand relatively simple behaviors which are under the volitional control of the actor (Fishbein & Ajzen, 1975).

Using condoms to prevent STD is a complex dyadic behaviour, which depends on the cooperation of one's sexual partner; nonetheless, the model is able to account for a substantial proportion of the variance in condom use intentions. Normative influences are clearly important, but attitudes toward condom use were the major predictors of intention to use condoms for both steady and casual partners. Intervention designers need to consider the differences in the beliefs that underlie attitudes with steady, as opposed to casual, partners in tailoring attitude-change messages to high risk teens.

Although the TRA variables were the major predictors of intention to use condoms, we do not suggest that researchers using this model should exclude variables from outside the model from consideration. In this study we found that for teens with steady partners, prediction is improved slightly by adding perceived efficacy for condom use and gender to the prediction model. These findings enhance our overall understanding of the behaviour under consideration and improve our ability to successfully intervene to change health-threatening behaviours. Teenagers may be at greater risk with their steady partners, given the shorter duration of their relationships, as compared to adults; their lower level of condom use; and the greater difficulty of introducing condom use into sex with a steady, as compared to a casual, partner.

Although attitudes and norms could account for over half of the variance in intention to use condoms, intention was not an impressive predictor of behaviour, accounting for only 23% of the variance in condom use with steady partners and less than 5% of condom use with casual partners. A number of factors may affect this disappointing result. Intentions may have changed during the three-month interval between the first and second measurements. Condom use is not a simple volitional behaviour; the intentions of the actor's sexual partner are also salient. The partner's attitude may cause a change in the actor's intention (i.e., by advocating for a different action) or may block the actor's ability to attain the goal (i.e., by refusing to cooperate).

Throughout this discussion we have noted how findings with this high risk sample of teenagers differ from findings with teens or adults recruited from other settings. While some of the differences reflect differences in measurement and research design, differences should not be dismissed simply as research artifacts. Fishbein and Middlestadt (1987) have suggested that theory should provide the framework for understanding behaviour, but that it is important to attend to the fact that the antecedents of behaviour are likely to vary by behaviour and by population under study. The context of sexuality for teens is considerably different from that of adults. Teens have less experience, may be less likely to anticipate sexual encounters, and have relationships of shorter duration than do adults. Further, the greater awareness of AIDS and STDs at a critical time in their sexual development may have influenced teens' attitudes about condoms in ways that have not occurred among adults.

AUTHOR NOTE

The research described in this paper was supported by grant AI29507 from the National Institute of Allergy and Infectious Diseases.

REFERENCES

Adler, N. E., Kegeles, S. M., Irwin, C. E., Jr., & Wibbelsman, C. (1990). Adolescent contraceptive behavior: An assessment of decision processes. *Journal of Pediatrics*, *116*, 463–471.

Ajzen, I. (1985). From intentions to actions: A theory of planned behavior. In J. Kuhl & J. Beckman (eds.), *Action Control: Cognition to Behavior* (pp. 11–39). New York: Springer Verlag.

Ajzen, I., & Fishbein, M. (1980). *Understanding Attitudes and Predicting Social Behavior*. Englewood Cliffs, NJ: Prentice Hall.

Ajzen, I., & Madden, T. J. (1986). Prediction of goal-directed behaviors: Attitudes, intentions and perceived behavioral control. *Journal of Experimental Social Psychology*, *22*, 453–474.

Albarracin, D., Fishbein, M., & Middlestadt, S. (1998). Generalizing behavioral findings across times, samples, and measures: A study of condom use. *Journal of Applied Social Psychology*, *28*, 657–674.

Baker, S. A., Morrison, D. M., Carter, W. B., & Verdon, M. S. (1996). Using the theory of reasoned action (TRA) to understand the decision to use condoms in an STD clinic population. *Health Education Quarterly*, *23*, 528–542.

Bandawe, C. R., & Foster, D. (1996). AIDS-related beliefs, attitudes and intentions among Malawian students in three secondary schools. *AIDS Care*, *8*, 223–232.

Bandura, A. (1977). Self-efficacy: Toward a unifying theory of behavioral change. *Psychological Review*, *84*, 191–215.

Bandura, A. (1989). Human agency in social cognitive theory. *American Psychologist*, *44*, 1175–1184.

Basen-Engquist, K., & Parcel, G. S. (1992). Attitudes, norms, and self-efficacy: A model of adolescents' HIV-related sexual risk behavior. *Health Education Quarterly*, *19*, 263–277.

Boyd, B., & Wandersman, A. (1991). Predicting undergraduate condom use with the Fishbein and Ajzen and the Triandis attitude-behavior models: Implications for public health interventions. *Journal of Applied Social Psychology*, *21*, 1810–1830.

Brooks-Gunn, J., Boyer, C. B., & Hein, K. (1988). Preventing HIV infection and AIDS in children and adolescents. *American Psychologist*, *43*, 958–964.

Carey, R. F., Herman, W. A., Retta, S. M., Rinaldi, J. E., Herman, B. A., & Athey, T. W. (1992). Effectiveness of latex condoms as a barrier to Human Immunodeficiency Virus-sized particles under conditions of simulated use. *Sexually Transmitted Diseases*, *19*, 230–234.

Carter, W. B. (1990). Health behavior as a rational process: Theory of reasoned action and multi-attribute utility theory. In K. Glanz, F. M. Lewis, & B. K. Rimer (eds.), *Health Behavior and Health Education: Theory, Research, and Practice* (pp. 63–91). San Francisco: Jossey-Bass.

Catania, J. A., Coates, T. J., & Kegeles, S. (1994). A test of the AIDS risk reduction model: Psychosocial correlates of condom use in the AMEN cohort survey. *Health Psychology*, *13*, 548–555.

Centers for Disease Control. (1988). Condoms for prevention of sexually transmitted diseases. *Morbidity and Mortality Weekly Report*, *37*, 133–137.

Chan, D. K., & Fishbein, M. (1993). Determinants of college women's intentions to tell their partners to use condoms. *Journal of Applied Social Psychology*, *23*, 1455–1470.

Cronbach, L. (1987). Statistical tests for moderator variables: Flaws in analyses recently proposed. *Psychological Bulletin*, *102*, 414–417.

Fishbein, M., Chan, D. K-S, O., Reilly, K., Schnell, D., Wood, R., Beeker, C., & Cohn, D. (1992). Attitudinal and normative factors as determinants of gay men's intentions to perform AIDS-related sexual behaviors: A multisite analysis. *Journal of Applied Social Psychology*, *22*, 999–1011.

Fishbein, M., & Middlestadt, S. E. (1987). Using the theory of reasoned to develop educational interventions: Applications to illicit drug use. *Health Education Research, 2,* 361–371.

Fisher, W. A., Fisher, J. D., & Rye, B. J. (1995). Understanding and promoting AIDS-preventive behavior: Insights from the theory of reasoned action. *Health Psychology, 14,* 255–264.

Galavotti, C., Cabral, R. J., Lansky, A., Grimley, D. M., Riley, G. E., & Prochaska, J. O. (1995). Validation of measures of contraceptive use among women at high risk for HIV infection and unintended pregnancy. *Health Psychology, 14,* 570–578.

Gillmore, M. R., Morrison, D. M., Lowery, C., & Baker, S. A. (1994). Beliefs about condoms and their association with intentions to use condoms among youths in detention. *Journal of Adolescent Health, 15,* 228–237.

Godin, G., Fortin, C., Michaud, F., Bradet, R., & Kok, G. (1997). Use of condoms: Intention and behavior of adolescents living in juvenile rehabilitation centres. *Health Education Research, 12,* 289–300.

Godin, G., Maticka-Tyndale, E., Adrien, A., Manson-Singer, S., Willms, D., & Cappon, P. (1996). Cross-cultural testing of three social cognitive theories: An application to condom use. *Journal of Applied Social Psychology, 26,* 1556–1586.

Hayes, C. D. (1987). *Risking the Future: Adolescent Sexuality, Pregnancy and Childbearing.* Washington, D. C.: National Academy Press.

Heckman, T. G., Sikkema, K. J., Kelly, J. A., Fuqua, R. W., Mercer, M. B., Hoffmann, R. G., Winett, R. A., Anderson, E. S., Perry, M. J., Roffman, R. A., Solomon, L. J., Wagstaff, D. A., Cargill, V., Norman, A. D., & Crumble, D. (1996). Predictors of condom use and human immunodeficiency virus test seeking among women living in inner-city public housing developments. *Sexually Transmitted Diseases, 23,* 357–365.

Holmes, K. K., Karon, J. M., & Kreiss, J. (1990). The increasing frequency of heterosexually acquired AIDS in the United States, 1983–1988. *American Journal of Public Health, 80,* 858–863.

Jaccard, J., Turrisi, R., & Wan, C. K. (1990). *Interaction Effects in Multiple Regression.* Newbury Park, CA: Sage.

Jemmott, L. S., & Jemmott, J. B. (1991). Applying the theory of reasoned action to AIDS risk behavior: Condom use among black women. *Nursing Research, 40,* 228–234.

Jemmott, J. B., III, Jemmott, L. S., & Hacker, C. I. (1992). Predicting intentions to use condoms among African-American adolescents: The theory of planned behavior as a model of HIV risk-associated behavior. *Ethnicity and Disease, 2,* 371–380.

Kelly, J. A., & Kalichman, S.C. (1995). Increased attention to human sexuality can improve HIV-AIDS prevention efforts: Key research issues and directions. *Journal of Clinical and Consulting Psychology, 63,* 907–918.

Kashima, Y., Gallois, C., & McCamish, M. (1993). The theory of reasoned action and cooperative behaviour: It takes two to use a condom. *British Journal of Social Psychology, 32,* 227–239.

Krahe, B., & Reiss, C. (1995). Predicting intentions of AIDS-preventive behavior among adolescents. *Journal of Applied Social Psychology, 25,* 2118–2140.

Morrison, D. M., Gillmore, M. R., & Baker, S. A. (1995). Determinants of condom use among high-risk heterosexual adults: A test of the theory of reasoned action. *Journal of Applied Social Psychology, 25,* 651–676.

Mosher, W. D., & Pratt, W. F. (1990). Contraceptive use in the United States, 1973–88. *Advance Data from Vital and Health Statistics,* Number 182.

Ozer, E. M. & Bandura, A. (1990). Mechanisms governing empowerment effects: A self-efficacy analysis. *Journal of Personality and Social Psychology, 58,* 472–486.

Reinecke, J., Schmidt, P., & Ajzen, I. (1996). Application of the theory of planned behavior to adolescents' condom use: A panel study. *Journal of Applied Social Psychology*, 26, 749–772.

Richard, R., & van der Pligt, J. (1991). Factors affecting condom use among adolescents. *Journal of Community and Applied Social Psychology*, 1, 105–116.

Rise, J. (1992). An empirical study of the decision to use condoms among Norwegian adolescents using the theory of reasoned action. *Journal of Community & Applied Social Psychology*, 2, 185–197.

Ross, M. W. (1990). Psychological determinants of increased condom use and safer sex in homosexual men: A longitudinal study. *International Journal of STD & AIDS*, 1, 98–101.

Ross, M. W., & McLaws, M.-L. (1992). Subjective norms about condoms are better predictors of use and intention to use than attitudes. *Health Education Research*, 7, 335–339.

Schaalma, H., Kok, G., & Peters, L. (1993). Determinants of consistent condom use by adolescents: The impact of experience with sexual intercourse. *Health Education Research*, 8, 255–269.

Sheeran, P., & Orbell, S. (1998). Do intentions predict condom use? Meta-analysis and examination of six moderator variables. *British Journal of Social Psychology*, 37, 231–250.

Shimp, T. A., & Kavas, A. (1984). The theory of reasoned action applied to coupon usage. *Journal of Consumer Research*, 11, 795–809.

St. Lawrence, J. S., Eldridge, G. D., Reitman, D., Little, C. E., Shelby, M.C., & Brasfield, T. L. (1998). Factors influencing condom use among African American women: Implications for risk reduction interventions. *American Journal of Community Psychology*, 26, 728.

Smetana, J. G., & Adler, N. E. (1980). Fishbein's value x expectancy model: An examination of some assumptions. *Personality and Social Psychology Bulletin*, 6, 89–96.

Stiffman, A. R., & Earls, F. (1990). Behavioral risks for human immunodeficiency virus infection in adolescent medical patients. *Pediatrics*, 85, 303–310.

Terry, D. J., & O'Leary, J. E. (1995). The theory of planned behaviour: The effects of perceived behavioural control and self-efficacy. *British Journal of Social Psychology*, 34, 199–220.

Valdiserri, R. O, Arena, V. C., Proctor, D., & Bonati, F. (1989). The relationship between women's attitudes about condoms and their use: Implications for condom promotion programs. *American Journal of Public Health*, 79, 499–501.

Wattleton, F. (1987). American teens: Sexually active, sexually illiterate. *Journal of School Health*, 57, 379–380.

Weisman, C. S., Plichta, S., Nathanson, C. A., Ensminger, M., & Robinson, J. C. (1991). Consistency of condom use for disease prevention among adolescent users of oral contraceptives. *Family Planning Perspectives*, 23, 71–74.

White, K. M., Terry, D. J., & Hogg, M. A. (1994). Safer sex behavior: The role of attitudes, norms, and control factors. *Journal of Applied Social Psychology*, 24, 2164–2192.

Wulfert, E., Wan, C., & Backus, C. (1996). Gay men's safer sex behavior: An integration of three models. *Journal of Behavioral Medicine*, 19, 345–366.

CHAPTER THREE

Can Protection Motivation Theory Predict Breast Self-Examination? A Longitudinal Test Exploring the Role of Previous Behaviour

Sarah E. MILNE and Sheina ORBELL

Breast Cancer and Breast Self-Examination

The present study concerns women's perceptions of the threat of breast cancer and their motivation to undertake breast self-examination to protect themselves against this threat. Breast cancer is the third most common tumour in the world, accounting for approximately 9% of all cancer mortalities. It is the most common form of cancer in women. In Britain, 1 in 4 of all female cancers are due to the disease (L. Tomatis, 1990). At present, 1 in 14 women in Britain can expect to develop breast cancer in her life time (Fallowfield & Clark, 1991; Pitts & Phillips, 1991), with around 13,000 UK women dying of the disease each year (Pitts & Phillips, 1991). Survival rates decrease rapidly with the progression of the disease. When the disease is localised there is a 91% five year survival expectation. Regional spread reduces this to 69%, with further spread decreasing the survival prognosis to only 19% (Kurtz et al., 1993). Breast self-examination (B.S.E.) is a process by which the breasts are manually palpated to check for any lumps which might be indicative of the early stages of breast cancer. B.S.E. is proposed to reduce the threat of breast cancer by ensuring that it is detected at a stage where it can be readily and effectively treated with minimum quality of life impact to the woman affected. There is documented evidence that regular practice of B.S.E. can significantly increase the chance of detection and diagnosis of breast cancer in its primary, localised stage (GIVO, 1991; Hill et al. 1988). Despite this the estimated number of British women practising B.S.E. on a regular basis ranges from 3 to 20 per cent (Fallowfield & Clark, 1991). This highlights the need to explore factors influencing adopting B.S.E. as a precautionary behaviour.

Protection Motivation Theory

Protection motivation theory (PMT) (Rogers, 1975; 1983; Maddux & Rogers, 1983) provides one of the most dominant accounts of precautionary behaviour in the health domain. The model accounts for the processes involved in determining whether or not an individual will respond to a threat, such as a threat to health, by adopting a recommended coping response. For example, whether or not an individual will be motivated to change their diet in response to the threat of heart disease and the recommendation that a low fat diet will reduce his or her risk of developing the disease. In the original formulation of the theory Rogers (1975) specifies two cognitive processes; threat and coping appraisal, which together determine motivation to take self-protective action. *Threat appraisal* is derived from perceptions that one is personally vulnerable to disease combined with beliefs that the disease in question would have severe consequences. Where *perceived vulnerability* and *perceived severity* are high, an individual is presumed to experience a significant degree of personal threat. The way in which a person responds to appraised threat is determined, in turn, by coping appraisal. In the original formulation of the theory Rogers (1975) identified *response efficacy* as the main determinant of coping appraisal. Response efficacy concerns beliefs that adopting a particular behavioural response will be effective in reducing disease threat.

In 1983 Rogers expanded the components of coping appraisal to include *self-efficacy* (Bandura, 1977, 1982), *perceived costs* of the protective response and *rewards* of not acting. Self-efficacy refers to beliefs about one's ability to perform the protective behaviour. Psychological costs associated with performing the protective behaviour, such as unpleasant emotional reactions, may serve to undermine protection motivation. Additional cognitive mediating processes were added, including an account of the appraisal processes leading to maladaptive coping responses, such as continuing or adopting cigarette smoking. Figure 3.1 shows the expanded model. This proposes that an individual will adopt a protective behaviour if he or she believes the disease is severe and likely to occur and perceives the protective behaviour to be effective in reducing threat, low in cost and something they feel capable of doing.

The Model's Structure and Variables

The structure of PMT was influenced by expectancy-value theory (Edwards, 1954). In expectancy-value theory the tendency to adopt a given behaviour is said to be a function of expectancies regarding the consequences of the behaviour and the value of those consequences. Hovland, Janis, and Kelley's (1953) expectancy-value theory suggested three main evaluations that are made by an individual contemplating whether or not to change a behaviour in the context of a threat, such as a threat to health; (a) the magnitude of noxiousness of a given event, (b) the probability that the given event will occur if no protective behaviour is adopted or existing behaviour modified and, (c) the availability and effectiveness of a coping response to reduce or eliminate the noxious stimulus (Rogers, 1975). Rogers adopted these three components as the basis for the original formulation of his model. He proposed that each of these constitutes a cognitive mediational process; the magnitude of noxiousness initiates perceived severity, probability of occurrence initiates perceived vulnerability and efficacy of the recommended response initiates perceived

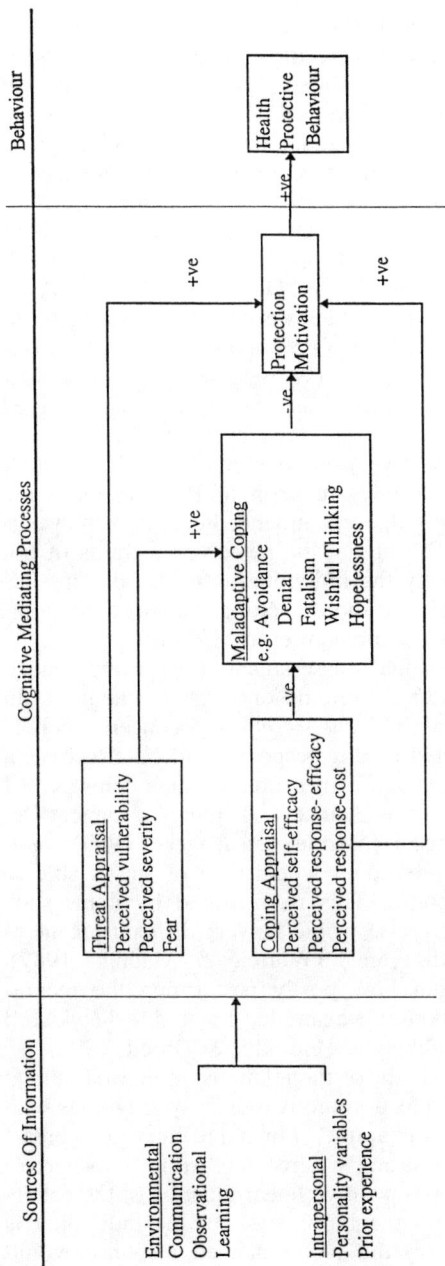

Figure 3.1 Schematic representation of protection motivation theory (adapted from Rogers, 1983)

response-efficacy. These cognitive mediational processes could be characterised as having two forms; threat appraisal and coping appraisal.

Threat appraisal concerns the process of evaluating an individual's perception of how threatened he or she feels as a result of the threat. For example, how threatened he or she feels by the thought of developing heart disease. The PMT variables involved in threat appraisal are perceived vulnerability, perceived severity and fear arousal. *Perceived vulnerability* assesses how personally susceptible an individual feels to the threat. It is typically measured by such items as 'Considering all of the different factors that may contribute to AIDS, including your own past and present behaviour, what would you say are your chances of getting AIDS?' (answered on a Likert scale with endpoints 'I am almost certain I will' to 'I am almost certain I will not') (Aspinwall, Kemeny, Taylor, Schneider, & Dudley, 1991). *Perceived severity* assesses how serious the individual believes the threat would be to their life. This is measured by items such as 'Osteoporosis is a very serious disease' ('strongly agree' to 'strongly disagree') (Wurtele, 1988). *Fear arousal* assesses how much fear is evoked by the individual's perceptions of perceived severity and perceived vulnerability and is measured by items such as 'The thought of breast cancer makes me feel' ('very anxious' to 'not at all anxious') (Hodgkins & Orbell, 1998). Roger's (1983) revision of PMT includes the appraisal of the *rewards* of not adopting the recommended coping response as part of the threat appraisal process. The higher the perceived rewards of not changing their behaviour, the less likely the individual is to do so. This has been measured by the item 'Sex would be more exciting without a condom' ('strongly agree' to 'strongly disagree') (Abraham et al., 1994).

Coping appraisal evaluates the individual's assessment of the recommended coping response to the threat. For example, should one change one's diet in response to the threat of heart disease? *Response-efficacy* concerns beliefs about whether or not the recommended coping response will be effective in reducing the threat felt by the individual and is measured by such items as 'If I quit smoking I will greatly increase my chances of living a longer life' ('strongly agree' to 'strongly disagree') (Maddux & Rogers, 1983). *Self-efficacy* concerns an individual's beliefs about whether he or she is able to adopt the recommended coping response. This is measured by items such 'Sticking with a regular program of exercise would be very difficult for me to do' ('strongly agree' to 'strongly disagree') (Wurtele & Maddux 1987). *Response costs* concerns beliefs about how costly performing the recommended response will be to the individual, for example, 'I would feel awkward examining my breasts' ('likely' to 'unlikely') (Hodgkins & Orbell, 1998).

Protection motivation is the key mediator of the relationship between threat and coping appraisal and behaviour. Protection motivation is synonymous with the intention to perform a behaviour, for example, 'I intend to carry out a breast self-examination in the next month' ('strongly agree' to 'strongly disagree') (Hodgkins & Orbell, 1998). Intention is a positive linear function of the beliefs that; (a) the threat would be severe to the individual, (b) the individual is personally vulnerable to the threat, (c) the recommended response would effective in reducing the threat, (d) the individual is able to perform the recommended response, and is a negative linear function of the belief that

(e) the perceived costs of the recommended coping response would be high. The model also permits the prediction of 'maladaptive coping responses'. When the perception of threat is high but coping appraisal is low, a person might adopt an avoidance response, such as denying the threat or actively avoiding information concerning the disease (Rippetoe & Rogers, 1987).

Although there have been 3 previous longitudinal tests of PMT to date on protection against earthquakes (Mulilis & Lippa, (1990), cancer prevention (Seydel, Taal & Weigman, 1990) and exercise participation (Wurtele & Maddux, 1987), none of these studies has included the cost component of coping appraisal or maladaptive coping responses. The first aim of the present study was to test the ability of the full PMT model to predict intention and future behaviour in a longitudinal study.

Protection Motivation Theory and Previous Behaviour

One way to establish the sufficiency of a model in accounting for future behaviour is by including a measure of previous behaviour in model tests (Ajzen, 1991). If the components of a model are sufficient to account for the behaviour in question the addition of previous behaviour into a regression analysis should not significantly improve prediction of subsequent behaviour. If previous behaviour is found to have a significant residual effect on the prediction of later behaviour, after entering all model components into a regression equation, this suggests that variables other than those being assessed may be required to fully account for behaviour. A number of studies have examined the role of previous behaviour in the theory of reasoned action (Azjen, 1991; Ajzen & Fishbein, 1980; Fishbein & Ajzen, 1975). A recent study by Bagozzi and Kimmel (1995) used previous behaviour to compare the sufficiency of the theory of reasoned action, the theory of planned behaviour (Ajzen, 1985, 1991), the theory of trying (Bagozzi & Warshaw, 1990) and the theory of self-regulation (Bagozzi, 1992) with respect to diet and exercise intention and behaviour. These authors found previous behaviour added significantly to the prediction of behaviour over and above the variables specified by the four theories. In addition, with the exception of the theory of trying in relation to diet behaviour, intention no longer predicted behaviour significantly when previous behaviour was added to the models. To date, only two studies have looked at the role of past behaviour in PMT (Abraham et al., 1994; Van der Velde & Van der Pligt, 1991). These authors found a direct effect of previous behaviour in predicting intention to take precautions against HIV. However, subsequent behaviour was not addressed in either study. The second aim of the present study was to examine the sufficiency of PMT in predicting future behaviour by assessing the effect of including previous behaviour in a test of the model.

Protection Motivation Theory and Breast Self-Examination

The present study will examine the sufficiency of PMT in accounting for women's intentions to perform B.S.E. and their subsequent behaviour. Previous studies indicate that PMT is of some use in predicting B.S.E. intentions and behaviour. Rippetoe and Rogers (1987) manipulated threat and coping appraisal within written persuasive messages. Participants were asked to read either; (i) a high versus low threat essay, where the level of vulnerability and severity of disease was manipulated, (ii) a high versus low response-efficacy essay, or, (iii) a high versus low self-efficacy essay. All the manipulations were found to be successful in changing beliefs about breast cancer and B.S.E. in the desired direction[1]. The effects of the different messages on intention to perform B.S.E. were compared. In addition, the effects of the persuasive messages on maladaptive coping with the threat of breast cancer such as; avoidance, wishful thinking, fatalism and hopelessness were explored. The high threat message was found to increase both intention to perform B.S.E. and maladaptive coping. The high response-efficacy and high self-efficacy messages increased intention to perform B.S.E. and reduced maladaptive coping. A path analysis showed high response-efficacy, self-efficacy and perceived severity to predict intention to perform B.S.E..

The role of PMT in predicting cancer-related protective behaviour, including B.S.E., was also explored by Seydel, Taal and Weigman (1990). Participants in an experimental group were shown a factual educational film about cancer with a control group watching a film on an unrelated topic. PMT variables, intention and concurrent behaviour were measured following the films. In addition, subsequent ordering of leaflets for further information on cancer was measured. Perceived severity, self-efficacy and response-efficacy were found to predict intention to perform B.S.E.. Self-efficacy and response-efficacy were found to predict concurrent B.S.E. behaviour with perceived severity, self-efficacy and response-efficacy predicting subsequent ordering of a leaflet about B.S.E..

Other studies have included individual PMT variables in studies exploring B.S.E.. For example, fear (Keller, 1978) and susceptibility (Kelley, 1979) have been found to be associated with B.S.E. performance. Lack of knowledge about B.S.E. procedure and lack of confidence in carrying it out, have been shown to act as barriers to B.S.E. performance (e.g. Alagna & Reddy, 1984; Kegeles, 1985). A number of authors have also found significant associations between perceived benefits of B.S.E. and its performance (e.g. Calnan & Rutter, 1986; Hill et al., 1985; Rutledge et al., 1988).

Main Objectives of the Present Study

The present study concerns the ability of social cognitive variables specified by PMT to account for practice of B.S.E.. We address the following specific aims. First, to determine which PMT variables are predictive of intention to perform B.S.E. and to test the sufficiency of PMT variables in accounting for the relation between previous performance and future intentions. Second, to examine the predictive sufficiency of the model in a longitudinal test over a one month period.

METHOD

Sample

Eighty-nine female psychology students and non-academic staff at an English university took part in the study. The age range was from 17 to 40 years (mean age = 21). Subjects took part in the study on a voluntary basis. The response rate was 63%. The use of personal numbers to couple the first questionnaires with the follow up ensured confidentiality and anonymity.

Design

The study took the form of a longitudinal survey. The first questionnaire incorporated the individual variables specified in PMT (Rogers, 1983) along with a measure of past B.S.E. behaviour. The follow-up questionnaire assessed B.S.E. performance in the month following the completion of the first questionnaire. Questionnaires were distributed in person during classes, or through the internal post. The follow up questionnaire was distributed one month following the deadline for the return of the first one. All measures were self-administered.

Measures

Protection motivation theory constructs. Salient cognitions concerning breast cancer and B.S.E. amongst an independent sample of 40 women typical of the study sample, were established in an elicitation survey. This consisted of a short questionnaire, comprising open ended questions on women's beliefs and fears about breast cancer and B.S.E., *e.g. In what way would you consider contracting breast cancer would affect your life?* Modal beliefs for each of the model variables were selected for the questionnaire.

The protection motivation theory constructs were measured by 7-point Likert scales, comprising belief statements or questions coupled with an appropriate response item. The number of items in each scale, the Cronbach's (1951) alpha coefficient of reliability, or the between item correlation in the case of two item scales, the mean and standard deviation for each variable included in the study are displayed in Table 3.1. All model constructs were found to form reliable scales.

Threat and coping appraisal cognitions. Perceived severity, perceived vulnerability and *fear* are the cognitions involved in *threat appraisal* (Rogers 1983). The elicitation survey indicated that *psychological severity* was more salient than *physical severity*. Therefore, *perceived severity* was operationalised in this way, for example; *Developing breast cancer would force me to change my goals in life (strongly agree – strongly disagree).* Perceived vulnerability was measured by 4 items, e.g.; *My chances of developing breast cancer in the future are (very low – very high).* The measure of *fear* was based on the most salient feelings associated with the thought of breast cancer, as demonstrated in the elicitation survey; *The thought of breast cancer makes me feel; very anxious – not at all anxious, not at all scared – very scared, very worried – not at all worried, not at all frightened – very frightened.*

Rogers (1983) outlines four components of *coping appraisal*; *response efficacy, self-efficacy, costs* of engaging in the suggested behaviour and *rewards* of not doing so. Rogers originally illustrated the concept of rewards with reference to smoking cessation, for example peer acceptance or enjoyment of taste. Not carrying out B.S.E. does not bring about reward in this way as it is not a behaviour that must be given up. This was confirmed by the elicitation study and so rewards were not included in the present study. *Response efficacy was* operationalised by 2 items, e.g.; *If I were to carry out B.S.E. I would ensure early detection of any abnormalities, (unlikely – likely). Self-efficacy* was measured by 5 items, e.g.; *I am discouraged from performing B.S.E. as I feel I do not know how, (strongly disagree – strongly agree). Psychological cost* was measured by 3 items, e.g.; *I would feel awkward examining my breasts, (likely – unlikely).*

Adaptive and maladaptive coping responses. Following Rogers (1983), *behavioural intention* was used as the *adaptive coping response* to *threat and coping appraisal.* This was measured by 3 items, e.g.; *I intend to carry out B.S.E. in the next month, (disagree – agree).* The elicitation survey highlighted *avoidance* as the most common *maladaptive coping response* to the threat of breast cancer. This was operationalised as avoiding thinking about breast cancer, e.g.; *I try not to let the thought of breast cancer enter my mind, (strongly disagree – strongly agree).*

Previous behaviour. Previous behaviour was measured by two items; *During the past year I have practised B.S.E. (never – once a week)* and; *During the past year I have carried out B.S.E. (never – very often).* Ajzen (1991) notes that shared method variance in measures of past and future behaviour may, in part, account for the residual effects of past behaviour in previous studies. In the present study previous behaviour was operationalised so as to be independent of the measure of future behaviour.

Follow up measures. B.S.E. performance was measured by one item; *Did you perform B.S.E. during the last month,(yes – no).* At time 2 participants were also asked if they had intended to perform B.S.E. during the past month.

Table 3.1   **Model constructs: reliabilities, means and standard deviations**

Measures	No. of Items	Cronbach's Alpha	Range	Mean	Standard Deviation
Threat Appraisal					
Perceived personal severity	3	.69	1–7	4.66	1.38
Perceived personal vulnerability	4	.86	1–7	4.11	0.75
Fear	4	.94	1–7	4.94	1.26
Coping Appraisal					
Response efficacy	2	.56*	1–7	5.73	1.01
Self efficacy	5	.86	1–7	4.34	1.52
Psychological costs	3	.76	1–7	2.55	1.45
Maladaptive Coping Behaviour					
Avoidance	3	.69	1–7	4.46	1.15
Adaptive Coping Behaviour					
Intention to perform B.S.E.	3	.90	1–7	3.03	1.89
Previous B.S.E. behaviour	2	.98*	1–6	2.09	1.26
B.S.E. Performance (reported in follow up)	1	–	1-2	1.16	0.36

* These constructs were assessed by 2 items, therefore correlations are reported rather than alphas

Table 3.2 Correlations between dependent and independent variables

	1.	2.	3.	4.	5.	6.	7.	8.	9.	10.
1. B.S.E. performance (point-biserial correlations)		.36**	−.27**	−.20*	.04	−.06	−.09	.30**	−.31**	.47**
2. Intention to perform B.S.E.			−.38**	−.07	.17	.11	.26**	.46**	−.35**	.74**
3. Avoidance				.09	−.13	−.18	−.20*	−.31**	.43**	−.42**
4. Perceived severity					−.04	.49**	.15	−.02	.22**	−.23**
5. Perceived vulnerability						.10	.18	−.19	−.10	−.01
6. Fear							.12	.003	−.02	.06
7. Response efficacy								.27	.03	.10**
8. Self-efficacy									−.39**	.55**
9. Psychological costs										−.52**
10. Previous B.S.E. behaviour										

* $p < .05$, ** $p < .01$

RESULTS

Descriptive Findings

Forty five per cent of the participants had never performed B.S.E. with 26% having done it only once. About a third performed B.S.E. on a regular basis. The majority (56%) of participants were undecided as to their chances of developing breast cancer, whilst 28% agreed that it was likely they would develop the disease. Twenty-five per cent saw breast cancer as a very severe threat, agreeing that it would their destroy chances of future happiness, and the majority (77%) felt that developing breast cancer would make a difference to their future. B.S.E. was generally (76%) seen as very effective in ensuring early detection of breast cancer. However, only 40% felt that they were capable of performing B.S.E. At follow-up 16% reported having performed B.S.E. during the last month.

Relationships Between Variables

Bivariate correlations were obtained between all variables in the study. Spearman point-biserial coefficients were calculated for correlations with behaviour and Pearson coefficients were calculated for all remaining correlations. The correlations ranged from .01 to .74 and are displayed in Table 3.2. Four of the PMT constructs were found to be significantly correlated with *intention to perform B.S.E.*. None of the threat appraisal measures were found to be related to intention. *Avoidance* (r = −0.38, p < 0.01) and *psychological costs* (r = –0.35, p < 0.01) were both inversely associated with B.S.E. intentions. Thus, women who felt that they did not want to think about breast cancer or felt that B.S.E. would cause them anxiety were less likely to intend to perform B.S.E. *Response efficacy* (r = 0.26, p < 0.01) and *self-efficacy* were positively related to *intention* (r = 0.46, p < 0.01), indicating that women who felt B.S.E. was useful in ensuring early detection of breast cancer and those who were confident in their ability to perform B.S.E. were more likely to intend to carry out B.S.E.. *Previous B.S.E. behaviour* was very strongly correlated with *intention* to do so in the next month (r = 0.74, p < 0.01).

Five of the PMT constructs were found to be significantly correlated with future B.S.E. performance. *Avoidance* (r = –0.27, p < 0.01) and *psychological costs* (r = –0.31, p < 0.01) were found to have negative associations with *future B.S.E. behaviour*. *Self-efficacy* (r = 0.30, p < 0.05) was positively associated with future behaviour, as was previous *behaviour* (r = 0.47, p < 0.01). Surprisingly, *perceived severity* (r = –0.20, p < 0.05) was also found to have a negative association with *future behaviour*. This was surprising as none of the threat appraisal components were found to have significant associations with intention, suggesting that participants who saw breast cancer as severe were less likely to engage in B.S.E., and that this association was independent of *intention*.

A path analysis (Bryman & Cramer, 1990) was conducted to establish the direct and indirect predictive relationships between the variables in the study. This followed the theoretical structure outlined by Rogers (1983). The path analysis was first conducted with only the PMT constructs and then repeated with the inclusion of previous B.S.E. performance. *Intention* was taken as the dependent variable. *Avoidance* was entered into the regression equation first. *Threat* and *coping appraisal* cognitions were entered together on the next stage of the analysis. *Previous B.S.E. performance* was entered as a final step in the second analysis.

Figures 3.2a and b show the significant pathways between the variables, with the corresponding standardised regression coefficients (betas), and their significance values. A construct will be said to 'predict' a dependent variable if it can account for a significant proportion of it's variance.

Predictors of Intention

The first aim of the study was to test the sufficiency of protection motivation theory as a model able to predict intention. *Self-efficacy* was the only construct found to predict intention when the protection motivation theory constructs were entered into the path analysis, (beta = 0.456, t = 4.785, p < 0.00001). *Psychological costs* predicted *avoidance* (beta = 0.433, t = 4.483, p < 0.00001). Overall, PMT variables explained 20% of variance in intention (model F = 22.896, p < 0.00001, Adjusted R Square = 0.199).

When *previous B.S.E. behaviour* was added to the model it became the only variable to directly predict *intention* (beta = 0.734, t = 8.252, p < 0.00001). *Previous behaviour* was also found to predict *perceived severity* (beta = –0.225, t = –2.154, p < 0.05), *self-efficacy* (beta = 0.546, t = 6.079,

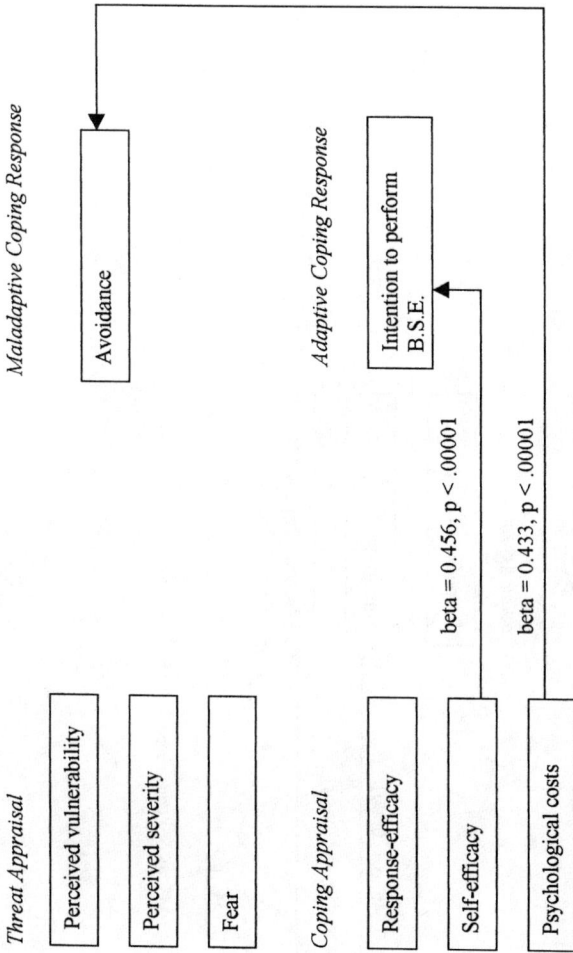

Figure 3.2a Path model of PMT theory constructs

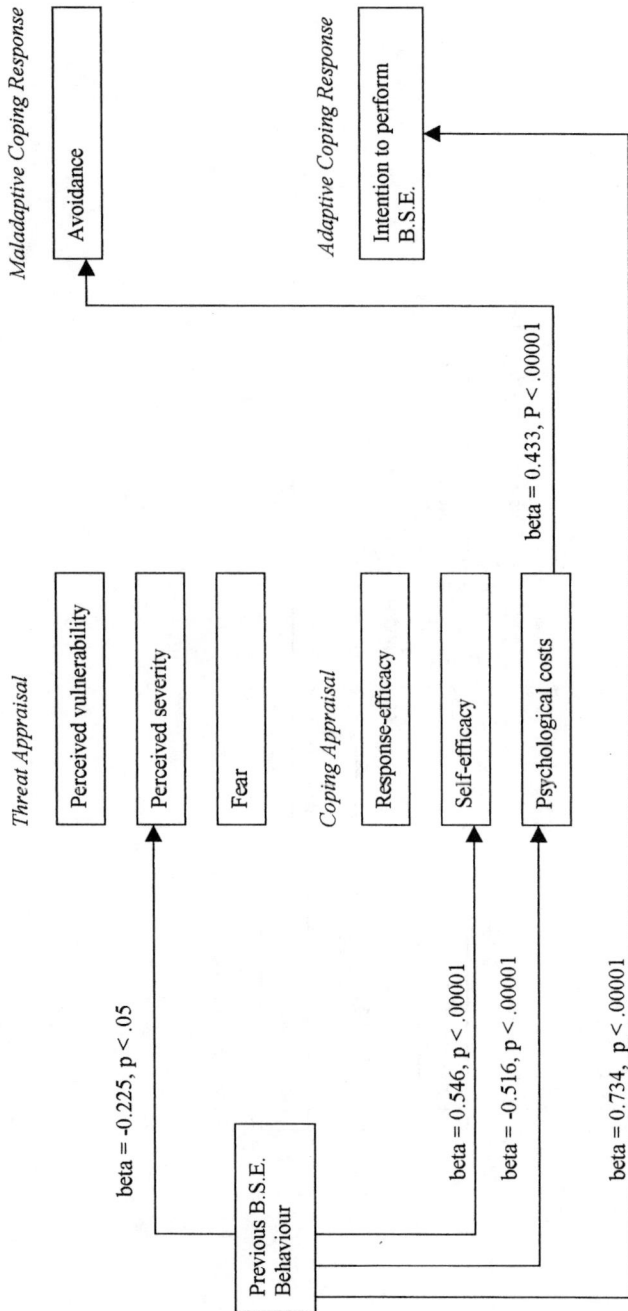

Figure 3.2b Path model of PMT theory constructs with previous behaviour

p < 0.00001) and *psychological costs* (beta $= -0.516$, t $= -5.617$ p < 0.00001). The model including previous behaviour explained 54% of variance in intention (model F $= 104.504$, p < 0.00001, Adjusted R Square $= 0.540$) The addition of previous behaviour resulted in an improvement of 34% in variance explained in intention.

Can Protection Motivation Theory Predict Intention to Initiate B.S.E. ?

Given the importance of previous behaviour in explaining intention as demonstrated by the path analysis, we conducted a further, post hoc analysis to determine whether PMT variables were able to explain the development of an intention to initiate routine B.S.E. amongst those who had not previously been regular B.S.E. performers. To address this question we first selected only those participants who had never previously performed B.S.E., or had performed it only once in the past. Our aim was to examine the ability of PMT variables to distinguish between women in this sub-sample, who subsequently reported an intention to perform B.S.E. and those who did not. Since none of the women in this sub-sample routinely practised B.S.E. at time 1 the intention measure at time 2 indicates intention to change one's behaviour.

Respondents who had not previously performed B.S.E., or had done so only once, were divided into four groups on the basis of their responses to the time 2 measure of intention. This was a dichotomous item measuring the intention to perform B.S.E. during the month between the first questionnaire and the follow up. Four sub-groups were identified; A – those who had never carried out B.S.E. and did not intend to (n $= 27$); B – those who had never carried out B.S.E. and now intended to (n $= 12$); C – those who had performed B.S.E. only once and did not intend to again (n $= 13$) and D – those who had performed B.S.E. once and now intended to do so again (n $= 10$).

The PMT variables were entered into a stepwise discriminant analysis to determine if the four groups could be distinguished on the basis of the model's components. Three discriminant functions were calculated with a combined Chi-square of 29.379 (df $= 15$, p < 0.05). After removal of the first function the association between the groups and predictors was reduced to non-significance (Chi-square $= 7.553$, df $= 8$, p $= 0.48$), indicating that only the first function was significant. This function was found to discriminate group C, those women who had performed B.S.E. once and did not intend to do so again, from the other groups (group C group centroid $= -1.261$, groups A, B and D group centroids $= 0.465$, 0.100 and 0.263 respectively). This function accounted for 77% of the between group variance. Inspection of Newman – Keuls *post hoc* pair wise comparisons of group means showed that those who had performed B.S.E. once and did not intend to do so again were distinguishable on the basis of two PMT variables. They scored lower than all the other groups on the measure of *psychological cost* (group C mean $= 5.54$ with groups A, B and D 9.96, 9.83, and 9.20 respectively. This indicates that women who had performed B.S.E. once and did not intend to do so again saw B.S.E. performance as being less likely to cause anxiety than those in the other three groups. However, they also perceived lower *response efficacy* than those who had never performed B.S.E. and did not intend to do so (group C mean = 9.92, group A mean = 11.41).This indicates that what distinguishes non-intenders who have tried B.S.E. once from those who have never tried it is a perception that it is unlikely to ensure early detection of breast cancer. It was not possible, on the basis of PMT variables, to discriminate between those who developed an intention and those who did not.

Predictors of Future Behaviour

The second aim of the study was to test the sufficiency of PMT in it's ability to predict future behaviour. A logistic regression was utilised as this is the preferred method where the dependent variable is dichotomous, thus violating the assumption, made by linear regression, of normally distributed errors. Logistic regression allows prediction of the probability of occurrence of an event from a set of independent variables. The PMT constructs were added on the first step of the logistic regression with *previous B.S.E. behaviour* added on a second step. The beta coefficients, and their corresponding Wald significance test results, obtained in both steps of the logistic regression are shown in Table 3.3.

The initial −2 Log-Likelihood value for the constant only model was 77.46. When the protection motivation theory constructs were added the −2 Log-Likelihood was reduced to 48.73 (df = 80), an improvement of 28.73. This was a significant change (Chi-square = 28.73, p < 0.001). *Intention* (beta = 0.24, p < 0.05) and *response efficacy* (beta = − 0.43, p < 0.05) were the only individual predictors of *subsequent behaviour*. In the second step *previous behaviour* was added to the model. The addition of *previous behaviour* resulted

Table 3.3   Logistic regression of protection motivation theory constructs and past behaviour on future B.S.E. performance

	Before addition of previous B.S.E. behaviour Beta	After addition of previous B.S.E. behaviour Beta
Intention	.24 *	.03 ns.
Avoidance	−.25 ns.	−.37 ns.
Perceived vulnerability	.01 ns.	.06 ns.
Perceived severity	−.13 ns.	−.10 ns.
Fear appraisal	−.10 ns.	−.20 ns.
Response efficacy	−.43 *	−.47 ns.
Self efficacy	.05 ns.	.01 ns.
Psychological costs	−.04 ns	.21 ns.
Previous B.S.E. behaviour		.90 *
− 2 log likelihood (initial value for model 77.46)	48.73 df = 80	37.80 df = 79
Improvement	28.73 df = 8 p = 0.0004	10.93 df = 1 p = 0.0009

* p < .05, ns. = not significant

in a significant improvement in the prediction of *future behaviour*, over and above the PMT variables. The value of the -2 Log-Likelihood value was reduced to 37.80 (df $=$ 79), An improvement of 10.93 (df $=$ 1). This change was also significant (Chi-square $=$ 10.93, p $<$ 0.001). *Previous behaviour* was the only significant independent predictor of *future behaviour* when both steps of the regression had been completed.

DISCUSSION

The present study is the first longitudinal test of the full PMT model. Rogers (1983) suggests that the combination of threat and coping appraisal processes determines the development of motivation to undertake health protective actions.

Predicting B.S.E. Intention

The first part of our analysis showed that coping appraisal but not threat appraisal was associated with intention to perform B.S.E.. Perceived self-efficacy was the single independent predictor of intention. The inclusion of previous behaviour in the regression model resulted in a dramatic improvement in variance explained in intention (a change from 20% to 54%), suggesting that PMT variables are not sufficient to explain *motivation* to enact B.S.E.. Although a significant path was obtained between previous behaviour and self-efficacy, suggesting that perceived competence partially mediated the effects of past behaviour, the analysis provides strong support for the contention that variables outside those specified by PMT may need to be addressed in order to acquire a fuller understanding of B.S.E. related motivation. Similar direct effects of previous behaviour on intention in PMT have been demonstrated by Abraham et al., (1994) and Van der Velde and Van der Pligt (1991).

The post hoc discriminant function analysis of predictors of B.S.E. intention amongst those who had not previously performed B.S.E. further supports the contention that PMT is insufficient to account for protection motivation, since it was not possible, on the basis of cognitions specified by PMT, to discriminate between those who developed an intention and those who did not. An interesting finding arising from this analysis was that women who had tried B.S.E. once and did not intend to do so again reported lower perceived response-efficacy than those who had never tried B.S.E.. A possible interpretation of this finding may be that response-efficacy plays a role in the *maintenance* of health behaviour routines. It may be that changes in perceived response efficacy are accountable for women not persisting with routine B.S.E. behaviour. Further research is required to examine this possibility.

Predicting Future B.S.E. Performance

The longitudinal analysis further demonstrated that whilst behavioural intention significantly predicted actual B.S.E. performance, the addition of previous behaviour to the logistic regression equation added significantly to the prediction of future behaviour. Whilst the addition of previous behaviour to the model reduced the effects of intention to non-significance, suggesting that the effects of previous behaviour were partially mediated by intention, the improvement in the -2 Log Likelihood indicates that previous behaviour had an effect over and above that attributable to intention.

Predicting Maladaptive Coping

Maladaptive coping, assessed in terms of cognitive avoidance, was predicted in the model by perceived psychological costs associated with B.S.E.. Clearly, women who felt uncomfortable about the act of B.S.E. or considered that it would make them anxious were motivated to deny or suppress thoughts of developing the disease. This finding is consistent with that from previous research on B.S.E. (e.g. Calnan & Rutter, 1986: Rutledge et al, 1988) and implies considerable uncertainty amongst women about whether the benefits of early detection outweigh the costs. Rippetoe and Rogers (1987) found avoidance to be predicted by fear of breast cancer. This finding was not supported in the present study. No significant associations were found between any of the threat appraisal variables and avoidance.

Sufficiency of Protection Motivation Theory

In sum, the findings indicate that the PMT variables are not sufficient to explain either the development of protection motivation, nor the translation of the motivational construct, intention into action. In discussing the effects of previous behaviour with respect to the theory of reasoned action Azjen (1991) notes that residual effects of previous behaviour might be explained by shared method variance in measures of past and future behaviour which is not shared by measures of intention. In the present study care was taken to ensure previous behaviour and future behaviour were completely independent, future behaviour was assessed by a dichotomous variable, whilst previous behaviour was measured in terms of the frequency with which behaviour had been performed in the past. It therefore seems unlikely that shared method variance accounted for the effects obtained. Thus, we can conclude that the PMT variables are not sufficient to account for future behaviour. This finding is consistent with Bagozzi and Kimmel's (1995) findings in relation to the theory of reasoned action, the theory of planned behaviour, the theory of trying and the theory of self-regulation. Future research might usefully address processes mediating the effects of previous behaviour on future behaviour. For example, when a behaviour has been frequently performed in the past it may be that it becomes habitual or routine and is no longer controlled by intention (see Sutton, 1993; Triandis, 1980). It may also be that frequent experience of a behaviour, such as B.S.E., leads to the development of skills which are not assessed by PMT model components.

Threat Appraisal

A number of interesting observations concerning the adoption of health-protective behaviour can be made on the basis of the present findings. Little support was obtained for the prediction that protection-motivation follows from perceptions of high vulnerability and high susceptibility. Breast cancer is a relatively salient threat to women since it is a very common disease. In fact only 22% of women in the présent sample endorsed the belief that it was unlikely that they would get breast cancer in the future. This supports the findings of Rippetoe and Rogers (1987) and Seydel et al., (1990). Clearly, perceptions of disease vulnerability may be less significant than is supposed by the structure of PMT, although it is also possible that, as Weinstein (1988) proposes, acceptance of vulnerability is a prerequisite of any health related action. Although Rippetoe and Rogers and Seydel et al., found perceived severity to predict intention to perform B.S.E. perceived severity was not associated with intention in the present study. However, it was interesting to note that those who had previously performed B.S.E. perceived breast cancer as less severe than those who had not done so. Perceived severity was not found to be associated with future behaviour in either the present study or in the study by Seydel et al.

This supports the view that threat appraisal is a poor predictor of intention and behaviour (Milne et al., in press). One possible reason why severity may appear to be a poor predictor of health-related intention and behaviour may be because it is often very difficult to obtain variability in the data for perceived severity (Harrison et al., 1992, Janz & Becker, 1984). For example, few people would disagree that contracting cancer would be serious for them. Ronis and Harel (1989) found that the effects of severity were not direct but were mediated by another variable. Their research combined components of the health belief model (Becker, 1974; Rosenstock, 1966) and subjective utility theory (Edwards, 1954) in a study of breast self-examination. They found that the effects of severity were entirely mediated by the benefits of adopting B.S.E.. It may be that the effects of threat appraisal variables in the present study were mediated by factors that were not measured. Another possibility is that perceived threat may be more strongly and consistently associated with intention and behaviour for some people but not others. For example, Brouwers and Sorrentino (1993) found that uncertainty orientation, an individual difference variable, moderated the impact of perceived threat on protective behaviour.

Coping Appraisal

Coping appraisal was a significant determinant of protection motivation and the path analysis demonstrated that self-efficacy was the only independent predictor of future intention. Clearly, the provision of information and instruction in B.S.E. by health educators would be valuable in increasing motivation. The importance of self-efficacy has been noted with respect to a range of health-protective behaviours including limiting number of sexual partners (Aspinwall et al, 1991), using condoms during sexual intercourse (Abraham et al., 1994: Van der Velde & Van der Pligt, 1991), taking exercise (Wurtele & Maddux, 1987) as well as in the context of B.S.E. (Alagna & Reddy, 1984: Kegeles, 1985). Wurtele and Maddux (1987) have suggested that self-efficacy may enhance performance even where perceived vulnerability is low.

Response efficacy was generally high, with the majority of women endorsing beliefs that B.S.E. would ensure early detection of breast cancer. However, response efficacy did not make a significant independent contribution to the prediction of B.S.E. intentions in the multiple regression analysis. The significant beta value obtained for this variable in the logistic regression is most likely due to the presence of a suppresser variable, since a non-significant correlation was obtained between response efficacy and future behaviour (Tabachnik & Fiddel, 1989, p. 161).

Practical Implications

This study has clear implications for health education interventions. The results support the view that self-efficacy is emerging as a major predictor of health-related behaviour (e.g. Milne et al., in press). Thus, an important issue for health education must be the development and testing of ways to enhance self-efficacy. The best way to increase self-efficacy is to provide practical experience of the behaviour (Bandura, 1991). Champion and Scott (1993) conducted an intervention study whereby four groups of women were randomly assigned to one of four groups; (i) a control group, (ii) a belief intervention group, (iii) a procedural intervention group or (iv) a procedural/belief intervention group. At follow-up one year later significant differences in self-reported proficiency were found between the procedural intervention and the control group and between the procedural/belief intervention and control group. Further research into methods of increasing self-efficacy in health education interventions is needed.

The results of the present study also highlight the importance of previous behaviour in predicting future behaviour. This suggests that health education programmes should stress the importance of repeating behaviours until they become habits and occur without the need for intentional control. Research should be conducted to explore methods of promoting the formation of 'healthy habits' in health education interventions.

The perception that B.S.E. would be high in cost was found to predict adopting the maladaptive coping strategy of avoidance when faced with the threat of breast cancer. Response-costs were not directly associated with B.S.E. intention or behaviour. However, health education interventions should aim to reduce perceived cost as a means of reducing the likelihood of maladaptive coping, such as avoidance.

Limitation

One limitation of this study which should be addressed is that the convenience sample is not necessarily representative of the female population. Therefore, the descriptive findings can only apply to this group of women and may not be generalisable to older samples.

Conclusion and Future Directions

In conclusion, the present study provides only limited support for Protection Motivation Theory in the prediction of breast self-examination. Previous regular performance was the single best predictor of intentions to carry out B.S.E. during the following month. PMT was found to be an insufficient model for the prediction of intention to perform B.S.E. and future performance. Thus, other variables need to be considered. A better model might be developed by investigating the self-regulatory beliefs which result from previous regular performance. Recently, a number of authors (e.g. Bagozzi, 1992; Gollwitzer, 1993 Schwarzer, 1992) have drawn attention to the neglect of volitional processes in accounts of goal directed behaviour. A useful framework for the prediction of B.S.E. behaviour has been suggested by Miller et. al. (1996) in which cognitive-social theory has been compiled to produce the C-SHIP, Cognitive-Social Health Information Processing model. This model incorporates self-regulatory steps between intention and behaviour, mainly concerned with the formation of behavioural scripts and procedural knowledge. More research is needed to establish the processes involved in the activation of behaviour. Understanding the role of previous behaviour and the mechanisms by which it acts on future behaviour would provide a useful starting point for this work.

NOTE

1. See Milne, Sheeran & Orbell (in press) for further discussion of experimental PMT studies.

REFERENCES

Abraham, S. C. S., Sheeran, P., Abrams, D., & Spears, R. (1994). Exploring teenagers adaptive and maladaptive thinking in relation to the threat of HIV infection. *Psychology and Health, 9,* 253–272.

Ajzen, I. (1985). From intention to action: A theory of planned behavior, In J. Kuhl and J. Beckmann (Eds.) *Action Control: From Cognition to Behavior.* New York: Springer-Verlag.

Ajzen, I. (1991). The Theory of Planned Behavior. *Organizational Behaviour And Human Decision Processes, 50,* 179–211.

Ajzen, I. & Fishbein, M. (1980). *Understanding Attitudes and Predicting Social Behavior.* Englewood Cliffs, N.J.: Prentice-Hall.

Alagna, S. W. & Reddy, D. M. (1984). The predictors of proficient techniques and successful lesion detection in breast self-examination. *Health Psychology, 3,* 113–127.

Aspinwall, L. G., Kemeny, M. E., Taylor, S. E., Schneider, S. G. & Dudley, J. P. (1991). Psychosocial predictors of gay men's AIDS risk – reduction behavior. *Health Psychology, 10,* 432–444.

Bagozzi, R. P. (1992). The self-regulation of attitudes, intention and behavior. *Social Psychology Quarterly, 55,* 178–204.

Bagozzi, R. P. & Kimmel, S. K. (1995). A comparison of leading theories for the prediction of goal-directed behaviours. *British Journal Of Social Psychology, 34,* 437–461.

Bagozzi, R. P. & Warshaw, P. R. (1990). Trying to consume. *Journal of Consumer Research, 17,* 127–140.

Bandura, A. (1977). Self-efficacy: Toward a unifying theory of change. *Psychological Review, 84,* 191–215.

Bandura, A. (1982). Self-efficacy mechanism in human agency. *American Psychologist, 37*, 122–147.

Bandura, A. (1991). Social cognitive theory of self-regulation. *Organisational Behaviour and Human Decision Processes, 50*, 248–287.

Becker, M. H. (1974). The health belief model and sick role behavior. *Health Education Monographs, 2*, 409–419.

Brouwers, M. C. & Sorrentino, R. M. (1993). Uncertainty orientation and protection motivation theory: The role of individual differences in health compliance. *Journal of Personality and Social Psychology, 65*, 102–112.

Bryman, A. & Cramer, D. (1990). *Quantitative Data Analysis for Social Scientists.* London: Routledge.

Calnan, M. & Rutter, D. R. (1985). Do health beliefs predict health behaviour? An analysis of breast self-examination. *Social Science and Medicine, 22*, 673–678.

Champion, V. & Scott, C. (1993). Effects of a procedural belief intervention on breast self-examination performance. *Research in Nursing and Health, 16*, 163–170.

Cronbach, L. J. (1951). Coeffcient alpha and the internal structure of tests. *Psychometrica, 16*, 296–334.

Edwards, W. (1954). The theory of decision making. *Psychological Bulletin, 51*, 380–417.

Fallowfield, L. & Clark, A. (1991). *Breast Cancer: The Experience of Illness Series.* London: Routledge.

Fishbein, M. & Ajzen, I. (1975). *Belief, Attitude, Intention and Behavior: An Introduction To Theory and Research.* M.A: Addison-Wesley.

Fruin, D. J., Pratt, C., & Owen, N. (1991). Protection Motivation Theory and adolescent's participation of exercise. *Journal of Applied Social Psychology, 22*, 55–69.

GIVO, Interdisciplinary Group For Cancer Care Evaluation (1991). Practise of breast self-examination: disease extent at diagnosis and patterns of surgical care. A report from an Italian study. *Journal of Epidemology and Community Health, 45*, 112–116.

Hill, D., Gardner, G., & Rassaby, J. (1985). Factors predisposing women to take precautions against breast and cervix cancer. *Journal of Applied Social Psychology, 15*, 59–79.

Hill, D., White, V., Jolley, D., & Mapperson, K. (1988). Self-examination of the breast: Is it beneficial? Meta-analysis of studies investigating breast self-examination and extent of disease in patients with breast cancer. *British Medical Journal, 297*, 271– 275.

Kegeles, S. S. (1985). Education for breast self-examination: why, who, what and how? *Preventative Medicine, 14*, 702–720.

Keller, K. (1978). Self-examination for breast cancer. *Today 's Clinician , May*, 49–52.

Kelly, P. T. (1979). Breast self-examination: Who does them and why? *Journal of Behavioral Medicine, 2*, 31–38.

Kurtz, M. E., Given, B., Given, C. W., & Kurtz, J. C. (1993). Relationships of barriers and facilitators to breast self-examination, mammography, and clinical breast examination in a worksite population. *Cancer Nursing, 16*, 251–259.

Maddux, J. E. & Rogers, R. W. (1983). Protection motivation and self-efficacy: A revised theory of fear appeals and attitude change. *Journal of Experimental Social Psychology, 19*, 469–479.

Miller, S. M., Shoda, Y. & Hurley, K. (1996). Applying Cognitive-Social Theory To Health- Protective Behaviour: Breast Self-Examination In Cancer Screening. *Psychological Bulletin, 119*, 70–94.

Milne, S. E., Sheeran, P. & Orbell, S. (in press). Prediction and intervention in health-related behaviour: A meta-analytic review of protection motivation theory. *Journal of Applied Social Psychology.*

Mulilis, J. P. & Lippa, R. (1990). Behaviour changes in earthquake preparedness due to negative threat appeals: A test of protection motivation theory. *Journal of Applied Social Psychology, 20,* 619–638.

Pitts, M. & Philips, K. (1991). *The Psychology of Health: An Introduction.* London: Routledge.

Rippetoe, P. A. & Rogers, R. W. (1987). Effects of components of protection motivation theory on adaptive and maladaptive coping with a health threat. *Journal of Personality and Social Psychology, 52,* 596–604.

Rogers, R. W. (1975). A protection motivation theory of fear appeals and attitude change. *The Journal of Psychology, 91,* 93–114.

Rogers, R. W. (1983). Cognitive and physiological processes in fear appeals and attitude change: A revised theory of protection motivation. In B. L. Cacioppo and L. L. Petty (Eds.). *Social Psychophysiology: A Sourcebook.* London:The Guildford Press.

Ronis, D. & Harel, Y. (1989). Health beliefs and breast self-examination behaviours: Analysis of linear structural relations. *Psychology and Health, 3,* 259–285.

Rosenstock, I. M. (1966). Why people use health services. *Millbank Memorial Fund Quarterly, 44,* 94–124.

Rutledge, D. N. & Davis, G. T. (1988). Breast self-examination compliance and the health belief model. *Oncology Nursing Forum, 251,* 175–179.

Schwarzer, R. (1992). Self-efficacy in the adoption and maintenance of health behaviours: Theoretical approaches and a new model. In R. Schwarzer (ed.) *Self-efficacy: Thought Control of Action.* (pp . 217–243). Washington: Hemisphere

Seydel, E., Taal, E. & Weigman, O. (1990). Risk appraisal, outcome and self-efficacy expectancies: Cognitive factors in previous behaviour related to cancer. *Psychology and Health, 4,* 99–109.

Sutton, S. (1994). The past predicts the future: Interpreting behaviour relations in social psychological models of health behaviours. In D. R. Rutter (ed.) *The Social Psychology of Health and Safety: European Perspectives.* Aldershot: Aldershot Publishers.

Tabachnick, B. G. & Fidell, L. S. (1989). *Using Multivariate Statistics (Second Edition).* New York: Harper and Row.

Tomatis, L., (Ed.) (1990). *Cancer: Causes, Occurrence and Control.* International Agency For Research On Cancer.

Triandis, H. C. (1980). Values, attitudes and interpersonal behavior. In H. C. Howe, Jr and M. M. Page (eds.) *Nebraska Symposium of Motivation (Vol. 27).* Lincoln University: Nebraska Press.

UK Trial Of Early Detection Of Breast Cancer Group (1988). First results on mortality reduction in the UK Trial of Early Detection of Breast Cancer. *The Lancet, ii,* 411–416.

Van der Velde, F. W. & Van der Pligt, J. (1991). AIDS-related health behavior: Coping, protection motivation and previous behavior. *Journal of Behavioral Medicine, 14,* 429–451.

Weinstein, N. D. (1988). The precaution adoption process. *Health Psychology, 7,* 335–386.

Wurtele, S. K. & Maddux, J. E. (1987) Relative contributions of protection motivation theory components in predicting exercise intentions and behavior. *Health Psychology, 6,* 453–466.

CHAPTER FOUR

Comparing the Theory of Planned Behaviour and the Health Belief Model: The Example of Safety Helmet Use Among Schoolboy Cyclists

Lyn QUINE, Derek R. RUTTER and Laurence ARNOLD

This paper reports a prospective, longitudinal comparison of the Health Belief Model (Rosenstock, 1966) and the Theory of Planned Behaviour (Ajzen, 1985) in which the models were used to predict and understand the use of protective helmets among schoolboy cyclists. In 1997 a total of 24,585 cyclists were injured in the United Kingdom, 2,707 aged between 8 and 11, 3,971 between 12 and 15, and 2,563 between 16 and 19; 354 of the 8–11 year olds, 511 of the 12–15 year olds, and 351 of the 16–19 year olds were *seriously* injured or killed (Department of Transport, 1998). These figures are consistent with research from around the world showing that child cyclists are over-represented in accident and casualty statistics (Weiss, 1986; Hoque, 1990; Stutts, Williamson, Whitley & Sheldon, 1990; Cooke, Margolius & Cadden, 1993). In a review presented in an earlier paper (Arnold & Quine, 1994) we showed that casualty rates for child cyclists are frequently under-reported (Cross & Fisher, 1977; Langley, Silva & Williams, 1987; Agran, Castillo & Winn, 1990; Harris, 1990; Stutts et al, 1990; Maimaris, Summers, Browning & Palmer, 1994); that casualties are age-related (Jones, 1989); and that boys are at particularly high risk (Stutts et al., 1990; Collins, Langley & Marshall, 1993; Thomas, Acton, Nixon, Battistutta, Pitt & Clark, 1994; Towner, Jarvis, Walsh & Aynsley-Green, 1994). Cycling accidents are frequently school related, occurring on weekdays on journeys to and from school (Taylor, 1989) and they often result in serious head injuries (McDermot & Klug, 1982; Wood & Milne, 1988; Stutts et al., 1990). A number of studies provide evidence that cycle helmets will help prevent or lessen the severity of head injury (Wood & Milne, 1988; Dorsch, Woodward & Somers, 1987; Pitt, Thomas, Nixon, Clark, Battistutta & Acton, 1994; Thomas et al., 1994).

Despite the beneficial effects, few child cyclists wear helmets in countries where helmet wearing is not legally mandatory. Cushman, Down, MacMillan and Waclawik (1990) report that only 2% of 568 injured child cyclists were wearing a helmet at the time of their injury although 13% claimed to own one.

Sissons-Joshi, Beckett and MacFarlane (1994) found that only 13% of their sample always wore a helmet and that rates of wearing decreased with increasing age. Other research seems to confirm this finding (DiGuiseppi, Rivara & Koepsall, 1990; Stutts et al., 1990; Maimaris et al., 1994). Although some schools encourage helmet use, the decision is left largely to the individual cyclist. From a social psychological perspective this makes the study of the cyclists' behaviour (wearing or not wearing a helmet) more interesting since it is likely to arise from cyclists' beliefs rather than from regulations or the insistence of others.

Social Cognition Models and Road Safety

There is growing evidence that expectancy-value models from social psychology such as the Theory of Reasoned Action (TRA), the Theory of Planned Behaviour (TPB), and the Health Belief Model (HBM) can provide valuable tools for predicting and understanding road user behaviours, for example wearing seatbelts (Wittenbraker, Gibbs & Kahle, 1983; Budd, North & Spencer, 1984; Budd & Spencer, 1986; Stasson & Fishbein, 1990; Thuen & Rise, 1994; Sutton & Hallett, 1989); using car seats and restraints for children (Gielen, Ericksen, Daltoy & Rost, 1984; Foss, 1985; Webb, Sanson–Fisher & Bowman, 1988); avoiding drink–driving (Åberg, 1994); driving safely (Parker, Manstead, Stradling, Reason & Baxter, 1992); and avoiding motorcycling accidents (Rutter, Quine & Chesham, 1995).

Budd and his colleagues (1984), for example, showed that the traditional components of the TRA all independently predicted intention to wear a seatbelt on long journeys. An addition to the model, past behaviour, was also an independent predictor. Gielen and her colleagues (1984) found that attitude was the most important variable in explaining parents' use of car seats for their children. Åberg (1994), in a LISREL analysis using the TRA, was able to predict drink-driving from attitudes, subjective norm, and a measure of drinking habits. Parker and her colleagues (1992) carried out a study to investigate whether the TRA or the TPB could better account for drivers' intentions to commit four specific driving violations: drinking and driving, speeding, close following, and overtaking in risky circumstances. Results showed that the addition of perceived behavioural control to the TRA led to significant increments in the variance explained in intentions. In addition, the relation between subjective norms and behavioural intentions was consistently stronger than that between attitudes towards behaviours and intentions. Rutter, Quine and Chesham (1995) used both the TRA and the HBM to predict safe riding and accidents in motorcyclists. They found that components in each model were able to predict safe riding behaviours, and that accident involvement was predicted by behaviour. Finally, a number of authors have begun to use social cognition models to investigate cycle helmet use. This may have resulted from the failure of promotional campaigns to have any appreciable impact on levels of helmet use – a failure that led researchers to consider the use of theory-driven models. Otis, Lesage, Godin, Brown, Farley and Lambert (1992), for example, used an expanded TRA to investigate the psychological correlations of intention to use helmets among children aged between 8 and 12 years. Attitude and subjective norm were assessed, as well as perceived risk of head injury when cycling without a helmet and potential severity of a head injury. Attitude and subjective norm were the only variables of statistical significance, accounting for 51% of the variance in intention. Sissons-Joshi et al., (1994), using components from both the HBM and the TPB in addition to a number of other variables, found that perceived vulnerability was the only component from either model to predict intention, but not behaviour. Other variables predicting both intention and behaviour were amount of active consideration given to the subject, anticipated regret, and desire to conform with friends' behaviour.

An earlier paper of our own (Arnold & Quine, 1994) reported a prospective study using the HBM to investigate the factors that influence cycle helmet use in a sample of schoolboy cyclists. The study addressed perceptions of vulnerability (to sustaining head injury in an accident) and injury severity, as well as the perceived benefits and barriers to helmet use. Multiple regression analysis showed that perceived benefits, barriers, vulnerability, and cues to action were significant predictors of helmet use four weeks later. Several individual beliefs discriminated significantly between helmet users and non-users, in particular the belief that helmet use would make parents worry less.

The results of the above studies show that the TRA, its extension the TPB, and the HBM have made a valuable contribution to understanding road safety behaviours, though the models have rarely been rigorously compared (for exceptions see Oliver & Berger, 1979; Conner & Norman, 1994). The aim of the present study was to compare the ability of two models, the TPB and the HBM, to predict and understand the factors determining helmet use in a new sample of schoolboy cyclists using a prospective design. We briefly describe the models and their differences below.

The Health Belief Model

The Health Belief Model (Rosenstock, 1966, 1974a, 1974b) proposes that people will be motivated to carry out preventive health behaviours such as wearing a cycle helmet in response to a perceived threat to their health (see Figure 4.1). Two classes of variables are important: '(1) the psychological state of readiness to take specific action, and (2) the extent to which a particular course of action is believed to be beneficial in reducing the threat' (Rosenstock, 1966, p. 98). Both variables, Rosenstock argued, are two-dimensional. The individual's state of readiness to act is determined by perceptions of personal susceptibility or *vulnerability* to a particular health threat, and perceptions of the *severity* with which that threat might affect his or her life. The extent to which a course of action is believed to be beneficial is the result of beliefs about the *benefits* to be gained by a particular action weighed against the costs of or *barriers* to action. Rosenstock (1966) believed that the level of readiness provided the energy or force to act and the perceptions of benefits less barriers provided a preferred path of action (p. 101). However, the combination of these could reach considerable levels of intensity without resulting in overt action unless some instigating event occurred to set the process in motion or trigger action in an individual psychologically ready to act (p. 102). Thus in addition

Perceptions of
Benefits

Perceptions of
Barriers

Cues to Action
measured at
Time 1

Perceptions of
Vulnerability

Perceptions of
Severity

Preventive Health
Behaviour

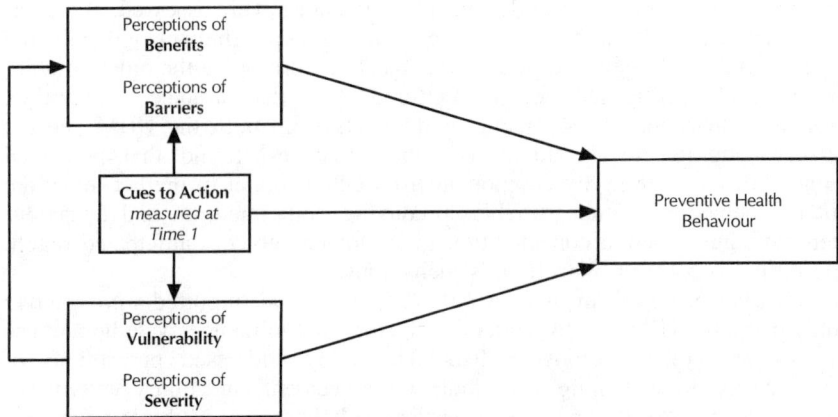

Figure 4.1   The Health Belief Model (HBM)

to the variables already described, a factor that serves as a cue or a trigger to appropriate action is necessary – such as having an accident oneself, in the present case, or recent media attention to the issue. This Rosenstock named the 'cue to action'. Some years later, Rosenstock and his colleagues also suggested that behavioural intention might be a mediating variable between the components of the HBM and behaviour (Becker, Haefner, Kasl, Kirscht, Maiman & Rosenstock, 1977). Other researchers have taken up this suggestion (King, 1982; Calnan, 1984; Norman & Fitter, 1989).

Despite its intuitive appeal, the HBM has conceptual difficulties. Rosenstock did not specify how different beliefs influence one another, or how the explanatory variables combine to influence behaviour. As a result, different studies have used different combinations of variables, and researchers have treated variables differently in the analysis. Some, for example, have used additive models in which the combined weight of the variables is used to predict outcome, while others have combined variables, either by adding vulnerability and severity (Witte, Stokols, Ituarte & Schneider, 1993; Wyper, 1990), or by multiplying them (Haefner & Kirscht, 1970; Hill, Gardner & Rassaby, 1985; Conner & Norman, 1994), or by subtracting barriers from benefits (Oliver & Berger, 1979; Rutledge, 1987; Wyper, 1990). A close inspection of Rosenstock's discussion of the model, however, seems to indicate that the dimensions are to be treated as separate influences on health behaviour and that an additive combination is consistent with the underlying theoretical principles (see Weinstein, 1988, for a discussion).

A second problem is that Rosenstock offered no operational definitions of the components of the model and therefore researchers use different ways of measuring them (Champion, 1984). Perceived vulnerability is assessed by measuring either personal vulnerability to a specific health threat or a general vulnerability to disease relative to other people. Barriers, which Rosenstock viewed as primarily psychological, are often assessed by investigating structural impediments instead (Hill et al., 1985; Melnyk, 1988; Simon,

Morse, Balson, Osofsky & Gaumer, 1993). Several revisions to the model have therefore been suggested (Becker, Drachman & Kirscht, 1972; Becker & Maiman, 1975; Becker et al., 1977). Becker (1974) has argued that the value placed upon their health by some individuals may predispose them to respond to the cues to action. Others have suggested that health locus of control beliefs should be included (Wallston & Wallston, 1981; Lau, Hartman & Ware, 1986; Arnold & Quine, 1994). Despite these theoretical and conceptual problems, the HBM has received sustained empirical support (see Harrison, Mullen & Green, 1992, for a meta-analysis and Sheeran & Abraham, 1996, for a review).

The Theory of Planned Behaviour

The Theory of Planned Behaviour (Ajzen, 1985, 1988) and its predecessor the Theory of Reasoned Action (Fishbein & Ajzen, 1975) are the most influential and widely used social cognition models of the attitude-behaviour relationship. The TPB represents an extension of the original TRA that is designed to allow for the fact that not all behaviours are entirely under volitional control. The TPB proposes that the immediate determinant of human behaviour is behavioural intention, which is in turn determined by the individual's attitude towards the behaviour in question and by his or her subjective norm (see Figure 4.2). Attitude towards the behaviour is itself a product of a small set of salient behavioural beliefs about the consequences of performing the behaviour, weighted by an evaluation of each of these consequences. Subjective norm is determined by a small set of salient normative beliefs, i.e. the person's beliefs about the perceived wishes of salient others weighted by his or her motivation to comply with these others' expectations. The product of each behavioural belief multiplied by the person's corresponding outcome evaluations gives a set of behavioural beliefs, the sum of which forms the overall attitude to the behaviour. Similarly, the summed product of each normative belief multiplied by the person's motivation to comply gives belief-based measures of subjective norm.

   To these two determinants of intention, Ajzen added a third component, perceived behavioural control, which refers to the degree to which a person feels that performance of the behaviour is under his or her volitional control (see Figure 4.2). Measurement of perceived behavioural control is designed to assess a person's beliefs about the ease or difficulty of performing the behaviour (Ajzen, 1988). According to Ajzen (1988), among the beliefs that determine intention and action is a set that deals with the presence or absence of requisite resources and opportunities (p. 135). The more resources and opportunities individuals think they possess and the fewer obstacles or impediments they anticipate, the greater their perceived control over the behaviour in question. These beliefs Ajzen termed 'control beliefs'. They may include both internal control factors (information, personal deficiencies, skills, abilities, emotions) and external control factors (opportunities, dependence on others, barriers). There is a certain amount of ambiguity about the way control beliefs should be operationalised (see Conner & Sparks (1996) for a discussion). Ajzen and Madden (1986) assessed perceived behavioural control both directly, by asking students how much control they thought they had over

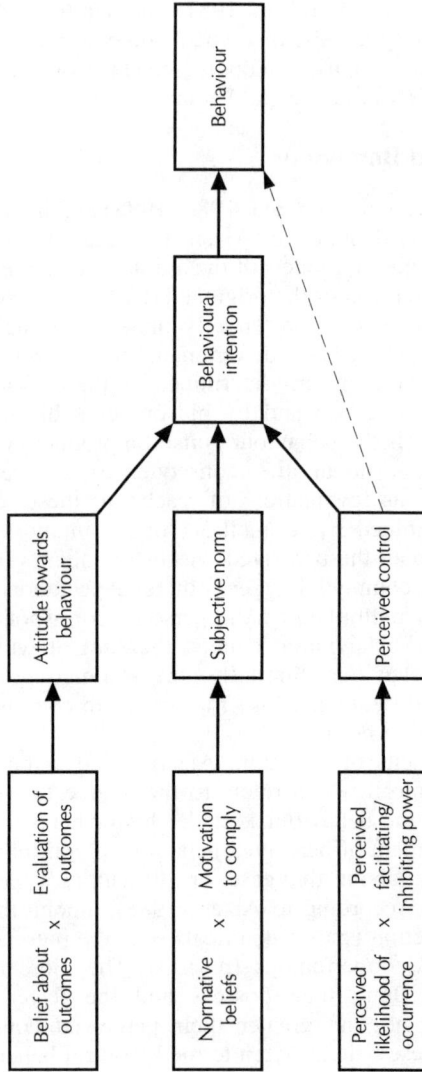

Figure 4.2   The Theory of Planned Behaviour (TPB)

regular class attendance using three questions añd summing the responses, and indirectly, by summing the frequency of occurrence of a number of factors likely to facilitate or interfere with the performance of the behaviour. Ajzen (1991), however, in the most comprehensive discussion of perceived behavioural control, suggests that each control belief is assessed by multiplying the frequency of likelihood of occurrence of the factor by the subjective perception of its power to facilitate or inhibit the performance of the behaviour. Perceived behavioural control is the summed product. As a result, Valois, Desharnis, Godin, Perron and Lecomte (1993) have computed perceived behavioural control as a multiplicative composite (in keeping with Ajzen's (1991) proposal), while a handful of others (eg. Ajzen & Driver, 1991; Kimiecik, 1992; Courneya, 1995; Norman & Smith, 1995; Parker, Manstead & Stradling, 1995) have assessed both belief-based and direct measures and examined the relationship between them. It is far more usual, however, for researchers only to assess variants of Ajzen and Madden's (1986) direct measures (see for example DeVellis, Blalock & Sandler, 1990; Netemeyer & Burton, 1990; Netemeyer, Burton & Johnston, 1991; Madden, Ellen & Ajzen, 1992; Reinecke, Schmidt & Azjen, 1996).

The introduction of perceived behavioural control is not the only amendment to the TRA. In the original theory the influence of beliefs and attitudes on behaviour was *always* mediated by behavioural intention. Ajzen (1985) departs from this by stating that in certain circumstances perceived behavioural control may influence behaviour directly: that is, it can be seen as a measure of people's confidence in their ability to carry out their intentions successfully. The Theories of Reasoned Action and Planned Behaviour have received extensive support in the health literature (see Conner & Sparks, 1996, for a review) and elsewhere (see the meta-analysis by Sheppard, Hartwick & Warshaw, 1988).

Differences Between the Models

There are a number of similarities and differences between the models, which have been ably reviewed by Conner and Norman (1994). We shall review the differences briefly here.

1. The HBM uses beliefs to predict actual probability of behaviour, while the TPB uses beliefs to predict behaviour indirectly via intentions. Some researchers, including Becker and Rosenstock themselves (Becker et al., 1977), have suggested that intention might mediate between the components of the model and behaviour (Cummings, Jette, Brock & Haefner, 1979; Hays, 1985; Champion, 1988).
2. The TPB examines individuals' evaluations of each of a set of consequences associated with performing a given behaviour (outcome evaluation) weighted by the strength of their belief that performing the behaviour will indeed lead to each of the consequences (belief strength). Attitude is made up of the summed products. The HBM has no mechanism by which to examine evaluation of consequences. The belief in a benefit or barrier itself signifies an outcome expectancy.

3. The TPB examines the individual's *subjective norm*: his or her normative beliefs (the belief that most of his or her important others think he or she should (or should not) perform the behaviour in question) weighted by the motivation to comply with those referents. In the TPB these are a major determinant of intentions, along with attitude and perceived behavioural control. The HBM has no equivalent measure. Normative influences are included in the cues to action construct among many other variables.

4. The TPB measures the degree of control a person believes he or she has over performing the behaviour. This factor is 'assumed to reflect past experience as well as anticipated impediments and obstacles' (Ajzen, 1988, p. 132). The greater the perceived behavioural control, the stronger should be the individual's intention to perform the behaviour under consideration. The HBM does not directly measure control beliefs. These are often included by researchers in the barriers construct.

5. The HBM measures individuals' perceptions of vulnerability to the health threat as separate from perceptions of the severity with which the threat may affect their lives. The TPB does not include measures of susceptibility and severity, assuming that such factors influence behaviour via their effects on behavioural and normative beliefs (Liska, 1984). It thus does not cater for emotional fear and arousal variables. This has led researchers such as Oliver and Berger (1979) to suggest that it is limited to the rational part of human decision-making.

6. The TPB does not include cues to action, the component that Rosenstock believed important for triggering the decision-making process. In the TPB these are assumed to influence behaviour via their effects on behavioural and normative beliefs.

The discussion above concerning the differences between the HBM and the TPB suggests that there is some reason to believe that the TPB might prove to have better predictive utility than the HBM, particularly for behaviours such as wearing a safety helmet where subjective norm may be particularly important. Our study was designed to compare the models.

METHOD

A prospective, longitudinal design was used. A sample of 162 schoolboys aged between 11 and 18 years who regularly cycled to school were given a questionnaire with items relating to the TPB and the HBM. Boys only were chosen since pilot work in schools carried out for our earlier study had revealed that few girls cycle to school. This is consistent with the casualty statistics we have reported, which show the predominance of boys. Agran and Winn (1993) make a distinction between using a bicycle for recreational purposes and using it for transportation. They propose that cycling to and from school is an example of what they term 'purposive bicycling', which is characterised by situational and behavioural factors that differentiate it from 'recreational cycling'. Children using a bicycle for transportation are likely to cycle longer distances from home than when play cycling and to use multi-lane roads – both of which expose the cyclist to motor vehicle traffic to a greater extent than when play cycling (see also Towner et al., 1994). For these reasons, we chose to focus on cycling to school as the criterion behaviour. The cyclists were drawn from six secondary schools in four different population centres, and so provided a representative sample of urban, semirural, and rural cycling conditions. Four weeks later they completed a second questionnaire which asked whether they had worn a helmet when riding to school in the last four weeks and, if so, how frequently. It was found that helmets were either worn every time the rider cycled to school or not at all. Helmet use was therefore construed as a dichotomous variable.

The questions were arranged in two booklets, the first for Time 1 and the second for Time 2. The first booklet contained the items relating to the HBM and TPB dimensions. The second contained measures for actual helmet use in the week leading up to the Time 2 questionnaire. When the questionnaires were handed out, the experimenter defined accident as 'any incident that involved minor or serious injury to yourself or another person or damage to another vehicle or the bicycle you were riding'.

THE MEASURES

The Health Belief Model

The investigation presented here kept closely to the original components described by Rosenstock (1966), but subsequently added a measure of intention to test for possible mediation between beliefs and behaviour. This is in line with Rosenstock's own suggestion (Becker et al., 1977) and allowed us to make direct comparisons with the TPB. Other researchers have also followed this procedure (Oliver & Berger, 1979; Champion & Miller, 1992; Conner & Norman, 1994; Sissons-Joshi et al., 1994). The questionnaire items addressed perceived vulnerability, severity, benefits and barriers, and cues to action. Examples of items from each of the components are given in Table 4.1. According to the model, the likelihood of cyclists adopting the preventive measure of wearing a safety helmet can be assessed by measuring their beliefs on each of the dimensions. Thus if a cyclist feels sufficiently vulnerable to any of the undesirable outcomes when not wearing a helmet (such as head injury or brain damage), and the consequences of nonuse. are recognised as sufficiently severe, then the readiness to act engendered by these perceptions of threat, augmented by an appropriate cue, should motivate him to evaluate the benefits and costs of wearing a helmet. If the perceived benefits outweigh the barriers, actual helmet use will follow.

Perceived vulnerability. Perceived vulnerability was measured by a seven-item scale. Each item was scored from 1 'Strongly disagree' to 5 'Strongly agree' (see Table 4.1). Scores for negatively worded items were reversed and the items were summed.

Severity. Severity was measured by four items (see Table 4.1). Each item was scored from 1 'Very little' to 5 'Very much'.

Benefits and barriers. Benefits and barriers were measured by five items each. These were phrased in such a way that they could also be used for the belief strength items in the TPB. Thus items measuring beliefs that wearing a helmet would lead to a given outcome were the same for both models, though of course in the TPB each belief strength was multiplied by an outcome evaluation to form a product, 'behavioural belief'. The items were scored from 1 'Extremely unlikely' to 7 'Extremely likely'. Examples are given in Table 4.1.

Cues to action. Cues to action were measured by simple Yes/No questions. The items were 'In the last year have you had an accident while cycling?' and 'In the last year has a friend, classmate, or relative had an accident while cycling?'.

Table 4.1   Reliability of scales from the Health Belief Model and Theory of Planned Behaviour and representative items from each scale

	Items	Alpha	Representative items	Scale/scoring
Vulnerability	6	0.74	If I had an accident while cycling to school and hit my head, I would be likely to suffer brain damage	1 = Strongly disagree 5 = Strongly agree
Severity	4	0.80	If you had a serious accident involving head injury and hospital treatment, how seriously do you think it would affect your ... school life/family life/physical and mental well-being	1 = Very little 5 = Very much
Benefits	5	0.82	My wearing a helmet while cycling to school would protect my head if I had an accident	1 = Extremely unlikely 7 = Extremely likely
Barriers	5	0.64	My wearing a helmet while cycling to school would make me look silly	1 = Extremely unlikely 7 = Extremely likely
Attitude[†]	10 × 10	0.82	My wearing a helmet while cycling to school would make me feel safe	1 = Extremely unlikely 7 = Extremely likely
			Feeling safe is ...	+3 = Extremely good −3 = Extremely bad
Subjective norm[‡]	6 × 6	0.90	My close friends think I should wear a helmet while cycling to and from school	1 = Extremely unlikely 7 = Extremely likely
			Generally speaking I want to do what my close friends think I should do	1 = Extremely unlikely 7 = Extremely likely
Perceived behavioural control	5	0.70	For me to wear a helmet while cycling to school would be ...	1 = Very difficult 7 = Very easy

[†]Each behavioural belief produced by multiplying a belief strength by an outcome evaluation. Attitude is the sum of the products.
[‡]Each subjective norm belief produced by multiplying a normative belief by a motivation to comply. Subjective norm is the sum of the products.

The Theory of Planned Behaviour

For the TPB, the operational procedures given by Ajzen and Fishbein (1980) and Ajzen (1985) were adhered to as closely as possible. The questionnaire used indirect belief-based measures of attitude, subjective norm, and perceived behavioural control. According to the model, cyclists should form an intention to wear a helmet if their overall attitude is influenced more by beliefs concerning the beneficial outcomes of wearing a helmet than by beliefs concerning negative outcomes, and if they are sufficiently motivated to comply with referent others perceived as supporting their intention to wear a helmet. This intention to wear should lead to helmet use. In addition, individuals will need to feel confident that they have the requisite skills, knowledge and resources to carry out their intentions at will and to overcome external barriers successfully, and will thus be able to wear a protective helmet whenever they desire. Anticipated control over the behaviour should enhance cyclists' intention to wear a helmet, and thus indirectly as well as directly increase the probability of the behaviour.

Attitude. Attitude was constructed from measures of belief strength and outcome evaluation in the following way. Ten salient beliefs were identified from our previous research (Arnold & Quine, 1994). Belief strength was assessed on seven-point unipolar scales scored from 1 'Extremely unlikely' to 7 'Extremely likely' and outcome evaluation was measured on bipolar scales from +3 'Extremely good' to –3 'Extremely bad' as Ajzen recommends (Ajzen, 1991, p. 193. See Ajzen, 1991, for a discussion of unipolar versus bipolar scaling). The product of each belief multiplied by its outcome evaluation produced a set of behavioural beliefs, the sum of which formed the overall attitude to the behaviour.

Subjective norm. Subjective norm was constructed from normative beliefs and motivation to comply. Six relevant referent groups were identified from our previous research (Arnold & Quine, 1994). They were close friends, parents, other family members, teachers, other cyclists, and road safety experts. Each normative belief and motivation to comply item was measured on a seven-point scale, from 1 'Extremely unlikely' to 7 'Extremely likely'. The summed product of each normative belief multiplied by the individual's motivation to comply gave an overall subjective norm.

Perceived behavioural control. Perceived behavioural control was measured by five items, which encompassed practical impediments scaled from 1 'Strongly disagree' to 7 'Strongly agree' (see Table 4.1 for example) and three items assessing the cyclists' confidence that they had the requisite skills, knowledge, and resources to carry out their intentions (Ajzen, 1988, p. 135). Factor analysis of these items revealed one interpretable factor and the items were therefore summed to form a single scale.

Prior behaviour. Prior behaviour (whether participants had worn a helmet in the previous four weeks) was also measured at Time 1 (Bentler & Speckart,

1979; Budd et al., 1984; Hill et al., 1985). Further examples of the items are given in Table 4.1.

Dependent Variables

In order to achieve correspondence between behavioural intention and behaviour, *intention* was assessed by a single item, 'I intend to wear a helmet while cycling to school in the next four weeks', scored from 1 'Extremely unlikely' to 7 'Extremely likely'. Actual *behaviour* was measured four weeks later by asking the questions 'In the past week have you worn a helmet while cycling to and from school?' and 'How many days out of five did you wear it?' (score 1–5). Behaviour was found to be dichotomous: cyclists either wore a helmet each time they cycled to school or not at all. This is consistent with the idea that helmet use is appropriately regarded as a routine – a sequence of behaviours that is repeated on a regular basis and which once it has been learned is likely to become habitual (Sutton, 1994). Other behaviours that can be seen as learned habits include seatbelt wearing, using children's carry cot restraints, and cleaning teeth. The relatively short time interval between the measurement of intention and behaviour – four weeks – was chosen to enhance the accuracy of the prediction of behaviour, as suggested by Ajzen and Fishbein (1980).

Analyses

Scales were constructed of all the major dimensions and components of the models and their reliabilities were investigated using Cronbach's alpha. One vulnerability item was discarded, giving a scale alpha of 0.74, and two perceived behavioural control items were discarded, yielding an alpha of 0.70. Satisfactory alphas were found for all other scales (see Table 4.1). Simple correlations and path analyses were then used to identify predictors of intention to wear a helmet and actual helmet use at Time 2.

RESULTS

One hundred and sixty two cyclists answered both the Time 1 and Time 2 questionnaires, giving a response rate of 88%. At Time 1, 52 boys (32.1%) reported wearing a helmet for cycling to and from school. At Time 2, 62 boys (38.3%) reported wearing a helmet. Only one wearer at Time 1 did not wear a helmet at Time 2. 37.1% of the boys at Time 1 reported some degree of intention to wear a helmet in the next four weeks while cycling to school. In this sense, the analyses reported below predict continuance of a habitual behaviour in many of the pupils as well as the start of a new behaviour in some.

Correlations Between Components of the Model, Intentions, and Behaviour

The first stage of our analysis was to examine relationships among the components of the models by simple correlation (Table 4.2). Intention was

Table 4.2 Correlations among components of the models, intention and behaviour

	Vulnerability	Severity	Benefits	Barriers	Own accident	Friend accident	Attitude	Subjective norm	Perceived control	Intention	Time 1 wearing	Time 2 wearing
Vulnerability	1.00											
Severity	0.08	1.00										
Benefits	0.28	0.06	1.00									
Barriers	-0.07	0.00	0.09	1.00								
Own accident	0.15	-0.08	0.01	-0.03	1.00							
Friend accident	0.13	0.04	-0.15	-0.14	0.29	1.00						
Attitude	0.25	-0.04	0.73	-0.27	0.06	-0.12	1.00					
Subjective norm	0.18	0.06	0.64	-0.10	0.02	-0.10	0.71	1.00				
Perceived control	0.22	-0.05	0.37	-0.18	0.06	-0.12	0.47	0.53	1.00			
Intention	0.16	-0.06	0.44	-0.15	0.03	-0.03	0.48	0.57	0.45	1.00		
Time 1 wearing	0.16	-0.09	0.32	-0.16	0.08	0.03	0.33	0.34	0.45	0.65	1.00	
Time 2 wearing	0.17	-0.06	0.38	-0.17	0.03	-0.01	0.40	0.41	0.42	0.63	0.85	1.00

For df = 150 r = 0.16 $p < 0.05$; r = 0.21 $p < 0.01$; r = 0.24 $p < 0.001$

strongly correlated with actual helmet use at Time 2 ($r = 0.63$; $p < 0.001$). It also correlated strongly with each component of the TPB – attitude ($r = 0.48$; $p < 0.001$), subjective norm ($r = 0.57$; $p < 0.001$), and perceived behavioural control ($r = 0.45$; $p < 0.001$). There were also significant correlations with three components of the HBM – perceived vulnerability ($r = 0.16$; $p < 0.05$), perceived benefits ($r = 0.44$; $p < 0.001$), and perceived barriers ($r = 0.15$; $p < 0.05$) – but they were all smaller. Time 1 helmet use was significantly correlated with all components of the TPB – attitude ($r = 0.33$; $p < 0.001$), subjective norm ($r = 0.34$; $p < 0.001$), and perceived behavioural control ($r = 0.45$; $p < 0.001$) – but with only three components of the HBM – vulnerability ($r = 0.16$; $p < 0.05$), barriers ($r = 0.16$; $p < 0.05$), and benefits ($r = 0.32$; $p < 0.001$). Time 2 helmet use was similarly significantly correlated with all components of the TPB – attitude ($r = 0.40$; $p < 0.001$), subjective norm ($r = 0.41$; $p < 0.001$), and perceived behavioural control ($r = 0.42$; $p < 0.001$) – but with only three components of the HBM – vulnerability ($r = 0.17$; $p < 0.05$), barriers ($r = 0.17$; $p < 0.05$), and benefits ($r = 0.38$; $p < 0.001$). The correlations were again stronger for the TPB than for the HBM. There were also significant correlations among the predictor variables *within* each of the models, as the models would expect, and *between* the HBM variables and the TPB variables.

Predicting Intention and Helmet Use

The second stage of our analysis was to test the two models by path analysis, for which we used SPSS. Each dependent measure was regressed on the predictor variables, and a second analysis was then conducted with just the significant predictors to determine the final beta weights and R^2 values. There were three sets of analyses. First, we tested the models in their original forms. The results are given in Figures 4.3 and 4.4. For the HBM, helmet use at Time 2 was predicted by just two variables: the perceived benefits of wearing the helmet and (negatively) perceived barriers. The variance explained by the six variables together was 18%. For the TPB, subjective norm and perceived behavioural control both predicted intention reliably – but attitude did not – and intention predicted Time 2 helmet use. There was also a direct path from perceived behavioural control to Time 2 helmet use. For intention the variance explained was 34%; for helmet use at Time 2 it was 43%.

In the second set of analyses, we tested whether intention, which is not included in the original HBM, might in fact mediate the links between the predictor variables and behaviour – as Oliver and Berger (1979) and Norman and Fitter (1989) have suggested. Our original analysis of the HBM was repeated, but with the six predictors allowed direct paths only to intention, which in turn went on directly to Time 2 helmet use. Perceived benefits and barriers both produced significant paths to intention (betas 0.46 $p < 0.001$ and 0.19 $p < 0.01$ respectively), and intention produced a significant path to behaviour (beta 0.64 $p < 0.001$). For intention the variance explained was 22%; for helmet use at Time 2 it was now 40%, against 18% for the original HBM without intention and 43% for the TPB.

In the third and final set of analyses, we examined the possible effects of prior behaviour, wearing or not wearing the helmet at Time 1. For the HBM,

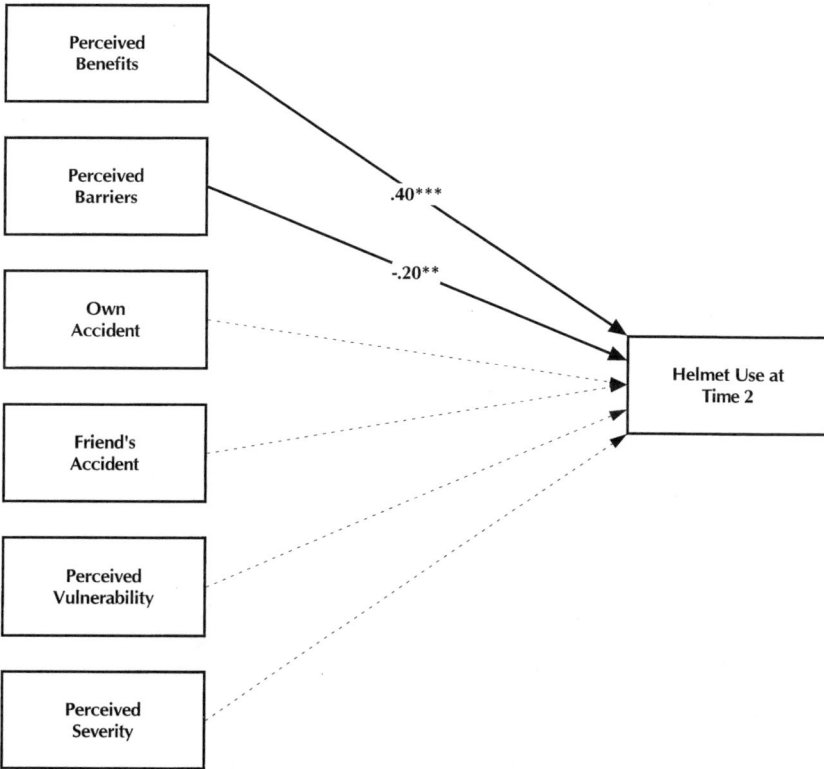

**p<0.01 ***p<0.001

Dotted lines denote non-significant paths

Figure 4.3 Path analysis for the Health Belief Model

Time 1 behaviour was added to the original six predictor variables at the same level. Perceived benefits and Time 1 helmet use both emerged as significant predictors of Time 2 helmet use (betas 0.13 $p < 0.01$ and 0.81 $p < 0.001$ respectively), and the overall variance explained was 73%. To test the 'intention' form of the model, all seven predictors were allowed direct paths to intention, and Time 1 helmet use was allowed a direct path to Time 2 use, alongside intention. Perceived benefits and Time 1 helmet use both produced reliable paths to intention (betas 0.26 $p < 0.001$ and 0.56 $p < 0.001$ respectively), and Time 1 helmet use produced a significant direct path to Time 2 use (beta 0.75 $p < 0.001$). For intention the variance explained was 47%; for helmet use at Time 2 it was 73%.

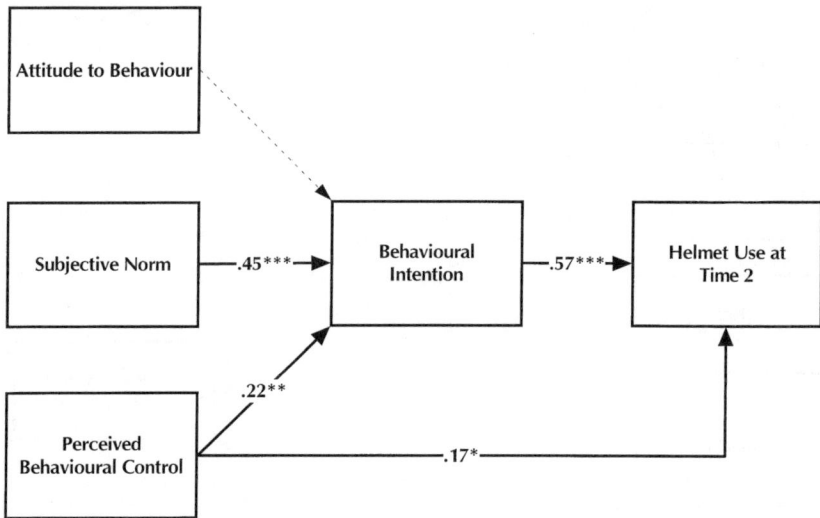

*p<0.05 **p<0.01 ***p<0.001

Dotted line denotes non-significant path

Figure 4.4   Path analysis for the Theory of Planned Behaviour

DISCUSSION

The study set out to examine the HBM and the TPB in a prospective longitudinal design to determine which model was better able to predict helmet use in schoolboy cyclists. For the HBM in its original form, the variance explained in Time 2 behaviour was 18%, against 43% for the TPB. Only two of the six paths produced reliable effects (perceived benefits and perceived barriers), and the path for perceived benefits was the stronger. For the TPB, however, four of the five paths were reliable, indicating greater economy and less redundancy than in the HBM. The leading predictor of intention was subjective norm. Perceived behavioural control influenced Time 2 behaviour directly as well as indirectly through intention.

Adding Intention to the Health Belief Model

In a second approach to the HBM, we tested whether intention might act as a mediator between the six original predictor variables and behaviour. The answer is that it did – as Cummings et al., (1979) also found, but Champion and Miller (1992) and Conner and Norman (1994) did not. Perceived benefits and barriers (but none of the four remaining variables) produced significant paths to intention, which then led to Time 2 behaviour. The variance explained in behaviour rose from the original 18% without intention to 40% with it, a slightly lower figure than for the TPB, and the four remaining variables still played no part. It should also be noted that the two significant predictors, perceived benefits and perceived barriers, in any case are conceptually close to attitude and perceived behavioural control in the TPB and that the *distinctive* components of the HBM (perceived vulnerability and severity, and cues to action) made no significant contribution. On that criterion too, therefore, the TPB emerges with the greater predictive utility.

Overall, then, even when intention was added to the model, our results provided only partial support for the HBM, since neither perceived vulnerability nor severity – said by Rosenstock (1966) to provide the readiness to act – were significant predictors of either intention to wear a helmet or actual helmet use. There was also no evidence that cues to action played any part in triggering behaviour. The findings are in accord with those of Conner and Norman (1994) and Abraham, Sheeran, Spears and Abrams (1992), who also found perceived benefits and barriers but not vulnerability or severity to be associated with intention. Witte et al. (1993), however, reported that perceived threat (vulnerability plus severity) significantly and positively influenced bicycle helmet attitudes, intention, and behaviour. One reason for differences in findings may be the lack of established procedures to measure the relevant concepts in the HBM and the fact that studies have differed widely in their operationalisation of concepts.

Attitude, Subjective Norm, and Perceived Behavioural Control in the Theory of Planned Behaviour

Perhaps the most interesting feature of the TPB analysis is that the strongest predictor of behavioural intention was subjective norm and that attitude had no reliable effect. This can be attributed to the strong performance of subjective norm rather than to attitude being unimportant, since the same set of beliefs (as benefits and barriers) were significantly associated with intention in the HBM analysis. The correlation between attitude and subjective norm was 0.71, suggesting that the effects of attitude on intention were absorbed by subjective norm.

Other studies have also found subjective norm to be the better predictor of intention (Lacy, 1981; Budd & Spencer, 1984; Harrison, Thompson & Rodgers, 1985; Hessing, Elffers & Weigel, 1988; Beck & Ajzen, 1991; Boyd & Wandersman, 1991; Vaile, Calnan, Rutter & Wall, 1993). A common link is that all of them have examined behaviours that are performed in the presence of a partner, with friends, or in public (e.g. condom use, illicit drug use, intention to drink) or are highly susceptible to prevailing standards of public morality (e.g. lying, tax evasion).[1] It may be that in general attitude is more important than subjective norm when the behaviour is performed in private (eg., breast/ testicular self-examination), but that the reverse is true when it is performed publicly, as in wearing a seatbelt (Wittenbraker et al., 1983), or where it is perceived that the consequences of failing to carry out the behaviour may profoundly affect the lives of referent others. Wearing a cycle helmet is very much a public behaviour and so is subject to a variety of normative influences, particularly those of parents. Examination of the univariate statistics in our study showed that the largest difference in normative beliefs between users and non-users was for the item 'My parents think that I should wear a helmet while cycling to school'. The mean for users was 6.4 (sd 1.1) while for non-users it was 4.8 (sd 1.9; $p < 0.001$). Children's attitude to helmet use is clearly strongly influenced by the views and behaviours of their parents (both by buying helmets and encouraging helmet use) and it may be that helmet use is partly due to a desire to allay parental anxieties. These findings are consistent with the work of Witte et al. (1993), who found parental attitudes to be a significant influence on helmet use, though Sissons-Joshi et al. (1994) found that users and non-users of cycle helmets shared the same norms, reporting that parents pressed them to wear a helmet but friends discouraged them.

Perceived behavioural control was also a predictor of intention, supporting Ajzen's (1985) claim that it increases the predictive power of the TRA (but see Conner & Norman, 1994, and Sissons-Joshi et al., 1994, who found that perceived behavioural control did not enter the regression equation). This suggests that cyclists *do* need to feel confident that they possess the requisite skills and resources to be able to carry out the behaviour and to feel that there are few practical impediments to helmet use.

Finally, both intention and perceived behavioural control were predictors of actual helmet use. Intention was the stronger predictor, with a beta weight of 0.57, while perceived behavioural control had a beta weight of 0.17, supporting Ajzen's argument that attitudes concerned with perceived behavioural control may also exert direct effects on behaviour (Ajzen, 1985). Forgetting to put the helmet on, or it being too much effort, or having nowhere to store the helmet once at school are factors likely to intervene between intention and behaviour. These results thus again provide good support for the TPB, suggesting that cyclists who perceive normative support for wearing a helmet and are confident that they have the requisite skills and resources to exercise personal control will formulate a strong intention to use a helmet, which in turn will predict actual helmet use. In addition, perceived behavioural control will influence helmet use directly.

Comparing the Models

Why does the TPB have the better predictive utility? As we have noted in our earlier discussion, there is considerable overlap between the two models. Concepts from the HBM – perceived susceptibility/vulnerability, perceived severity, and perceived benefits and barriers to carrying out the behaviour – are also part of the subjective cost-benefit analysis that determines an individual's overall attitude in the TPB. Perceived barriers are also closely related to the concept of perceived behavioural control. As Van der Pligt (1994) notes, one reason for the superior predictive power of Ajzen's model may be the rigorously defined procedures for measuring the relevant concepts. For example, the HBM does not state how vulnerability and severity should be combined to arrive at perceived threat. Consequently, researchers have operationalised the components very differently from study to study (Oliver & Berger, 1979; Conner & Norman, 1994). In addition, as we have noted, researchers tend to extend the HBM to include other components which have their own effects on the analysis (and make comparisons more difficult). To our knowledge there has been no previously published attempt to compare the two models using only the original components.

A further difference between the two models, of course, is the presence of the concept of normative beliefs in the TPB. For schoolboy cyclists, the perceived views of significant others and their motivation to comply with these views are the most powerful influence on behavioural intention. In the HBM normative beliefs are not measured explicitly, though they may be included in the 'cues to action' concept.

Adding Prior Behaviour to the Models

The final theoretical issue to consider is the role of prior behaviour in the two models. Prior behaviour is included in neither of the original statements of the models, though Fishbein and Ajzen (1975) do acknowledge that it may influence subsequent behaviour through effects on behavioural and normative beliefs. Bentler and Speckart (1979) argued, however, and demonstrated, that prior behaviour often influences subsequent behaviour directly, and we were able to show exactly the same in the present analyses. For the HBM, the addition of prior behaviour (wearing or not wearing a helmet at Time 1) alongside the six predictors of Time 2 behaviour increased the overall variance explained to 73%, but the original effect of perceived barriers dropped out, leaving perceived benefits as the only significant predictor apart from prior behaviour. In the TPB, the addition of paths from prior behaviour direct to Time 2 behaviour and indirectly through intention increased the variance explained in Time 2 behaviour to 73%. Two of the original paths were lost – perceived behavioural control to intention and Time 2 behaviour – but the effects of subjective norm remained intact. Most of the cyclists who were wearing helmets at Time 2 were also doing so at Time 1, which means that the behaviour for most of the respondents was what Sutton (1994) has called a routine. When we perform a routine we know from experience that we are likely to be able to continue doing so. For that reason our estimate of perceived behavioural control over the behaviour becomes redundant, and the variable drops out of the analysis.

Practical Implications

We now turn to the practical implications of our results. Both the TPB and the HBM can be used to identify variables that are important predictors of intention and behaviour, thus offering useful indicators as to how effective behaviour change interventions should be planned. For example, Van der Pligt and Eiser (1984) reported findings that showed that smoking and non-smoking adolescents evaluated the consequences of smoking very differently. The writers argued that in order to be effective in influencing behaviour, promotional campaigns need to focus on beliefs about consequences that are seen as important by the target group, and also to try to increase the importance of beliefs about consequences that are seen as less relevant. Evaluation of the univariate statistics in our study showed us that for certain behavioural beliefs there were significant differences between belief strengths but not outcome evaluations, indicating that while users are more likely to subscribe, for example, to the belief that wearing a cycle helmet while cycling to school will make them feel safe and make their parents worry less, they do not evaluate each consequence significantly more or less favourably than non-users. For other beliefs such as 'make me look silly' and 'make me physically uncomfortable' the reverse is true. Both users and non-users believe that wearing a helmet will lead to these consequences, but differ in their evaluation of the consequences: for non-users, looking silly and being physically uncomfortable are significantly more likely to be perceived negatively. For other beliefs such as 'make me take care' and 'protect my head if I had an accident' there are significant differences both for belief strength and outcome evaluation, showing that users and non-users not only differ in the strength of their beliefs about whether wearing a helmet will lead to each consequence, but also on the importance of the consequences. Information of this kind concerning the reasons for the different attitudes of users and non-users may be used to inform promotional campaigns by indicating the beliefs that are seen as important by the target group, which provides a focus for attempts to influence attitudes and change behaviour. They may also indicate which consequences are seen as less relevant so that attempts may be made to increase their importance to the target group.

We have carried out one such intervention study, with promising results (Quine, Rutter & Arnold, 1998a). The intervention was designed to increase the use of protective helmets among schoolboy cyclists. Principles described in the Elaboration Likelihood Model of Persuasion (Petty & Cacioppo, 1986) provided the framework. Beliefs known from our previous work (Quine, Rutter & Arnold, 1998b) to discriminate between helmet users and non-users were used to inform a series of persuasive messages intended to influence beliefs and behaviour. Ninety-seven young cyclists who did not wear a helmet were randomly assigned to experimental or control conditions, in which they were asked to read and respond to persuasive messages focusing on either the use of cycle helmets or other (neutral) behaviour. Results showed that the experimental subjects became significantly more positive than controls in behavioural, normative, and control beliefs and intentions. Five months later the differences remained. Moreover, there was a significant effect on behaviour: none of the 49 control children had taken up helmet wearing, whilst 12 (25%) of the 45 experimental children had.

Future Directions

How might future research in predicting health behaviours proceed? Fruitful directions may lie in attempting to increase the predictive power of the TPB – perhaps by the separation of personal and social norm to reflect the individual's internalised moral rules, as several researchers have suggested (Gorusch & Ortberg, 1983; Beck & Ajzen, 1991). At present the TPB takes no account of the individual's personal beliefs about what is right and wrong (although in Fishbein's original formulation of the TRA personal and social influences were distinguished (Fishbein, 1967)). One example might be anticipatory affective reactions to having behaved in a certain way, such as *anticipated regret*. Sissons-Joshi et al. (1994), in a study of cycle helmet wearing among teenagers, found that anticipated regret distinguished between wearers and non-wearers. Van der Pligt and Richard (1994) have shown that anticipated regret is an important predictor of behavioural expectations in the context of sexual and contraceptive behaviour, while Parker, Manstead and Stradling (1995) have shown that both anticipated regret and 'moral norm' substantially improve the prediction of intention to commit driving violations. An intervention to modify drivers' behavioural intentions on the road went on to demonstrate that anticipated regret and normative pressure were the most important variables to focus on (Parker, Stradling & Manstead, 1996).

A second group of affective responses to behaviour that are conceptually distinct from personal norm concern the effects that the individual expects to experience while performing the behaviour in question. Examples include the sense of personal freedom a cyclist might experience when not wearing a helmet or the 'thrill' of riding in a 'risky' way. Manstead and Parker (1995) have called these responses 'affective evaluations', and they too might help to shape intentions and behaviour and so improve the predictive power of the model.

NOTES

1. In a study by Tedesco, Keffer and Fleck-Kandath (1991), although subjective norms were a better predictor of intention to use dental floss than attitudes, the reverse was true of intention to brush. However, until flossing becomes as widely accepted as brushing, it is likely to be affected more by normative influences.

REFERENCES

Åberg L. (1994). Relations among variables influencing drivers' intentions to drive after drinking. In D. R. Rutter and L. Quine (Eds), *Social Psychology and Health: European Perspectives*. Aldershot: Avebury, 89–100.

Abraham C., Sheeran P., Spears R. & Abrams D. (1992). Health beliefs and promotion of HIV-preventive intentions among teenagers: A Scottish perspective. *Health Psychology, 11*, 363–370.

Agran P. F., Castillo D. N. & Winn D. G. (1990). Limitations of data compiled from police accident reports on pediatric pedestrian and bicycle motor vehicle events. *Accident Analysis and Prevention, 22*, 361–370.

Agran P. F. & Winn D. G. (1993). The bicycle: A developmental toy versus a vehicle. *Pediatrics, 91*, 752–755.

Ajzen I. (1985). From intentions to actions: A theory of planned behavior. In J. Kuhl and J. Beckman (Eds.), *Action Control: From Cognition to Behavior*. Heidelberg: Springer.

Ajzen I. (1988). *Attitudes, Personality and Behavior*. Milton Keynes: Open University Press.

Ajzen I. (1991). The Theory of Planned Behavior. *Organizational Behavior and Human Decision Processes, 50*, 179–211.

Ajzen I. & Driver B. L. (1991). Prediction of leisure participation from behavioral, normative and control beliefs: An application of the theory of planned behavior. *Leisure Sciences, 13*, 185–204.

94 *Lyn Quine, Derek R. Rutter and Laurence Arnold*

Ajzen I. & Fishbein M. (1980). *Understanding Attitudes and Predicting Social Behavior.* Englewood Cliffs, N.J.: Prentice-Hall.

Ajzen I. & Madden T. J. (1986). Prediction of goal-directed behaviour: Attitudes, intentions, and perceived behavioural control. *Journal of Experimental Social Psychology, 22,* 453–474.

Arnold L. & Quine L. (1994). Predicting helmet use among schoolboy cyclists: An application of the Health Belief Model. In D. R. Rutter and L. Quine (Eds), *Social Psychology and Health: European Perspectives.* Aldershot: Avebury, 101–130.

Beck L. & Ajzen I. (1991). Predicting dishonest actions using the Theory of Planned Behavior. *Journal of Research in Personality, 25,* 285–301.

Becker M. H. (1974). The Health Belief Model and sick role behavior. In M. H. Becker (Ed.) *The Health Belief Model and Personal Health Behavior.* Thorofare, NJ: Charles B. Slack, 82–92.

Becker M. H., Drachman R. H. & Kirscht J. P. (1972). Motivations as predictors of health behavior. *Health Services Reports, 87,* 852–62.

Becker M. H. & Maiman L. A. (1975). Socio-behavioral determinants of compliance with health and medical care recommendations. *Medical Care, 13,* 10–14.

Becker M. H., Haefner D. P., Kasl S. V., Kirscht J. P., Maiman L. A. & Rosenstock I. M. (1977). Selected psychosocial models and correlates of individual health-related behaviors. *Medical Care, 15* (supplement), 27–46.

Bentler P. M. & Speckart G. (1979). Models of attitude-behavior relations. *Psychological Review, 86,* 452–464.

Boyd B. & Wandersman A. (1991). Predicting undergraduate condom use with the Fishbein and Ajzen and the Triandis Attitude-Behaviour models: Implications for public health interventions. *Journal of Applied Social Psychology, 21,* 1810–1830.

Budd R. J. & Spencer C. P. (1984). Predicting undergraduates' intentions to drink. *Journal of Studies on Alcohol, 45,* 179–183.

Budd R. J. & Spencer C. P. (1986). Lay theories of behavioural intention: A source of response bias in the theory of reasoned action? *British Journal of Social Psychology, 25,* 109–117.

Budd R. J., North D. & Spencer C. (1984). Understanding seat belt use: A test of Bentler and Speckart's extension of the 'theory of reasoned action'. *European Journal of Social Psychology, 14,* 69–78.

Calnan M. (1984). The health belief model and participation in programmes for the early detection of breast cancer: A comparative analysis. *Social Science and Medicine, 19,* 823–830.

Champion V. L. (1984). Instrument development for Health Belief Model constructs. *Advances in Nursing Science, 6,* 73–85.

Champion V. L. (1988). Attitudinal variables related to intention, frequency and proficiency of breast self-examination in women 35 and over. *Research in Nursing and Health, 11,* 283–291.

Champion V. L. & Miller T. K. (1992). Variables related to breast self-examination: Model generation. *Psychology of Women Quarterly, 16,* 81–96.

Collins B. A., Langley J. D. & Marshall S. W. (1993). Injuries to pedal cyclists resulting in death and hospitalisation. *New Zealand Medical Journal, 106,* 514–516.

Conner M. & Norman P. (1994). Comparing the Health Belief Model and the Theory of Planned Behaviour in health screening. In D. R. Rutter and L. Quine (Eds.), *Social Psychology and Health: European Perspectives.* Aldershot: Avebury, 1–24.

Conner M. & Sparks P. (1996). The theory of planned behaviour and health behaviours. In M. Conner and P. Norman (Eds.), *Predicting Health Behaviour,* 121–162. Buckingham: Open University Press.

Cooke C. T., Margolius K. A. & Cadden G. A. (1993). Cycling fatalities in Western Australia. *Medical Journal of Australia, 159,* 783–785.

Courneya K. S. (1995). Understanding readiness for regular physical activity in older individuals: An application of the Theory of Planned Behavior. *Health Psychology, 14*, 80–87.

Cross K. D. & Fisher G. (1977). *Identification of Specific Problems and Counter-Measure Approaches to Enhance Bicycle Safety.* Santa Barbara, CA: Anacapa Sciences.

Cummings K. M., Jette A. M., Brock B. M. & Haefner D. P. (1979). Psychosocial determinants of immunisation behavior in a swine influenza campaign. *Medical Care, 17*, 639–649.

Cushman R., Down J., MacMillan N. & Waclawik H. (1990). Bicycle-related injuries: A survey in a paediatric emergency department. *Canadian Medical Association Journal, 143*, 108–112.

Department of Transport (1998). *Road Accidents Great Britain 1997.* London: HMSO.

DeVellis B. M., Blalock S. J. & Sander R. S. (1990). Predicting participation in cancer screening: The role of perceived behavioral control. *Journal of Applied Social Psychology, 20*, 639–660.

DiGuiseppi C. G., Rivara F. P. & Koepsall T. D. (1990). Attitudes toward bicycle helmet ownership and use by school-age children. *American Journal of Diseases of Children, 144*, 83–86.

Dorsch M., Woodward A. J. & Somers R. L. (1987). Do bicycle safety helmets reduce the severity of head injuries in real crashes? *Accident Analysis and Prevention, 20*, 447–58.

Fishbein M. (1967). Attitude and prediction of behavior. In M. Fishbein (Ed.), *Readings in Attitude Theory and Measurement*, 477–492. New York: Wiley.

Fishbein M. & Ajzen I. (1975). *Belief, Attitude, Intention and Behavior: An Introduction to Theory and Research.* Reading, MA: Addison-Wesley.

Foss R. D. (1985). Psychosocial factors in child safety restraint use. *Journal of Applied Social Psychology, 15*, 269–285.

Gielen A. C., Ericksen M. P., Daltoy L. H. & Rost K. (1984). Factors associated with the use of child restraint devices. *Health Education Quarterly, 11*, 195–206.

Gorusch R. L. & Ortberg J. (1983). Moral obligations and attitudes: Their relation to behavioural intentions. *Journal of Personality and Social Psychology, 44*, 1025–1028.

Haefner D. P. & Kirscht L. P. (1970). Motivational and behavioral effects of modifying health beliefs. *Public Health Reports, 85*, 478–484.

Harris S. (1990). The real number of road traffic accident casualties in the Netherlands: A year long survey. *Accident Analysis and Prevention, 22*, 371–378.

Harrison J. A., Mullen P. D. & Green L. W. (1992). A meta-analysis of studies of the Health Belief Model with adults. *Health Education Research, 7*, 107–116.

Harrison W., Thompson V. D. & Rogers J. L. (1985). Robustness and sufficiency of the Theory of Reasoned Action in longitudinal prediction. *Basic and Applied Social Psychology, 6*, 25–40.

Hays R. (1985). An integrated value-expectancy theory of alcohol and other drug use. *British Journal of Addiction, 80*, 379–384.

Hessing D. J., Elffers H. & Weigel R. H. (1988). Exploring the limits of self-reports and reasoned action: An investigation of the psychology of tax evasion behavior. *Journal of Personality and Social Psychology, 54*, 405–413.

Hill D., Gardner G. & Rassaby J. (1985). Factors predisposing women to take precautions against breast and cervix cancer. *Journal of Applied Social Psychology, 15*, 59–79.

Hoque M. M. (1990). An analysis of fatal bicycle accidents in Victoria (Australia) with a special reference to nighttime accidents. *Accident Analysis and Prevention, 22*, 1–11.

Jones D. (1989). Child casualties in road accidents. In Department of Transport, *Road Accidents Great Britain 1989: The Casualty Report*, 37–40. London: HMSO.

Kimiecik J. (1992). Predicting vigorous physical activity of corporate employees: Comparing the theories of reasoned action and planned behavior. *Journal of Sport and Exercise Psychology, 14*, 192–206.

King J. B. (1982). The impact of patients' perceptions of high blood pressure on attendance at screening: An extension of the health belief model. *Social Science and Medicine, 16*, 1079–1091.

Lacy W. B. (1981). The influence of attitudes and current friends on drug use intentions. *Journal of Social Psychology, 113*, 65–76.

Langley J., Silva P. A. & Williams S. M. (1987). Cycling experiences and knowledge of the road code of nine-year-olds. *Accident Analysis and Prevention, 19*, 141–145.

Lau R. R., Hartman K. A. & Ware J. E. (1986). Health as a value: Methodological and theoretical considerations. *Health Psychology, 5*, 25–43.

Liska A. E. (1984). A critical examination of the causal structure of the Fishbein/Ajzen attitude-behavior model. *Social Psychology Quarterly, 47*, 61–74.

Madden T. J., Ellen P. S. & Ajzen I. (1992). A comparison of the theory of planned behavior and the theory of reasoned action. *Personality and Social Psychology Bulletin, 18*, 3–9.

Maimaris C., Summers C. L., Browning C. & Palmer C. R. (1994). Injury patterns in cyclists attending an accidents and emergency department: A comparison of helmet wearers and non-wearers. *British Medical Journal, 308*, 1537–1540.

Manstead A. S. R. & Parker D. (1995). Evaluating and extending the theory of planned behaviour. In W. Stroebe and M. Hewstone (Eds.), *European Review of Social Psychology, 6*, 69–95. Chichester: Wiley.

McDermot F. T. & Klug G. L. (1982). Differences in head injuries of pedal cyclist and motor cyclist casualties in Victoria. *Medical Journal of Australia, 2*, 30–32.

Melnyk K. A. M. (1988). Barriers: A critical review of recent literature. *Nursing Research, 37*, 196–201.

Netemeyer R. G. & Burton S. (1990). Examining the relationship between voting behaviour, intention, perceived behavioural control, and expectation. *Journal of Applied Social Psychology, 20*, 661–680.

Netemeyer R. G., Burton S. & Johnston M. (1991). A comparison of two models for the prediction of volitional and goal-directed behaviors: A confirmatory analysis approach. *Social Psychology Quarterly, 54*, 87–100.

Norman P. & Fitter M. (1989). Intentions to attend a health screening appointment: Some implications for general practice. *Counselling Psychology Quarterly, 2*, 261–272.

Norman P. & Smith L. (1995). The theory of planned behaviour and exercise: An investigation into the role of prior behaviour, behavioural intentions and attitude variability. *European Journal of Social Psychology, 25*, 403–415.

Oliver R. L. & Berger P. K. (1979). A path-analysis of preventive health care decision models. *Journal of Consumer Research, 6*, 113–122.

Otis J., Lesage D., Godin G., Brown B., Farley C. & Lambert J. (1992). Predicting and reinforcing children's intentions to wear protective helmets while bicycling. *Public Health Reports Hyatsville, 107*, 283–287.

Parker D., Manstead A. S. R. & Stradling S. G. (1995). Extending the Theory of Planned Behaviour: The role of personal norm. *British Journal of Social Psychology, 34*, 127–137.

Parker D., Manstead A. S. R., Stradling S. G., Reason J. T. & Baxter J. (1992). Intention to commit driving violations: An application of the Theory of Planned Behavior. *Journal of Applied Psychology, 77*, 94–101.

Parker D., Stradling S. G. & Manstead A. S. R. (1996). Modifying beliefs and attitudes to exceeding the speed limit: an intervention study based on the Theory of Planned Behaviour. *Journal of Applied Social Psychology, 26*, 1–19.

Petty R. E. & Cacioppo J. T. (1986). The elaboration likelihood model of persuasion. In L. Berkowitz (Ed.), *Advances in Experimental Psychology, 19*, 123–205. London: Academic Press.

Pitt W. R., Thomas S., Nixon J., Clark R., Battistutta D. & Acton C. (1994). Trends in head injuries among child bicyclists. *British Medical Journal, 308*, 177–8.

Quine L., Rutter D. R. & Arnold L. (1998a). Use of the Elaboration Likelihood Model of Persuasion to promote helmet wearing in school age cyclists. British Psychology Society Division of Health Psychology Annual Conference, Bangor, July 1998.

Quine L., Rutter D. R. & Arnold L. (1998b). Predicting and understanding safety helmet use among schoolboy cyclists: A comparison of the Theory of Planned Behaviour and the Health Belief Model. *Psychology and Health, 13*, 251–269.

Reinecke J., Schmidt P. & Ajzen I. (1996). Application of the Theory of Planned Behaviour to adolescents' condom use: A panel study. *Journal of Applied Social Psychology, 26*, 749–772.

Rosenstock I. M. (1966). Why people use health services. *Millbank Memorial Fund Quarterly, 44* (supplement), 94–127.

Rosenstock I. M. (1974a). Historical origins of the Health Belief Model. In M. H. Becker (Ed.) *The Health Belief Model and Personal Health Behavior*. Thorofare, NJ: Charles B. Slack, 1–8.

Rosenstock I. M. (1974b). The Health Belief Model and preventive health behavior. *Health Education Monographs, 2*, 354–386.

Rutledge D. N. (1987). Factors related to women's practice of breast self-examination. *Nursing Research, 36*, 117–121.

Rutter D. R., Quine L. & Chesham D. J. (1995). Predicting safe riding behaviour and accidents: Demography, beliefs, and behaviour in motorcycling safety. *Psychology and Health, 10*, 369–386.

Sheeran P. & Abraham C. (1996). The health belief model. In M. Conner and P. Norman (Eds.), *Predicting Health Behaviour*, 23–61. Buckingham: Open University Press.

Sheppard B. H., Hartwick J. & Warshaw P. R. (1988). The Theory of Reasoned Action: A meta-analysis of past research with recommendations for modifications and future research. *Journal of Consumer Research, 15*, 325–339.

Simon P. M., Morse E. V., Balson P. M., Osofsky H. J. & Gaumer H. R. (1993). Barriers to human immunodeficiency virus related risk reduction among male street prostitutes. *Health Education Quarterly, 20*, 261–273.

Sissons-Joshi M., Beckett K. & MacFarlane A. (1994). Cycle helmet wearing in teenagers – do health beliefs influence behaviour? *Archives of Disease in Childhood, 71*, 536–539.

Stasson M. & Fishbein M. (1990). The relation between perceived risk and preventive action: A within-subject analysis of perceived driving risk and intentions to wear seatbelts. *Journal of Applied Social Psychology, 20*, 1541–1557.

Stutts J. C., Williamson J. E., Whitley T. & Sheldon F. C. (1990). Bicycle accidents and injuries: A pilot study comparing hospital- and police-reported data. *Accident Analysis and Prevention, 22*, 67–78.

Sutton S. (1994). The past predicts the future: Interpreting behaviour-behaviour relationships in social psychological models of health behaviours. In D. R. Rutter and L. Quine (Eds.), *Social Psychology and Health: European Perspectives*, 71–88. Aldershot: Avebury.

Sutton S. & Hallett R. (1989). Understanding seat-belt intentions and behavior: A decision-making approach. *Journal of Applied Social Psychology, 19*, 1310–1325.

Taylor S. (1989). Pedal cycle casualties. In Department of Transport, *Road Accidents Great Britain 1989: The Casualty Report*, 41–46. London: HMSO.

Tedesco L. A., Keffer M. A. & Fleck-Kandath C. (1991). Self-efficacy, reasoned action, and oral health behaviour reports: A social cognitive approach to compliance. *Journal of Behavioural Medicine, 14*, 341–355.

Thomas S., Acton C., Nixon J., Battistutta D., Pitt W. R. & Clark R. (1994). Effectiveness of bicycle helmets in preventing head injury in children: Case-control study. *British Medical Journal, 308,* 173–6.

Thuen F. & Rise J. (1994). Young adolescents' intention to use seatbelts: The role of attitudinal and normative beliefs. *Health Education Research, 9,* 215–223.

Towner E. M. L., Jarvis S. N., Walsh S. S. M. & Aynsley-Green A. (1994). Measuring exposure to injury risk in schoolchildren aged 11–14. *British Medical Journal, 308,* 449–452.

Vaile M. S. B., Calnan M., Rutter D. R. & Wall B. (1993). Breast cancer screening services in three areas: Uptake and satisfaction. *Journal of Public Health Medicine, 15,* 37–45.

Valois P., Desharnais R., Godin G., Perron J. & Lecomte C. (1993). Psychometric properties of a perceived behavioural control multiplicative scale developed according to Ajzen's Theory of Planned Behavior. *Psychological Reports, 72,* 1079–1083.

Van der Pligt J. (1994). Risk appraisal and health behaviour. In D. R. Rutter and L. Quine (Eds.), *Social Psychology and Health: European Perspectives.* Aldershot: Avebury, 131–151.

Van der Pligt J. & Eiser J. R. (1984). Dimensional salience, judgement and attitudes. In J. R. Eiser (Ed.), *Attitudinal Judgement.* New York: Springer Verlag.

Van der Pligt J. & Richard R. (1994). Changing adolescents' sexual behaviour: Perceived risk, self-efficacy and anticipated regret. *Patient Education and Counselling, 23,* 187–196.

Wallston K. A. & Wallston B. S. (1981). Health locus of control scales. In H. M. Lefcourt (Ed.), *Research with the Locus of Control Constant I: Assessment Methods.* New York: Academic Press.

Webb G. R., Sanson-Fisher R. W. & Bowman J. A. (1988). Psychosocial factors related to parental restraint of pre-school children in motor vehicles. *Accident Analysis and Prevention, 20,* 97–94.

Weinstein N. D. (1988). The precaution adoption approach. *Health Psychology, 7,* 355–386.

Weiss B. D. (1986). Bicycle helmet use by children. *Pediatrics, 77,* 677–679.

Witte K., Stokols D., Ituarte P. & Schneider M. (1993). Testing the Health Belief Model in a field study to promote bicycle safety helmets. *Communication Research, 20,* 564–586.

Wittenbraker J., Gibbs B. L. & Kahle L. R. (1983). Seat belt attitudes, habits, and behaviors: An adaptive amendment to the Fishbein model. *Journal of Applied Social Psychology, 13,* 406–421.

Wood T. & Milne P. (1988). Head injuries to pedal cyclists and the promotion of helmet use in Victoria, Australia. *Accident Analysis and Prevention, 20,* 177–85.

Wyper M. A. (1990). Breast self-examination and the Health Belief Model: Variations on a theme. *Research in Nursing and Health, 13,* 421–428.

Section 3 –
Extensions to Social Cognition Models

CHAPTER FIVE

Attitudinal and Normative Processes in Health Behaviour

David TRAFIMOW

Given that one of the major goals of psychologists is to understand, predict and change behaviour, it is not surprising that many theories have been proposed to do so. What is more surprising, however, is that most of these theories assume a distinction between attitude and subjective norm. An attitude is an evaluation of the behaviour under consideration and a subjective norm is a person's opinion about what his/her important others think he/she should do. This distinction was first assumed by Fishbein (Fishbein, 1967; Fishbein & Ajzen, 1975; Fishbein, 1980) as a component of what eventually became the 'theory of reasoned action.' According to this theory (e.g., Ajzen & Fishbein, 1980; Fishbein, 1980), behaviours are determined by intentions to behave which, in turn, are determined by attitudes and subjective norms. Attitudes are determined by beliefs about the consequences of performing the behaviour and subjective norms are determined by beliefs about the opinions of specific others. More recently, some researchers have added variables to the theory. For example, Triandis (1980) added affect and habit, Ajzen (1988) added perceived behavioural control, and Fazio (1990) added a spontaneous process to the more 'reasoned' one proposed by Fishbein (1980).[2] But suppose, as Miniard and Cohen (1981) and Liska (1984) have argued, that the attitude-subjective norm distinction is not a correct one. In that case, the various theories that assume the distinction (e.g., Ajzen, 1988; Fazio, 1990; Fishbein, 1980; Taylor & Todd, 1995; Triandis, 1980 and others) would be invalid. Further, the intervention programs that have been based on these theories would be similarly invalid. Consequently, one important task for researchers has been to definitively support or disconfirm the distinction. However, although the first criticisms against the distinction were levelled over 15 years ago, it was not until recently that they were dealt with in a satisfactory manner. And, congruent with the theme of this book, some of the crucial contributions were rooted in basic social cognition research. Thus, the goal of this chapter is to review the relevant research, with emphasis on important experiments derived from the social cognition tradition.

EVIDENCE AGAINST THE DISTINCTION

There are four kinds of arguments that have been used to criticise the attitude-subjective norm distinction. Firstly, there is a conceptual issue. Theoretically, the supposed determinants of attitudes and subjective norms are beliefs about the consequences of the behaviour (hereafter, behavioural beliefs) and beliefs about the opinions of particular important others (hereafter, normative beliefs), respectively (e.g., Fishbein, 1980). However, Miniard and Cohen (1981) argued that behavioural and normative beliefs are not really different. For example, the normative belief that 'My father thinks that I should not perform the behaviour' is not very different from the behavioural belief that 'Performing the behaviour will cause my father to disagree with me.' Thus, if behavioural and normative beliefs are not different from each other, then there is no justification for assuming that attitudes are distinguishable from subjective norms.

A second criticism is based on the fact that researchers who have studied attitudes and subjective norms have used correlational paradigms. Not only does correlation generally fail to prove causation, but, in addition, a large correlation has often been obtained between attitudes and subjective norms. This large correlation suggests that 'attitude' and 'subjective norm' are really different names for the same underlying construct (but see Fishbein & Ajzen, 1981).

A third criticism stems from findings of 'crossover' effects between attitudes and subjective norms (Grube, Morgan, & McGree, 1986; Oliver & Bearden, 1985; Shimp & Kavas, 1984; Vallerand, Deshaies, Cuerrier, Pelletier, & Mongeau, 1992). These crossover effects refer to the fact that arrows connecting attitudes and subjective norms to each other often result from 'causal modelling' approaches. Such data can be interpreted in a variety of ways. One interpretation is that attitudes and subjective norms affect each other (or that whatever affects attitudes affects subjective norms and/or vice versa). In contradiction to the attitude-subjective norm distinction, however, an alternative interpretation is that attitudes and subjective norms are really the same construct. Consequently, they are highly correlated with each other even when other variables are statistically taken into account.

Finally, Budd (1987) found that the strengths of the relationships between attitudes, subjective norms, and other variables they are supposed to predict, change depending on the order in which they are measured. Thus, previously obtained support for the distinction (to be presented shortly) might be eliminated simply by changing the order of the measures.

EVIDENCE IN FAVOUR OF THE DISTINCTION

Despite the previous arguments, there are several kinds of evidence in favour of the attitude-subjective norm distinction. One kind of evidence is based on patterns of correlations. For example, attitudes and subjective norms have often been found to correlate more highly with intentions than with each other (Bowman & Fishbein, 1978; Jaccard & Davidson, 1972). Attitudes and subjective norms have also sometimes been shown to predict intentions independently of each other (Shepherd, 1987). Further, attitudes are generally more highly correlated with behavioural beliefs than are subjective norms, and the reverse is true for normative beliefs (Fishbein, 1980; Fishbein & Ajzen,

1975; Trafimow & Miller, 1996). Finally, for some behaviours, intentions have been shown to be positively associated with attitudes, but negatively associated with subjective norms (Taylor & Todd, 1995).

A second kind of evidence concerns variations in the size of attitude-intention and subjective norm-intention correlations as a function of individual differences. For example, Miller & Grush (1986) found that people who were both high in private self-consciousness and low in self-monitoring displayed high attitude-behaviour correspondence, but people with other combinations of these traits displayed high subjective norm-behaviour correspondence. Arie, Durand, & Bearden (1979) performed a study using American employees at a large southeastern university as subjects. They found that opinion leaders' (those whose opinions others seek for advice about products and services) intentions to patronise credit unions were under attitudinal control, but non-leaders' intentions were under normative control. Finally, Bagozzi, Baumgartner, and Yi (1992) found a greater attitude-intention than subjective norm- intention correlation for action-oriented subjects, but the reverse was true for state-oriented subjects.

A third way to address this problem is to use a paradigm involving experimental manipulations of attitudes and subjective norms for different types of behaviours. Evidence for the distinction would be obtained if the importance of attitudinal and normative manipulations in affecting intentions changed depending on the behaviour. In other words, if some behaviours could be shown to be primarily under attitudinal control (AC behaviours) and some could be shown to be under normative control (NC behaviours), then the attitude-subjective norm distinction would receive strong support. This support would be especially strong if the AC and NC behaviours used were chosen on the basis of beta weights obtained from previously performed multiple regression paradigms. If such beta weights give a valid picture of the AC-NC distinction, then the attitude manipulation should have a greater effect on intentions to perform the AC (large attitude beta weight) behaviour than on intentions to perform the NC (large normative beta weight) behaviour. Further, analogous effects should result if subjective norms are manipulated.

It is interesting to note that although the problem of distinguishing between AC and NC behaviours has been with us for a long time (e.g., Miniard & Cohen, 1981), it was not until recently that the solution described above was explored. One possible reason is that it is difficult and/or time consuming to manipulate attitudes towards behaviours with which people are familiar (possibly because they already have well-formed attitudes towards such behaviours). In addition, such attitude change is likely to be small (even if statistically significant) and ephemeral. Fortunately, a social cognition perspective suggests some ways around this difficulty. For example, attitudes towards extremely *unfamiliar* behaviours can be easily manipulated. Further, the concept of an AC or NC behaviour can be *primed* (made cognitively accessible). The AC-NC distinction implies that if attitudes are manipulated in the presence of either an AC behaviour prime or NC behaviour prime, the manipulation should have a greater effect on intentions under the AC behaviour prime than under the NC behaviour prime.

A social cognition perspective implies an additional experiment. Even if it is difficult to change people's actual attitudes towards a familiar behaviour, it is easy to request them to *imagine* that they had a different attitude. According to the AC-NC distinction, if subjects are asked to imagine that they had a positive or negative attitude towards performing an AC or NC behaviour (seat belt use in a safe or risky situation, see Stasson & Fishbein, 1990), the manipulation should have a greater effect on intentions to perform the AC than the NC behaviour. In fact, Trafimow and Fishbein (1994a) performed all of these experiments and obtained findings that supported the validity of the distinction. Further, Trafimow and Fishbein (1994b) performed a set of analogous experiments where subjective norms towards AC or NC behaviours were manipulated, and they obtained analogous effects. In sum, the distinction between AC and NC behaviours has received strong support.

Finally, Trafimow and Fishbein (1995) performed a test based on research in the person memory and event memory areas indicating that when people consider items in relation to each other, associations tend to get formed between the items (Srull, 1981; Wyer & Srull, 1989; Trafimow & Wyer, 1993). More specifically, they argued that if behavioural beliefs are compared with each other in order to form an attitude, and normative beliefs are compared with each other to form a subjective norm, then behavioural beliefs should become associated with each other and normative beliefs should become associated with each other. However, because behavioural and normative beliefs tend not to be compared with each other, associations between the two types of beliefs should be unlikely to get formed. When people retrieve their beliefs, the order in which the beliefs are retrieved should be a function of the associations that had been previously formed. Therefore, during retrieval, people can traverse associative pathways from behavioural beliefs to other behavioural beliefs, and from normative beliefs to other normative beliefs, but not from behavioural to normative beliefs, nor from normative to behavioural beliefs. Consequently, behavioural beliefs should tend to be retrieved together and normative beliefs should likewise tend to be retrieved together. Thus, people's recall protocols should be cognitively clustered by belief type. In fact, Trafimow & Fishbein (1995) performed a set of three experiments that strongly supported this prediction. In addition, similar methodology has been recently employed to distinguish between evaluative and affective beliefs (Trafimow & Sheeran, 1998) and between positively and negatively valenced behavioural beliefs (Duran & Trafimow, in press).

Overall, then, the evidence seems to favour the distinction. Two of the findings against the distinction were (1) large attitude-subjective norm correlations and (2) crossover effects. Note that although each of these findings *suggests* that 'attitudes' and 'subjective norms' are different names for the same construct, they do not *prove* that this is the case. It is possible to argue (Fishbein and Ajzen, 1981) that attitudes and subjective norms are different constructs that are correlated with and/or affect each other.[3] This brings us to the criticism by Miniard and Cohen (1981) that the distinction is philosophically untenable. However, it does not matter if a philosopher of logic would agree or disagree with the distinction, only that people do or do not process information in the hypothesised manner; there is no imperial decree stating that people must be logical![4] Consequently, there is some justification for Fishbein and Ajzen's (1981) argument that if attitudes and subjective norms are differentially correlated with other variables, then such discriminant validity should be taken as support for the distinction. To be sure, Budd's (1987) demonstration that the pattern of correlations may depend on the order in which subjects complete the items mitigates the impact of the correlational evidence, but there seems to be no reasonable way of accounting for the experimental data (Trafimow & Fishbein, 1994a; 1994b) or the cognitive clustering of recall protocols (Trafimow & Fishbein, 1995) except by virtue of the attitude-subjective norm distinction. In addition, research exploring further implications of the distinction provides even more impressive support for its validity, as will be discussed presently.

FURTHER ISSUES AND IMPLICATIONS

The establishment of the distinction between attitudes and subjective norms has both practical and theoretical implications. One such implication concerns people's intentions to use condoms. Previous research (Fishbein, Middlestadt, & Trafimow, 1993; Fishbein, Trafimow et al., 1993; Fishbein et al., 1995) has shown that although both attitudes and subjective norms predict condom use, only subjective norms account for unique variance ($r = .58$, $r^2 = .34$). Note that although a correlation of .58 is certainly respectable, their data failed to account for 66% of the variance.

Based on social cognition research pertaining to the cognitive processes underlying how people make confidence judgements (e.g., Trafimow & Sniezek, 1994), Trafimow (1994) suggested that people might vary in their confidence that their perceptions of normative pressure are accurate. Given this assumption, Trafimow argued that people who are confident in their perceptions of normative pressure should be more likely to behave (or intend to behave) consistently with those perceptions than should people who are not confident. In one study, confidence in the accuracy of perceptions of normative pressure was varied experimentally, and, consistent with expectations, intentions to use a condom were more consistent with subjective norms when subjects were confident than when they were not. In a second study, Trafimow (1994) measured intentions to use a condom, subjective norms, attitudes, and confidence in the accuracy of perceptions of normative pressure to see if the relationships between subjective norms and intentions would vary depending on confidence. In fact, the results were striking in their support for the conceptualisation. When extremely confident subjects were analysed, subjective norms were highly correlated with intentions to use a condom ($r = .88$, $r^2 = .77$); but when subjects low in confidence were analysed, the correlation was essentially zero. Further, the prediction of intentions from attitudes was not moderated by confidence. Finally, these results were recently replicated (Trafimow, in press). It is worth pointing out that this prediction could not have been made had the distinction between attitudes and subjective norms not been previously established.

Social Identity Theory and Perceived Norms

The assumption of the distinction between attitudes and subjective norms can be fruitfully combined with other ideas. For example, Terry and Hogg (1996) used social identity theory (Hogg & Abrams, 1988; Tajfel & Turner, 1979) to make an interesting prediction about two health behaviours. According to social identity theory, two processes come into play when people evaluate themselves in terms of a group. These are categorisation (people accentuate similarities among in-group members and differences between in-group versus out-group members) and self-enhancement (the in-group is favoured over the out-group with a resultant gain for the person due to his or her group membership). Terry and Hogg pointed out that although subjective norms have generally been found to be relatively poor predictors of intentions relative to attitudes, conceptualising subjective norms in terms of group identity might increase the prediction of intentions. They performed two experiments to test their hypothesis. In Study 1, they found that perceived norms strongly influenced intentions to exercise, but only for subjects who identified strongly with their in-group. In Study 2, females' intentions to engage in sun-protective behaviour were highly affected by perceived norms, but only for those who highly identified themselves with their in-group. They also found that perceived norms affected attitudes more for high than for low identifiers. Their research suggests that much can be gained by considering the attitude-subjective norm distinction within the context of theories other than those in which the distinction is usually employed.

Normatively Controlled People, the Collective Self, and Intentions

In spite of the large subjective norm-intention correlation (.88) obtained by Trafimow (1994) for the behaviour of condom use, the vast majority of behaviors seem to be more under attitudinal than normative control (see Ajzen & Fishbein, 1980; Farley, Lehmann, & Ryan, 1981; Fishbein & Ajzen, 1975 for reviews). Nevertheless, subjective norm usually accounts for a small, but statistically significant, proportion of variance in intention above and beyond that which can be accounted for by attitude alone. Why should subjective norm account for a small, but significant, proportion of variance in intention across a wide variety of behaviours? There are at least two explanations. First, perhaps most behaviours are substantially under attitudinal control and slightly under normative control across a range of individuals. Second, perhaps most people are under attitudinal control but a minority of people are under normative control, and it is the normatively controlled minority that causes the effect.

How can one show that there are individual differences in the extent to which people are under normative control across a wide range of behaviours? Trafimow and Finlay (1996) argued that at least three criteria should be met for a convincing demonstration. First, it must be shown that attitudes and/or subjective norms are capable of predicting behavioural intentions across a range of behaviours using a within-subjects analysis. Otherwise it makes no sense to talk about whether people are attitudinally or normatively controlled. Second, there must be a subset of the subject sample for whom the within-subjects prediction of intentions is better from subjective norms than from attitudes. Finally, the relationship between subjective norms and intentions should be demonstrated to vary predictably with some other individual difference variable. In their study, Trafimow and Finlay used the strength of the collective self as this 'other' individual difference variable.

The Collective Self. According to Trafimow, Triandis, and Goto (1991), people have a separate private self (where thoughts about one's own states and traits are stored) and collective self (where thoughts about group membership are stored), but the relative accessibility of these selves depends, in part, upon whether the target person has an individualistic or collectivist cultural background. In support of this 'two-location' theory, Trafimow et al. found that the private self and the collective self of both American and Chinese people could be primed independently of each other. They further found that people are more likely to retrieve two cognitions in a row from the same self-structure than from different self-structures. Moreover, Trafimow, Silverman, Fan, and Law (1997) replicated these findings in an experiment performed in Hong Kong.

Singelis (1994) used a factor analytic paradigm to further test the theory. He constructed a set of 'independent' and 'interdependent' items and pointed out that the Trafimow et al. theory makes a prediction that is at odds with traditional Cross-Cultural literature. Traditionally, 'independence' and 'inter-dependence' have been thought of as opposite poles of the same dimension. Thus, both types of items should load on the same factor (of course, half of the items should get negative loadings). In contrast, if people really have a distinct private self and collective self in memory, then the items pertaining to each self should load on separate factors. In fact, Singelis's confirmatory factor analyses strongly demonstrated that a two factor solution provides a much better account of the data than a one factor solution. In addition, these factors were not correlated with each other (see Bontempo, 1993 for similar findings).

The support for the two location theory suggests the possibility that the strength of the collective self (which can be measured using the Singelis scale) should be related to the tendency for a person to be under normative control. People who have a strong collective self, for example, should be more likely than those who do not to behave in accordance with the opinions of those who are important to them (Triandis, 1994).

Fulfilling the Three Criteria. In order to meet the three criteria for demonstrating that there are individual differences in the extent to which people are under normative control, Trafimow and Finlay (1996) measured attitudes, subjective norms, and intentions across 30 behaviours. They also measured the strength of the collective self. When traditional multiple regression analyses (between-subjects) were run on the 30 behaviours, the results paralleled those obtained by previous researchers; attitudes were more related to intentions than were subjective norms for 29 of the 30 behaviours (median multiple correlation = .69, median attitude-intention correlation = .68, and median subjective norm-intention correlation = .40). Less traditional within-subjects analyses were also conducted across the 30 behaviours. Like the between-subjects analyses, the within-subjects analyses also indicated that attitudes were more related to intentions than were subjective norms (median within-subjects multiple correlation = .82, median within-subjects attitude-intention correlation = .77, and median within-subjects subjective norm-intention correlation = .64). These within-subjects analyses fulfilled the first criterion (i.e., obtaining good within-subjects prediction of intentions from attitudes and subjective norms). In addition, although most of the subjects seemed to be under attitudinal control across the 30 behaviours (79%), 21% of the subjects had a larger within-subjects subjective norm-intention correlation than attitude-intention correlation (and these subjects were deemed to be under normative control). More interestingly, however, when the normatively controlled subjects were removed from the sample, and the traditional between-subjects analyses were re-run, the median unique variance in intentions accounted for by subjective norms was .00, indicating that the previous effects of subjective norms on intentions were completely due to the normatively controlled subjects in the sample. Thus, the second criterion (obtaining better within-subjects prediction of intentions from subjective norms than from attitudes for a subset of the sample) was fulfilled, and the importance of normatively controlled subjects for traditional between-subjects analyses was demonstrated. Finally, in order to fulfill the third criterion (demonstrating a correlation with an outside variable), within-subjects normative beta weights were calculated as a measure of the extent to which subjects were under normative control (as opposed to attitudinal control). Consistent with expectations, subjects' degree of normative control was significantly correlated with the strength of the collective self. In sum, there is now considerable evidence that although most people are under attitudinal control across a range of behaviours, an important and substantial minority of people are under normative control. Thus, researchers must not only consider characteristics of the behaviour in their studies, but also characteristics of the subjects.

Several implications of this research may be of interest to health psychologists. For example, the findings imply that people with an accessible collective self are more likely than others to be under normative control. Ybarra and Trafimow (1998) obtained some evidence that bears on this point. They primed the private self or the collective self and measured attitudes, subjective norms, and intentions towards using a condom during sex. When the private self was primed, the attitude beta weight (for predicting intentions) was greater than the subjective norm beta weight. But when the collective self was primed, the reverse was true. Further, this pattern of findings was replicated in a second experiment where a much more subtle priming manipulation was employed. These findings suggest that the effectiveness of attitudinal or normative interventions may be significantly enhanced in the presence of the 'appropriate' prime.

The Trafimow and Finlay findings also suggest the possibility that there might be individual differences *within the domain of health behaviours* in the extent to which people are under attitudinal or normative control. In order to test this, Finlay, Trafimow, and Jones (1997) attempted a replication of the Trafimow and Finlay (1996) experiment, but using 32 behaviours specifically pertaining to health. Their findings indicate that a substantial percentage (15%) of people are under normative control across the domain of health behaviours, as well as across the domain of behaviours not specifically pertaining to health. The implications of this work for health psychology are only beginning to be explored.

PRACTICAL IMPLICATIONS

The distinction between attitudes and subjective norms, particularly in the area of condom use, has had implications for intervention. For example, Middlestadt, Fishbein, Albarracin, Francis, and Eustace (1995) implemented a radio campaign in three nations (St. Lucia, St. Vincent and the Grenadines, and Grenada) to decrease the spread of AIDS. Consistent with previously cited research, the central theme of the radio campaign was a normative one. Middlestadt et al. (1995) then compared respondents who were or were not exposed to the campaign and obtained a statistically significant impact for exposure, thereby indicating that a mass media campaign based on the distinction 'can be an effective tool in the battle to prevent the spread of AIDS (p. 21).' In addition, Kelly et al. (1991) and Kelly et al. (1992) have found normatively based programs to be surprisingly effective. Of course, it is possible that interventions based on other variables might have been just as good. But Boyer, Barrett, Peterman, & Bolan (1997) tested a cognitive/ behavioural skills-building intervention and obtained no effect on acquisition of sexually transmitted diseases compared to a control group. Thus, the fact that normatively based interventions have repeatedly been shown to be effective (Middlestadt et al., 1995; Kelly et al., 1991; Kelly et al., 1992) supports the practical utility of distinguishing subjective norms from attitudes. It is also worth noting that condom use is not the only domain where normative interventions are particularly effective. Bruvold (1993) conducted a meta-analysis of 94 adolescent smoking prevention programs. He found that behavioural effect sizes were largest for programs with a 'social reinforcement' (i.e., normative) orientation (p. 872). There are also numerous cases where interventions based on attitudes (or the beliefs underlying attitudes) have been shown to be effective (see Eagly & Chaiken, 1993; Chaiken, Wood, & Eagly, 1996 for reviews). But this tradition long predated the distinction between attitudes and subjective norms, so it will not be discussed further here.

The distinction between attitudinally and normatively controlled people suggests an additional point about interventions that, to my knowledge, has never been tested. I suggested earlier that interventions should focus on attitudes for AC behaviours and subjective norms for NC behaviours. An analogous point can be made about people: interventions should focus on attitudes for AC people, and they should focus on subjective norms for NC people. It follows that health researchers should perform preliminary studies to determine if the behaviours and/or persons of concern are of the AC or NC variety before designing intervention programs. There is little point in spending resources on attitudinal interventions for NC people and/or behaviours, or on normative interventions for AC people and/or behaviours.

CONCLUSION

I have attempted to show that (1) although there are reasons to question the attitude-subjective norm distinction, the available evidence strongly supports it; (2) much of the evidence, particularly that obtained in my own investigations

(Finlay, et al., 1997; Trafimow, 1994; in press; 2000; Trafimow & Finlay, 1996; Trafimow & Fishbein, 1994a; 1994b; 1995; Trafimow et al., 1991; Trafimow et al., 1997; Ybarra & Trafimow, 1998), was strongly influenced by a social cognition perspective; and (3) several recent advances in both basic social psychology and application to interventions could not have been made without the assumption that the distinction is valid. Thus, it not only accounts for a large amount of data, but it has heuristic value as well. However, there remain some theoretical issues to be settled. For example, do people distinguish between different kinds of behavioural beliefs when they form an attitude towards a behaviour? If so, what are these distinctions? Recent research suggests that the answer to the former question may be 'yes,' and that some candidates for these distinctions are affective-evaluative (Trafimow & Sheeran, 1998) and positive-negative (Duran & Trafimow, 1998). There are also issues regarding subjective norms. For example, the research by Terry and Hogg (1996) suggests that in-group norms, and the extent to which people are high or low identifiers, should be considered in future research. In addition, other research (Finlay et al., 1997; Trafimow & Finlay, 1996) suggests that individual differences in the degree to which people are under normative control, and the relative accessibility of the collective versus private self also need to be considered. Finally, because of the potential importance of culture in influencing the relative accessibility of the private and collective selves, and therefore the relative emphasis placed on attitudes and subjective norms in forming intentions, it seems likely that future investigations of attitudes and subjective norms will be studied within the context of Cross-Cultural research paradigms.

AUTHOR NOTE

I thank Sabine Trafimow, Annie Duran, Karen Kaufman, Paul Norman, and two anonymous reviewers for their valuable comments on a previous draft.

NOTES

1. I thank an anonymous reviewer for suggesting this title.
2. Actually, these are only a few of the additions people have suggested. Others include moral values (Gorsuch & Ortberg, 1983), previous behavior (Bentler & Speckart, 1981; Fredricks & Dossett, 1983), behavioral norms (Grube, Morgan, & McGree, 1986), confidence in the correctness of normative perceptions (Trafimow, 1994), and reasons theory (Westaby & Fishbein, 1996).
3. Theoretically, attitudes can affect subjective norms by influencing the normative beliefs upon which subjective norms are based, and subjective norms can affect attitudes by influencing the behavioural beliefs upon which attitudes are based.
4. Actually, Fishbein and Ajzen (1981) argued that it is logical for people to distinguish between behavioural and normative beliefs. My point is not that it is either logical or illogical, only that people do it

REFERENCES

Ajzen, I. (1988). *Attitudes, Personality, and Behavior.*, Chicago: The Dorsey Press.
Ajzen, I., & Fishbein, M. (1980). *Understanding Attitudes and Predicting Social Behavior.* Englewood Cliffs, NJ: Prentice Hall.

Arie, O. G., Durand, R. M., & Bearden, W. O. (1979). Attitudinal and normative dimensions of opinion leaders and nonleaders. *The Journal of Psychology, 101,* 305–312.

Bagozzi, R. P., Baumgartner, H., & Yi, Y. (1992). State versus action orientation and the theory of reasoned action: An application to coupon usage. *Journal of Consumer Research, 18,* 505–518.

Bentler, P. M., & Speckart, G. (1981). Attitudes 'cause' behavior: A structural equation analysis. *Journal of Personality and Social Psychology, 40,* 226–238.

Bontempo, R. (1993). Translation fidelity of psychological scales. *Journal of Cross-Cultural Psychology, 24,* 149–166.

Bowman, C. H., & Fishbein, M. (1978). Understanding public reactions to energy proposals: An application of the Fishbein Model. *Journal of Applied Social Psychology, 8,* 319–340.

Boyer, C. B., Barrett, D. C., Peterman, T. A., & Bolan, G. (1997). Sexually transmitted disease (STD) and HIV risk in heterosexual adults attending a public STD clinic: Evaluation of a randomized controlled behavioral risk-reduction intervention trial. *AIDS, 11,* 359–367.

Bruvold, W. H. (1993). A meta-analysis of adolescent smoking prevention programs. *American Journal of Public Health, 83,* 872–880.

Budd, R. J. (1987). Response bias and the action. *Social Cognition, 5,* 95–107.

Duran, A., & Trafimow, D. (1998). Cognitive organization of beliefs for and against performing a behavior. *The Journal of Social Psychology,* in press.

Eagly, A. H., & Chaiken, S. (1993). *The Psychology of Attitudes.* New York: Harcourt Brace Jovanovich College Publishers.

Farley, J. U., Lehmann, D. R., & Ryan, M. J. (1981). Generalizing from 'imperfect' replication. *Journal of Business, 54,* 597–610.

Fazio, R. H. (1990). Multiple processes by which attitudes guide behavior: The MODE model as an integrative framework. In M. P. Zanna (Ed.), *Advances in Experimental Psychology* (Vol. 23, pp. 75–109). San Diego: Academic Press.

Finlay, K., Trafimow, D., & Jones, D. (1997). Predicting health behaviors: Between-subjects and within-subjects analyses. *Journal of Applied Social Psychology, 27,* 2015–2031.

Fishbein, M. (1980). Theory of reasoned action: Some applications and implications. In H. Howe & M. Page (Eds.), *Nebraska Symposium on Motivation, 1979* (pp. 65–116). Lincoln, NE: University of Nebraska Press.

Fishbein, M., & Ajzen, I. (1975). *Belief, Attitude, Intention and Behavior: An Introduction to Theory and Research.* Reading, MA: Addison-Wesley.

Fishbein, M., & Ajzen, I. (1981). On construct validity: A critique of Miniard and Cohen's paper. *Journal of Experimental Social Psychology, 17,* 340–350.

Fishbein, M., Middlestadt, S. E., & Trafimow, D. (1993). Social norms for condom use: Implications for HIV prevention interventions of a KABP survey with heterosexuals in the eastern Caribbean. *Advances in Consumer Research, 20,* 292–296.

Fishbein, M., Trafimow, D., Francis, C., Helquist, M., Eustace, M. A., Ooms, M., & Middlestadt, S. E. (1993). AIDS knowledge, attitudes, beliefs, and practices (KABP) in two Caribbean countries: A comparative analysis. *Journal of Applied Psychology, 23,* 687–702.

Fishbein, M., Trafimow, D., Middlestadt, S. E., Helquist, M., Francis, C., & Eustace, M. A. (1995). Using an AIDS KABP Survey to identify determinants of condom use among sexually active adults from St. Vincent and The Grenadines, *Journal of Applied Social Psychology, 25,* 1–20.

Fredricks, A. J., & Dossett, D. L. (1983). Attitude-behavior relations: A comparison of the Fishbein-Ajzen and the Bentler-Speckart models. *Journal of Personality and Social Psychology, 45,* 501–512.

Gorsuch, R. L., & Ortberg, J. (1983). Moral obligation and attitudes: Their relation to behavioral intentions. *Journal of Personality and Social Psychology, 44,* 1025–1028.

Grube, J. W., Morgan, M., & McGree, S. T. (1986). Attitudes and normative beliefs as predictors of smoking intentions and behaviours: A test of three models. *British Journal of Social Psychology, 25,* 81–93.

Hogg, M. A., & Abrams, D. (1988). *Social Identifications: A Social Psychology of Intergroup Relations and Group Processes.* London: Routledge & Kegan Paul.

Jaccard, J. J., & Davidson, A. R. (1972). Toward an understanding of family planning behaviors: An initial investigation. *Journal of Applied Social Psychology, 2,* 228–35.

Kelly, J. A., Lawrence, J. S., Stevenson, L. Y., Hauth, A. C., Brasfield, T. L., Kalichman, S. C., Smith, J. E., & Andrew, M. E. (1991). HIV risk behavior reduction following intervention with key opinion leaders of population: An experimental analysis. *American Journal of Public Health, 81,* 168–171.

Kelly, J. A., Lawrence, J. S., Stevenson, L. Y., Hauth, A. C., Kalichman, S. C., Diaz, Y. E., Brasfield, T. L., Koob, J. J., & Morgan, M. G. (1992). Community AIDS/HIV risk reduction: The effects of endorsements by popular people in three cities. *American Journal of Public Health, 82,* 1483–1489.

Middlestadt, S. E., Fishbein, M., Albarracin, D., Francis, C., Eustace, M. A., Helquist, M., Schneider, A. (1995). Evaluating the impact of a national AIDS prevention radio campaign in St. Vincent and the Grenadines. *Journal of Applied Social Psychology, 25,* 21–34.

Miller, L. E., & Grush, J. E. (1986). Individual differences in attitudinal versus normative determination of behavior. *Journal of Experimental Social Psychology, 22,* 190–202.

Miniard, P. W., & Cohen, J. B. (1981). An examination of the Fishbein behavioral intentions model's concept and measures. *Journal of Experimental Social Psychology, 17,* 309–329.

Oliver, R. L., & Bearden, W. O. (1985). Crossover effects in the theory of reasoned action: A moderating influence attempt. *Journal of Consumer Research, 12,* 324–340.

Shepherd, G. J. (1987). Individual differences in the relationship between attitudinal and normative determinants of behavioral intent. *Communication Monographs, 54,* 221–230.

Shimp, T. A., & Kavas, A. (1984). The theory of reasoned action applied to coupon usage. *Journal of Consumer Research, 11,* 795–809.

Singelis, T. M. (1994). The measurement of independent and interdependent self-construals. *Personality and Social Psychology Bulletin, 20,* 580–591.

Srull, T. K. (1981). Person memory: Some tests of associative storage and retrieval models. *Journal of Experimental Psychology: Human Learning and Memory, 7,* 440–463.

Stasson, M., & Fishbein, M. (1990). The relation between perceived risk and preventive action: Within-subjects analysis of perceived driving risk and intentions to wear seat belts. *Journal of Applied Social Psychology, 20,* 1541–1557.

Tajfel, H., & Turner, J. C. (1979). An integrative theory of intergroup conflict. In W. G. Austin & S. Worchel (Eds.), *The social psychology of intergroup relations* (pp. 33–147). Pacific Grove, CA: Brooks/Cole.

Taylor, S., & Todd, P. (1995). An integrated model of waste management behavior: A test of household recycling and composting intentions. *Environment and Behavior, 27,* 603–630.

Terry, D. J., & Hogg, M. A. (1996). Group norms and the attitude-behavior relationship: A role for group identification. *Personality and Social Psychology Bulletin, 22,* 776–793.

Trafimow, D. (1994). Predicting intentions to use a condom from perceptions of normative pressure and confidence in those perceptions. *Journal of Applied Social Psychology, 24,* 2151–2163.

Trafimow, D. (in press). Predicting condom use: The importance of confidence in normative and attitudinal perceptions. The Journal of Social Psychology.

Trafimow, D. (2000). A theory of attitudes, subjective norms, and private versus collective self-concepts. In D. J. Terry and M. A. Hogg (Eds.) *Attitudes, Behavior, and Social Context: The Role of Norms and Group Membership*, (pp. 47–65). Hillsdale, NJ:Lawrence Erlbaum Associates, Inc., Publishers.

Trafimow, D., & Finlay, K. (1996). The importance of subjective norms for a minority of people. *Personality and Social Psychology Bulletin, 22*, 820–828.

Trafimow, D., & Fishbein, M. (1994a). The importance of risk in determining the extent to which attitudes affect intentions to wear seat belts. *Journal of Applied Social Psychology, 24*, 1–11.

Trafimow, D., & Fishbein, M. (1994b). The moderating effect of behavior type on the subjective norm-behavior relationship. *Journal of Social Psychology, 134*, 755–763.

Trafimow, D., & Fishbein, M. (1995). Do people really distinguish between behavioral and normative beliefs? *British Journal of Social Psychology, 34*, 257–266.

Trafimow, D., & Miller, A. (1996). Predicting and understanding mental practice. *The Journal of Social Psychology, 136*, 173–180.

Trafimow, D., & Sheeran, P. (1998). Some tests of the distinction between cognitive and affective beliefs. *Journal of Experimental Social Psychology, 34*, 378–397.

Trafimow, D., Silverman, E. S., Fan, R. M., & Law, J. S. F. (1997). The effects of language and priming on the relative accessibility of the private self and the collective self. *Journal of Cross-Cultural Psychology, 28*, 107–123.

Trafimow, D., & Sniezek, J. A. (1994). Perceived expertise and its effect on confidence. *Organizational Behavior and Human Decision Processes, 57*, 290–302.

Trafimow, D., Triandis, H. C., & Goto, S. G. (1991). Some tests of the distinction between the private self and the collective self. *Journal of Personality and Social Psychology, 60*, 649–655.

Trafimow, D., & Wyer, R. S. (1993). Cognitive representation of mundane social events. *Journal of Personality and Social Psychology, 64*, 365–376.

Triandis, H. C. (1980). Values, attitudes, and interpersonal behavior. In H. E. Howe & M. M. Page (Eds.), *Nebraska Symposium on Motivation 1979* (pp. 195–259). Lincoln, Nebraska: University of Nebraska Press.

Triandis, H. C. (1994). *Culture and Social Behavior*, New York: McGraw-Hill, Inc.

Wyer, R. S., & Srull, T. K. (1989). *Memory and Cognition in its Social Context*. Hillsdale, NJ: Lawrence Erlbaum Associates, Publishers.

Ybarra, O., & Trafimow, D. (1998). How priming the private self or the collective self affects the relative weights of attitudes and subjective norms. *Personality and Social Psychology Bulletin, 24*, 362–370.

CHAPTER SIX

Behavioural and Normative Beliefs About Condom Use: Comparing Measurement Alternatives Within the Theory of Reasoned Action

Christopher R. Agnew

INTRODUCTION

Cognitive approaches to understanding health behaviour tend to focus on the specific beliefs held by a person. For example, the Health Belief Model (cf. Rosenstock, 1990; Janz & Becker, 1984), Protection Motivation Theory (cf. Rippetoe & Rogers, 1987; Prentice-Dunn & Rogers, 1986), and the Transtheoretical Model of Change (cf. Prochaska, DiClemente, & Norcross, 1992) all hold that the beliefs held by a person are critical in determining whether or not that individual will enact specific health behaviours. While each of these cognitive models places different degrees of emphasis on specific types of beliefs (e.g., perceived threat or self-efficacy), beliefs are central to all of these theoretical approaches.

The most general and most utilised social psychological model for understanding the enactment of health behaviour is similarly belief-based, Fishbein and Ajzen's (1975; Ajzen & Fishbein, 1980) theory of reasoned action (TRA). The theory is concerned with the immediate antecedents of behaviour and places beliefs within a more comprehensive theoretical framework. According to the theory, behavioural intention is seen as the most proximal determinant of an individual's behaviour. That is, given volitional control, a person is said to be very likely to enact a behaviour that he or she has a strong intention to enact and very unlikely to enact a behaviour that he or she has a weak intention to enact. Behavioural intention is held to be determined by two independent constructs, one personal in nature (an individual's attitude toward the behaviour) and the other social in nature (the subjective norm regarding the behaviour). These two constructs, in turn, are determined by the salient behavioural and normative beliefs held by the individual. According to Fishbein and Ajzen, the relative weights of the two independent constructs in predicting behavioural intention are determined empirically and depend on the specific behaviour under investigation.

Over the years TRA has been shown to predict a broad range of health behaviours, including donating blood (Zuckerman & Reis, 1978), having an additional child (Vinokur-Kaplan, 1978), obtaining a swine flu shot (Oliver & Berger, 1979), smoking marijuana (Pomazal & Brown, 1977), and using various contraceptive methods (e.g., Jaccard & Davidson, 1972). In addition to the results of literally hundreds of individual empirical tests, two recent meta-analyses provide strong and converging empirical evidence in support of the theory. Sheppard, Hardwick, and Warshaw (1988), in a review of 87 tests of the intention-behaviour relation, found a frequency-weighted average correlation of .53. The overall intention-attitude toward behaviour/subjective norm link was also found to be robust, with a frequency-weighted average correlation of .66. Similarly, Van den Putte's meta-analytic review (1993) found the correlation between behavioural intention and behaviour to be .62 and the relationship between intention and attitude/subjective norm to be .68.

Belief Underpinnings of the Theory of Reasoned Action

According to TRA, attitude toward behaviour is a function of two elements: (1) the perceived consequences of performing a behaviour, and (2) the evaluation of those consequences. Algebraically, attitude toward behaviour (A_B) is represented as

$$A_B = \sum_{I=1}^{n} b_i e_i$$

where b_i is the belief that enacting the behaviour is likely to lead to consequence i, e_i is the person's evaluation of consequence i, and n is the total number of behavioural beliefs held by the individual. The $b \times e$ products are calculated and then summed to form the overall attitude toward the behaviour. The A_B construct can be traced back to work in the expectancy-value tradition of attitudes (Peak, 1955; Rosenberg, 1956; Fishbein, 1963; for a comprehensive review, see Feather, 1982).

Like A_B, subjective norm is also theorised to be a function of two elements: (1) the perceived expectations concerning the behaviour held by others who are important to the individual, and (2) the general motivation to comply with these important others. Algebraically, subjective norm (SN) is represented as

$$SN = \sum_{j=1}^{n} b_j m_j$$

where b_j is the belief that enacting the behaviour would be approved by specific important referent j, m_j is the general motivation to comply with that referent, and n is the total number of important referents. The $b \times m$ products are computed for each important referent and summed to form the overall subjective norm.

Operationally, Fishbein and Ajzen have advocated measuring the A_B construct in two ways. Consistent with its theoretical components, they have used behavioural belief-based ratings. For example, subjects are asked about the likelihood of specific consequences resulting from performing a behaviour and then whether they consider each consequence to be positive or negative. Fishbein and Ajzen have also endorsed a more 'global' technique that uses semantic differential attitudinal measures. The global measure is viewed as equivalent to the belief-based attitude measure and the two kinds of measures have been found to be highly correlated (cf. Ajzen & Fishbein, 1980), with the measurement of specific beliefs allowing for increased insight into the underlying roots of the behaviour under investigation. In practice over the years, however, the belief-based measures are often not collected or are disregarded once a significant correlation with the global A_B measure has been established.

Operationally, Fishbein and Ajzen also measure the SN construct in two ways. Consistent with its theoretical origins, they have used normative belief-based ratings. For example, subjects are asked whether specific important others favour the subject performing a behaviour and then the degree to which the subject generally follows each referent's advice. Fishbein and Azjen have also utilised a 'global' normative rating which uses a single item to assess overall normative support for behavioural enactment (i.e., 'Most people who are important to me think that I should perform behaviour x.'). This single item is then multiplied by a general motivation to comply measure (i.e., 'Generally speaking, how much do you want to do what important others think you should do?'). The global norm measurement approach is viewed as equivalent to the belief-based norm measure. As with the measurement of A_B, the normative belief-based measures, if collected, are often dropped once a significant correlation with the global SN measure has been established.

Examining Measurement Criticisms of the Theory of Reasoned Action

Over the years, TRA has been criticised and questioned on a number of grounds (cf. Bentler & Speckart, 1979; Budd, North, & Spencer, 1984; Liska, 1984; Warshaw & Davis, 1984). The most common criticisms revolve around the measurement of the theory's various elements.

Assessing Modal versus One's Own Behavioral and Normative Beliefs

Although TRA is an individual-level model that attempts to explain the determinants of an individual's behaviour, it often relies on the operational use of *modal* beliefs in the measurement of attitude toward behaviour and subjective norm. In tests of TRA, a preliminary sample from the population of interest (tested prior to and separate from the principal study sample) is asked to list the advantages and disadvantages of engaging in a specific behaviour, and also to provide the names of any individuals or groups who are perceived as influential regarding the behaviour. From the list of behavioural beliefs, the most frequently occurring responses are then incorporated into closed-ended questions that tap the expectancy-value formulation underlying Fishbein and Ajzen's A_B concept. Similarly, the most frequently mentioned individuals and groups are used to create closed-ended questions assessing normative influence for inclusion in the main study.

There is some controversy regarding the idea of using modal beliefs rather than each subject's own beliefs to measure the model's constructs (cf. Towriss, 1984; O'Keefe, 1990). In an early paper on the measurement of attitude toward objects, Kaplan and Fishbein (1969) presented empirical support for the equivalence of predictive validity when modal or an individual's own beliefs were used to estimate attitude. Although not explicitly stated in either of their books (Fishbein & Ajzen, 1975; Ajzen & Fishbein, 1980), Fishbein and Ajzen appear to accept and follow the logic that what has been found true for attitude toward objects should hold true for attitude toward behaviour and subjective norm. Therefore, the use of modal beliefs appears to have been offered as a practical and valid method for assessing the underlying roots of the theory.

There are clearly advantages to the modal measurement approach. By providing all subjects with a standard set of modal beliefs to evaluate, uniformity of measure content is assured. Although subjects are not necessarily responding to items that are personally salient, the modal approach avoids administrative difficulties associated with the collection and use of personally-held beliefs. As Ajzen and Fishbein maintain, the use of own belief measures 'usually produces sets of beliefs that differ from respondent to respondent in terms of content and number. This makes it difficult to compare the beliefs of different individuals and to submit their responses to quantitative analyses' (1980, p. 68). However, while analyses are made more difficult, they are far from impossible. Some investigators (e.g., Crawford & Boyer, 1985) have used individually-derived belief measures in their tests of the reasoned action model. Others (e.g., Jaccard & Wood, 1985; Conner, 1993) discuss the merits of adopting an idiographic analysis of the attitude-behaviour relation.

In a theoretical critique of Fishbein and Ajzen's measurement approach, Towriss (1984) argued that the use of modal beliefs represents a compromise between research expediency and accuracy. Specifically, the use of modal salient beliefs assumes homogeneity of beliefs within a given population, an assumption that may or may not be true. Rutter and Bunce (1989) empirically examined Towriss's position in their study of the predictors of milk consumption. These researchers tested the use of modal behavioural beliefs (which they called the 'Fishbein and Azjen condition') versus the use of subject-generated behavioural beliefs (called the 'Towriss' condition) in the prediction of intentions and present behaviour. Using a between-subjects design, they found that subject-generated behavioural beliefs were a stronger predictor of intention and present behaviour than were modal behavioural beliefs. It is important to note, however, that these researchers did not assess subjects' own *normative* beliefs and their relative predictive power versus ratings of modal normative referents. Moreover, these researchers relied on a between-subject experimental design that did not allow for a direct within-subject comparison of the predictive ability of modal versus individually-derived beliefs.

How Many and Which Beliefs are 'Salient'?

Fishbein and Ajzen (1975, Ajzen & Fishbein, 1980) also hold that it is a person's *salient* beliefs which contribute to his or her attitude and subjective norm. The exact number and relative importance of these salient beliefs are matters of considerable theoretical speculation. Consistent with early findings from cognitive psychology (e.g., Miller, 1956; Mandler, 1967), Ajzen and Fishbein state that 'although a person may hold a large number of beliefs about any given object, it appears that he can attend to only a relatively small number of beliefs – perhaps five to nine – at any give moment' (1980, p. 63). Consistent with this position, Budd (1986) found that the sum of the five modal behavioural beliefs which were rated as most important by subjects was more predictive of a semantic differential measure of that person's attitude toward cigarette smoking than was the sum that included all rated behavioural beliefs. However, Budd provided the subjects with a list of modal behavioural beliefs (derived from a pilot sample) and had them choose five that they saw as 'most important' rather than eliciting subjects' *own* beliefs and their perceived importance or order of generation. It is, therefore, unclear as to whether or not a subset of a subject's own beliefs also provide a stronger prediction to general attitude and/or behavioural intention. Furthermore, like Rutter and Bunce (1989), no assessment of subjects' own normative beliefs was included.

It seems reasonable to propose that, regardless of how many beliefs are considered 'salient,' some beliefs will be more *important* in determining one's attitude toward a behaviour than will others. However, Ajzen and Fishbein argue that it is not necessary to include a separate assessment of belief importance because such a measure would serve as a redundant measure of the evaluation of each individual outcome (the 'e' in the $b_i e_i$ attitude equation). That is, they hold that 'importance' is effectively being tapped by using only 'salient' beliefs and that the relative extremity of a subject's rating of 'e' for each belief would render a separate measure of belief importance repetitive. In contrast, Eiser and van der Pligt (1988; van der Plight & Eiser, 1984) favour an approach which incorporates a separate measure of belief salience into expectancy-value models of attitude. Similarly, and consistent with work by Fazio (e.g., Fazio & Williams, 1986), it also seems reasonable to posit that those beliefs that are more accessible in memory (i.e., beliefs that a subject generates first or relatively early in a listing) may be more predictive of general attitude and overall subjective norm than are all generated beliefs.

The Present Study

The current chapter reports the findings from an empirical comparison of various methods for assessing the behavioural and normative beliefs that underlie the theory of reasoned action. The present study was designed in part to test whether one's own behavioural and normative beliefs or a rated set of modal behavioural and normative beliefs are better predictors of attitude toward behaviour, subjective norm, and behavioural intentions. Moreover, the present study was designed to gather measures of the perceived importance, order (accessibility), and cumulative serial sums of subject-generated behavioural and normative beliefs in order to test each of these measures separately as predictors of the more global theory constructs as well as behavioural intention.

Beliefs that support or undermine condom use by young, sexually-active adults were investigated. Condom use was selected for examination because of its importance from both a theoretical and an applied perspective. From a theoretical perspective, understanding the determinants of sexual and contraceptive behaviours is of tremendous value. Sexual and contraceptive behaviours combine a number of individual and interpersonal processes of longstanding social psychological interest, including self-regulation, communication, decision-making, negotiation, and power dynamics (cf. Agnew, 1999; Agnew & Loving, 1998; Pryor & Reeder, 1993; Terry, Gallois, & McCamish, 1993). Moreover, because condom use occurs in the context of sexual activity, the degree to which this behaviour can be considered to be under the conscious control of the actor, particularly a young person, has come into question (e.g., Loewenstein & Furstenberg, 1991). Given the behavioural context, it is entirely plausible that very few, if any, beliefs reliably predict general attitude toward the behaviour, subjective norms regarding condom use, or intention to use a condom. Thus, a detailed examination of condom use beliefs will help to elucidate their role in guiding the enactment of this important health behaviour.

Beyond the theoretical advantages, the application of social psychological knowledge to pregnancy and disease prevention efforts is extremely important, especially in light of the rising numbers of unwanted pregnancies and cases of sexually-transmitted disease, including AIDS, throughout the world (cf. Poppen & Reisen, 1994; Aral & Holmes, 1991). While contraceptive practices continue to receive attention from population and public health researchers (e.g., Miller & Pasta, 1995), such behaviours receive relatively scant attention from social psychological researchers (with some notable exceptions, e.g., Davidson & Morrison, 1983; Fisher & Fisher, 1992; Jemmott & Jones, 1993). This is an unfortunate oversight. Many of today's most pressing social problems (overpopulation, unwanted children, sexual abuse, AIDS) are, at least in part, behaviourally-based. Understanding the determinants of condom use may yield knowledge that will help alleviate a number of current social problems (cf. Pryor & Reeder, 1993). In a recent statement concerning uses of TRA, Fishbein (1993, p. xxi) acknowledges the appropriateness of using his theory to understand AIDS-relevant behaviours: 'I can think of no better use of the theory of reasoned action than for it to be employed in the battle against AIDS.' Therefore, for both theoretical and applied reasons, condom use was chosen as the behaviour to be examined.

METHOD

Pilot Study

Belief-based Measures

Fishbein and Ajzen provide detailed instructions on TRA construct measurement in the appendix to their 1980 book. In constructing all of the measures for the current study, these instructions were followed as closely as possible. Consistent with Fishbein and Ajzen's measurement approach, all study measures were matched in terms of their specification of the behaviour (i.e., using a condom during sexual intercourse over the next month).

Eliciting Modal Behavioural and Normative Beliefs About Condom Use

To construct a list of modal salient behavioural beliefs, the following three questions (suggested by Ajzen & Fishbein, 1980) were asked of a pilot sample of subjects from the same population as the main study ($N = 90$ North American university students, 51 females and 39 males): (1) 'What do you see as the advantages of using a condom during sexual intercourse over the next month?'; (2) 'What do you see as the disadvantages of using a condom during sexual intercourse over the next month?'; (3) 'List anything else you associate with using a condom during sexual intercourse over the next month.' [1]

To construct the list of modal salient referents (i.e., normative beliefs), the following three questions (also suggested by Ajzen & Fishbein, 1980) were asked of the pilot sample: (1) 'List any people or groups who would approve of your using a condom during sexual intercourse over the next month'; (2) 'List any people or groups who would disapprove of your using a condom during sexual intercourse over the next month'; (3) 'List any other people or groups who come to mind when you think about using a condom during sexual intercourse over the next month.'

Ajzen and Fishbein note that there is no definitive method for determining which elicited beliefs should be considered 'modal.' They offer several suggestions, including using 'those beliefs that exceed a certain frequency' (1980, p. 70). In this study, a belief was considered to be modal if it was mentioned by a minimum of 20% of the overall pilot sample.[2] Table 6.1 provides the modal salient behavioural and normative beliefs concerning condom use.

Main Study

Subjects

Ninety-seven North American university students (48 females and 49 males) involved in romantic relationships participated in this study in order to fulfil an introductory psychology course research experience requirement. Seventy-four subjects (78%) were in exclusive relationships (with neither partner dating other people), 15 subjects were in bilaterally casual relationships (with both partners dating other people), 5 subjects were in unilaterally casual relation-ships (with one partner dating other people), and 1 subject was engaged to be married. Median relationship duration was 10 months. The mean age of subjects was 19.4 ($SD = 1.5$). The ethnicity of the sample approximated that of the university: 87% White, 7% Black, 5% Asian, and 1% Hispanic. Eighty-three of these subjects (86%) had engaged in sexual intercourse at least once prior to the study, although not necessarily with their current relationship partner. Only those subjects who had engaged previously in sexual intercourse ($N = 83$) were included in the analyses, since condom use requires exposure to intercourse.

Table 6.1 Modal salient behavioural and normative beliefs about using a condom

Behavioural Beliefs about Using a Condom

> Creates emotional detachment from my partner (F)
> Reduces spontaneity and ruins the moment
> Does not provide 100% protection
> Makes me feel responsible (M)
> Reduces my pleasure
> Prevents disease acquisition
> Expensive (M)
> Prevents pregnancy

Normative Beliefs (i.e., Referents) about Using a Condom

> My partner
> My church, religious groups, priests, ministers
> My parents
> My friends
> My siblings (my brothers and/or sisters)
> Doctors and other medical professionals
> Myself

Note. (F) indicates that the belief was noted by 20% or more of females, but not males; (M) indicates that the belief was noted by 20% or more of males, but not females. In either case, however, 20% or more of the *overall* sample noted the belief.

Rating Modal Behavioural and Normative Beliefs About Condom Use

Subjects were asked to rate the valence and likelihood of each of the eight modal behavioural beliefs, derived from the pilot sample, shown in Table 6.1. The valence of each belief was rated on a 7-point scale (1 = 'Extremely Bad' to 7 = 'Extremely Good'). The likelihood of each belief was also rated on a 7-point scale (1 = 'Extremely Unlikely' to 7 = 'Extremely Likely'). After recoding (described below), the valence and likelihood ratings for each belief were multiplied together and the sum of these products served as the measure of 'Total Modal Behavioural Beliefs' ($\Sigma b_i e_i$).

Subjects also rated each of the seven modal normative referents shown in Table 6.1 on a 7-point scale (anchored by 1 = 'Think(s) I Definitely Should Not' and 7 = 'Think(s) I Definitely Should'). In addition, general motivation to comply with each specific referent was assessed using a 7-point scale (1 = 'Definitely Do Not Do What They Want' and 7 = 'Definitely Do What They Want'). After recoding (see below), these two measures for each normative referent were multiplied together and the sum of these products served as the measure of 'Total Modal Normative Beliefs' ($\Sigma b_j m_j$).

Eliciting and Rating Individually-derived Behavioural and Normative Beliefs About Condom Use

Each subject provided his or her own behavioural beliefs regarding condom use. Instructions provided for this task were as follows:

> 'Everyone has their own beliefs about engaging in certain behaviours. We'd like you to tell us your beliefs concerning using a condom during sexual

intercourse over the next month. What do you believe are the advantages and disadvantages of using a condom during sexual intercourse over the next month? Using the numbered spaces below, please list up to 9 beliefs you have concerning using a condom during sexual intercourse over the next month.'

Subjects were provided with nine two-line spaces to list their own beliefs.[3] After writing down their beliefs, subjects then were instructed to rate each one on a 7-point evaluative scale (anchored by 1 = 'Extremely Bad' and 7 = 'Extremely Good'). Subjects recorded this evaluative rating for each belief in a box located to the left of each of the two-line spaces provided for belief listings. Next, subjects were instructed to rate each thought on a 7-point likelihood scale (anchored by 1 = 'Extremely Unlikely' and 7 = 'Extremely Likely'). Subjects recorded this likelihood rating for each belief in a box located to the right of each of the spaces provided for belief listings. After recoding (described below), the valence and likelihood ratings for each belief were multiplied together and the sum of these products served as the measure of 'Total Own Behavioural Beliefs' ($\Sigma b_i e_i$). Finally, to assess the role of perceived belief importance, subjects were instructed to 'circle the number(s) of the belief(s) that you feel are the most important in determining whether you would use a condom during sexual intercourse over the next month.' The valence and likelihood ratings for these beliefs were separately multiplied together and the sum of these products served as the measure of the 'Most Important Own Behavioural Belief(s)'.

Subjects also listed up to nine of their own normative referents regarding condom use. After writing down their normative referents, subjects were instructed to rate each one on a 7-point scale (anchored by 1 = 'Thinks I Definitely Should Not' and 7 = 'Thinks I Definitely Should'). Subjects recorded this referent approval rating for each referent in a box located to the left of each of the spaces provided for referent listings. Next, subjects were instructed to indicate their motivation to comply with each referent concerning condom use. For this question, subjects were provided with a 7-point scale (anchored by 1 = 'Definitely Do Not Do What They Want' and 7 = 'Definitely Do What They Want'). Subjects recorded this motivation to comply rating for each referent in a box located to the right of each of the spaces provided for referent listings. After recoding (see below), these two measures for each normative referent were multiplied together and the sum of these products served as the measure of 'Total Own Normative Beliefs' ($\Sigma_j m_j$). Finally, subjects were asked to 'please circle the number(s) of the people or groups whom you feel are the most important in determining whether you use a condom during sexual intercourse over the next month.' The two measures for each of these most important normative referents were multiplied together and the sum of these products served as the measure of 'Most Important Own Normative Belief(s)'

Scoring the Belief-based Measures

There is controversy regarding the appropriate method for scoring the multiplicative belief-based measures (cf. Hewstone & Young, 1988). As

Fishbein (1993, p. xvii) points out, this scoring controversy is largely 'the result of Evans' (1991) demonstration that cross-products are not invariant with respect to scoring systems.' In this study, behavioural and normative beliefs were scored in accordance with the procedure advocated by Ajzen and Fishbein (1980). That is, specific components of the behavioural and normative beliefs measures were rescored in a bipolar fashion, from –3 ('Extremely Bad' / 'Extremely Unlikely') to +3 ('Extremely Good' / 'Extremely Likely') and the motivation to comply measures were scored as they appeared in the questionnaire (i.e., from 1 to 7).

Global Measures

Intention to Use a Condom

Three items assessed intention to use a condom during sexual intercourse over the next month: (1) 'I intend to use a condom during sexual intercourse over the next month' (anchored by 1 = 'Definitely Do Not' and 7 = 'Definitely Do'); (2) 'I will make an effort to use a condom during sexual intercourse over the next month' (anchored by 1 = 'Definitely False' and 7 = 'Definitely True'); and (3) 'I will try to use a condom during sexual intercourse over the next month' (1 = 'Definitely Will Not' and 7 = 'Definitely Will'). Because the responses to these three items were highly intercorrelated (Cronbach's α = .98), an average behavioural intention measure was computed and used in the analyses.

Attitude Toward Condom Use

Attitude toward using a condom during sexual intercourse over the next month was measured globally through the use of three 7-point semantic differential scales. The scales were anchored by (1) pleasant and unpleasant, (2) good and bad, and (3) useful and useless. Because the three items were found to be significantly intercorrelated (Cronbach's α = .77), an average global attitude measure was computed and used in the analyses.

Subjective Norm Regarding Condom Use

Consistent with Ajzen and Fishbein's (1980) approach, a global measure of subjective norm regarding condom use was collected from subjects. Provided with a 7-point scale, subjects were asked how likely or unlikely it was that 'Most people who are important to me think I should use a condom during sexual intercourse over the next month' (1 = 'Extremely Unlikely' and 7 = 'Extremely Likely'). Responses were recoded in a bipolar fashion, from –3 ('Extremely Unlikely') to +3 ('Extremely Likely').

A general motivation to comply measure was also collected. Provided with a 7-point scale, subjects were asked: 'Generally speaking, how much do you want to do what important others think you should do?' (1 = 'Definitely Do Not Do What They Think I Should Do' and 7 = 'Definitely Do What They Think I Should Do'). Consistent with Fishbein and Ajzen's theory, this item was used to weight the global subjective norm measure (i.e., the two measures were multiplied together).

Procedure

Subjects completed questionnaires in groups ranging in size from 5 to 15 and were isolated from each other as much as possible in order to assure privacy. Two separate questionnaire packets were administered. The first packet contained the measures which allowed subjects to provide their own beliefs (behavioural and normative) regarding condom use. The second packet contained the global measures of intention, attitude, and subjective norm. Items in this second packet were mixed such that the multiple measures of model constructs were separated from one another so as not to artifactually inflate their combined relationship (e.g., every fourth item was an intention item). It also contained the modal behavioural and normative belief items.[4] Finally, subjects were asked a number of personal background and demographic questions, including questions about their own past experience with sexual and contraceptive behaviours.

RESULTS

Descriptive Statistics

Of the 83 sexually active subjects in the sample, 73 completed all necessary behavioural belief measures and 63 completed all necessary normative belief measures.[5] Table 6.2 provides the descriptive statistics for these subjects for the respective variables concerning condom use. On average, subjects intended

Table 6.2   Descriptive statistics

Global Variables	Mean	SD	Possible Range Min.	Possible Range Max.
Intention to Use a Condom	4.33	2.51	1	7
Attitude Toward Condom Use	4.84	1.46	1	7
Subjective Norm Regarding Condom Use	7.49	7.21	−21	21
Belief-Based Variables				
Behavioural Beliefs				
Total Modal Behavioural Beliefs ($\Sigma\, b_i e_i$)	15.21	19.02	−72	72
Number of Own Behavioural Beliefs Listed	4.68	1.50	0	9
Total Own Behavioural Beliefs ($\Sigma\, b_i e_i$)	6.11	13.39	−81	81
Most Important Own Behavioural Belief(s) ($\Sigma\, b_i e_i$)	4.62	11.22	−81	81
First Listed Own Behavioural Belief ($b_1 e_1$)	4.07	5.07	−9	9
First 2 Listed Own Behavioural Beliefs ($\Sigma\, b_{1-2} e_{1-2}$)	6.45	9.01	−18	18
First 3 Listed Own Behavioural Beliefs ($\Sigma\, b_{1-3} e_{1-3}$)	6.52	11.49	−27	27
Normative Beliefs				
Total Modal Normative Beliefs ($\Sigma\, b_j m_j$)	45.92	56.72	−147	147
Number of Own Normative Beliefs Listed	5.41	1.74	0	9
Total Own Normative Beliefs ($\Sigma\, b_j m_j$)	53.92	49.85	−189	189
Most Important Own Normative Belief(s) ($\Sigma\, b_j m_j$)	19.94	28.53	−189	189
First Listed Own Normative Belief ($b_1 m_1$)	11.11	9.59	−21	21
First 2 Listed Own Normative Beliefs ($\Sigma\, b_{1-2} m_{1-2}$)	20.65	17.33	−42	42
First 3 Listed Own Normative Beliefs ($\Sigma\, b_{1-3} m_{1-3}$)	29.41	25.54	−63	63

Table 6.3   **Correlations between behavioural belief-based measures of condom use, global attitude toward condom use (A_B), and behavioural intention (BI)**

	A_B	BI
Total Modal Behavioural Beliefs ($\Sigma\ b_i e_i$)	.38	.33
Total Own Behavioural Beliefs ($\Sigma\ b_i e_i$)	.46	.42
Most Important Own Behavioural Belief(s) ($\Sigma\ b_i e_i$)	.41	.43
First Listed Own Behavioural Belief ($b_1 e_1$)	.36	.31
First 2 Listed Own Behavioural Beliefs ($\Sigma b_{1-2} e_{1-2}$)	.42	.43
First 3 Listed Own Behavioural Beliefs ($\Sigma b_{1-3} e_{1-3}$)	.42	.45

Note   All correlations are significant at the .01 level or less.

to use a condom during sexual intercourse over the next month ($M = 4.33$, on a 1 to 7 scale with higher numbers indicating stronger intention). Consistent with this intention, they expressed a positive global attitude toward condom use ($M = 4.84$). Moreover, subjects were relatively positive in their global normative beliefs, tending to believe that their important referents were in favour of their using condoms ($M = 7.49$, on a –21 to 21 scale). Finally, Table 6.2 shows that subjects tended to generate between four and six of their own behavioural and normative beliefs about using a condom.

Comparing Modal versus Own Behavioral Beliefs

Table 6.3 provides the correlations between the various behavioural belief-based measures and the global attitude toward behaviour measure (A_B). As can be seen, the measure of subjects' Total Own Behavioural Beliefs was descriptively more strongly correlated with the global attitude measure than was the measure of Total Modal Behavioural Beliefs ($r = .46$ versus .38). This difference in correlational strength is marginally significant ($p_{\text{diff}} < .10$). Similarly, for behavioural intention (BI), subjects' Total Own Behavioural Beliefs correlated more strongly than did the Total Modal Behavioural Beliefs ($r = .42$ versus .33); this difference was also marginally significant ($p_{\text{diff}} < .10$).

Importance, Accessibility, and Cumulative Serial Sums of Behavioural Beliefs

Subjects were given the opportunity to circle those behavioural beliefs that they considered to be 'the most important in determining whether you would use a condom during sexual intercourse over the next month.' This meant that subjects could circle as few as one of their beliefs or as many as the total they had generated. Table 6.3 shows the correlations of this behavioural belief importance measure with global attitude and behavioural intention. The Most Important Own Behavioural Belief(s) measure did not correlate descriptively as strongly with global attitude as did the Total Own Behavioural Beliefs measure, nor did it demonstrate a significantly stronger relationship with attitude than did the Total Modal Behavioural Beliefs measure. However, the

Most Important Own Behavioural Belief(s) measure was found to be marginally more correlated with behavioural intention than the Total Modal Behavioural Beliefs measure ($r = .43$ versus $.33$, $p_{\text{diff}} < .10$)

The procedure used to collect subjects' own beliefs also allowed for an assessment of the relationship between belief accessibility, attitude toward behaviour, and behavioural intention. Table 6.3 contains the correlations obtained between the first listed behavioural belief, the totals from increasing sums of serially listed behavioural beliefs (up to the first three), attitude toward behaviour, and behavioural intention. The most accessible behavioural belief (i.e., the First Listed Own Behavioural Belief) did not correlate stronger than either of the Total Belief-based measures with either attitude toward behaviour or behavioural intention. The sum of the first two and the first three behavioural beliefs provided a descriptively higher correlation with both attitude and intention than did the Total Modal Behavioural Beliefs measure but this difference in correlational strength was only significant for behavioural intention ($p_{\text{diff}} < .05$).[6]

Comparing Modal versus Own Normative Beliefs

Table 6.4 provides the correlations between the various normative belief-based measures and the global subjective norm measure. Subjects' Total Own Normative Beliefs measure was no more strongly correlated with the global subjective norm measure than was the measure of Total Modal Normative Beliefs ($r = .34$ for both). Similarly, subjects' Total Own Normative Beliefs were no more strongly correlated with behavioural intention than was the measure of Total Modal Normative Beliefs ($r = .70$ versus $.73$, $p_{\text{diff}} = $ ns).

Importance, Accessibility, and Cumulative Serial Sums of Normative Beliefs

As with behavioural beliefs, subjects were given the opportunity to circle those normative referents that they considered to be 'the most important in determining whether you would use a condom during sexual intercourse over the next month.' This meant that subjects could circle as few as one of their normative referents or as many as the total they had generated. Table 6.4 shows the results for this importance measure. The Most Important Own Normative Belief(s) measure resulted in a correlation that was statistically equivalent to that obtained by either of the Total Beliefs measures in relation to both global subjective norm and behavioural intention.

The procedure used to collect subjects' own normative beliefs also allowed for an assessment of the relationship between belief accessibility, global subjective norm, and behavioural intention. Table 6.4 displays the correlations obtained between the first listed normative referent, the totals from increasing sums of serially listed normative beliefs (up to three), global subjective norm, and behavioural intention. The First Listed Own Normative Belief measure correlated descriptively higher with the global norm measure than did either the Total Modal or Total Own measures but this difference in correlational strength was not statistically significant. The sum of increasing numbers of normative beliefs (up to

Table 6.4   Correlations between normative belief-based measures of condom use, global subjective norm regarding condom use (SN), and behavioural intention (BI)

	SN	BI
Total Modal Normative Beliefs ($\Sigma b_j m_j$)	.34	.73
Total Own Normative Beliefs ($\Sigma b_j m_j$)	.34	.70
Most Important Own Normative Belief(s) ($\Sigma b_j m_j$)	.35	.63
First Listed Own Normative Belief ($b_1 m_1$)	.41	.59
First 2 Listed Own Normative Beliefs ($\Sigma b_{1-2} m_{1-2}$)	.39	.65
First 3 Listed Own Normative Beliefs ($\Sigma b_{1-3} m_{1-3}$)	.41	.70

Note   All correlations are significant at the .01 level or less.

the first three) yielded similar correlations with the global subjective norm measure. For behavioural intention, none of the measures of subject-generated normative beliefs correlated higher than the measure of Total Modal Beliefs.[7]

Assessing Belief Homogeneity

One reason why individually-derived beliefs may not have proven to be consistently superior to modal beliefs in the prediction of the global TRA constructs involves the issue of belief homogeneity. Recall that an assumption underlying the use of modal beliefs is that they will accurate reflect the beliefs held by the sample of primary interest (cf. Towriss, 1983). That is, subjects in the main sample are assumed to hold beliefs identical to those generated by the pilot sample. To determine the degree to which the content of the beliefs generated by the main subjects was similar to the content of the beliefs generated by the pilot subjects (i.e., the modal beliefs), the percentage of each main subject's own beliefs that did not appear among the modal beliefs was calculated. Specifically, two separate percentages were calculated, one assessing behavioural belief listing overlap and another assessing normative belief listing overlap. Substantial overlap in belief content was found between the modal and individual listings. For behavioural beliefs, the mean percentage of own, non-modal beliefs was only 20.2% ($SD = 17.5$). For normative beliefs, the mean percentage of own, non-modal referents was 18.8% ($SD = 17.0$).[8] Furthermore, 35.6% of subjects failed to list *any* idiosyncratic behavioural beliefs and 34.9% of subjects failed to list any idiosyncratic normative referents (i.e., all individually-derived beliefs were among the modal beliefs). In essence, it appears that the pool of modal beliefs derived from the pilot sample adequately captured the kinds of beliefs that subjects in the main study sample tended to possess. This overlap in belief content helps explain the relatively small differences obtained between individually-derived and modal condom use beliefs.

Predicting Condom Use Intention from Modal versus Individually-Derived Beliefs

To determine the relative empirical weights of behavioural versus normative beliefs in the prediction of condom use intention, and to examine the overall

Table 6.5   Multiple regression analyses employing modal belief measures and individually-derived belief measures to predict intention to use a condom

Predicting Intention to Use a Condom			
Modal Belief Measures:	b	$p <$	R^2
Total Modal Behavioural Beliefs ($\Sigma\ b_i e_i$)	.10	.23	
Total Modal Normative Beliefs ($\Sigma\ b_j m_j$)	.71	.01	.56
Individually-Derived Measures:	b	$p <$	R^2
Total Own Behavioural Beliefs ($\Sigma\ b_i e_i$)	.23	.01	
Total Own Normative Beliefs ($\Sigma\ b_j m_j$)	.64	.01	.54

Note b = standardized beta coefficient.

ability of modal versus individually-derived belief measures to predict this behavioural intention, two separate multiple regression equations were computed. Table 6.5 provides the results from these regression analyses. Two points are particularly noteworthy. First, as suggested by the patterns of correlations in Tables 6.3 and 6.4, the normative belief measures proved to be substantially stronger predictors of condom use intention than did the behavioural belief measures. In fact, the modal normative belief measure was so strongly related to intention that it effectively 'prevented' the modal behavioural belief measure from attaining statistical significance. Second, the modal belief model and the individual belief model fared equally well in their respective prediction of condom use intention, with each set of variables predicting about 55% of the variance in behavioural intention.

DISCUSSION

This study tested several different measurement approaches for assessing the cognitive underpinnings of the theory of reasoned action. Having subjects rate a set of modal beliefs concerning condom use versus having subjects generate and rate their own beliefs about this important health behaviour were compared as methods for predicting the respective global theory constructs. Overall, subjects' ratings of their own behavioural and normative beliefs tended to provide marginally higher correlations with global measures of attitude toward behaviour and subjective norm, although the relative magnitude of the differences among the various correlations in most cases was modest.

Intention to Use a Condom: The Primacy of Normative Beliefs

In the prediction of condom use intention, subject-generated behavioural beliefs were found to correlate more strongly than ratings of modal behavioural beliefs but this was not found for normative beliefs. Subjects' ratings of a list of modal referents yielded an equivalent correlation with intention than did their ratings of their own listing of referents, with both correlations being quite robust ($r = .73$ and $.70$, respectively). The magnitude of the relation between the various measures of normative beliefs and behavioural intention indicates that subjects' concerns about the opinions of others were particularly powerful determinants of motivation to use a condom. Multiple regression analyses further support the relative importance of normative beliefs over behavioural beliefs in the prediction of condom use intention. This finding is consistent with those of other recent tests of the reasoned action model in the context of AIDS-relevant behaviours (cf. Terry et al., 1993).[9]

Comparing Modal versus Individually-Derived Beliefs

There are several possible reasons why subject-generated beliefs did not achieve higher correlations overall with the various TRA constructs than those reported here. As suggested by the analysis of belief homogeneity, the pool of modal beliefs derived from the pilot sample closely mirrored those listed by subjects in the main sample, with 80% or more overlap on average. While a notable percentage of listed beliefs were idiosyncratic, the lack of wide divergence between own and modal beliefs helps account for the relative modest findings. It also provides support for Towriss's (1983) position that if one assumes belief homogeneity between pilot and main sample, use of modal beliefs should result in little measurement error.

Furthermore, with respect to normative beliefs, it is possible that being provided with a complete listing of possible referents (see Table 6.1) *after* having generated their own referent listing increased subjects' awareness of potentially overlooked sources of normative influence and that this increased awareness resulted in a more complete and accurate overall assessment of the modal referents. Second, regarding behavioural beliefs, it is possible that subjects had difficulty in understanding the relatively cumbersome task of providing both evaluative and likelihood ratings for all of their own beliefs. Moreover, the relatively straightforward procedure of rating a set of modal beliefs may have been facilitated by subjects' initial experience of providing their own beliefs. Since the modal belief measures were collected *after* the self-generated belief measures, subjects may have gained valuable experience and information on how to properly complete the measures. Alternatively, subjects may have been more certain of their true beliefs and feelings as the result of the thought required to complete the 'own' belief measures. Such possible order effects cannot be ruled out or avoided entirely without risking other potential confounds (e.g., see note 4). Although use of a within-subject design in the current study allowed for a powerful and useful direct comparison of the predictive ability of individually-derived versus modal beliefs, future research might counterbalance the order in which subjects complete the different belief measures in order to provide evidence in possible support of one or more of the above suppositions. As they stand, the present findings provide an important partial replication and extension of Rutter and Bunce's (1989) between-subject findings.

Utility of Individually-Derived Beliefs

The modest increase in correlation obtained via individually-derived beliefs might reasonably lead one to question the relative utility of this measurement approach. Indeed, overall, the modal beliefs worked quite well, calling into question whether the extensive amount of questionnaire preparation, administration, and analysis required are worth the effort. However, one must also consider the time and expense associated with obtaining relevant modal beliefs from a preliminary sample, a requirement of the 'standard Fishbein and Ajzen' approach. In support of collecting ratings of individually-generated beliefs, it was found that subjects' most accessible behavioural and normative belief (i.e., the first belief listed) significantly correlated with the respective global construct measures. In fact, the first listed normative belief was the strongest predictor of the global subjective norm measure. These findings have important implications from a data collection perspective. Researchers who have time or space constraints may want to have subjects simply list and rate a single behavioural and normative belief to gain some insight into the belief structure underlying the more proximal and general theory constructs.

An additional comment concerning the possibility of sample reduction is also in order. The procedure employed to generate the various individually-derived belief measures required subjects to complete a number of separate steps including (a) generating several beliefs, both behavioural and normative, and (b) determining and circling those considered 'most important.' Despite the seeming simplicity of these requirements, a moderate number of subjects either failed to list more than two beliefs or failed to indicate which belief or beliefs they considered to be most important (see Footnote 5). Because of the sensitive nature of the behaviour under investigation in this study, subjects were not monitored as to their full compliance with the questionnaire instructions. Future researchers who utilise a subject-generated belief procedure with no monitoring are cautioned to anticipate similar loss of sample size.

Practical Implications

Condom use was selected for examination in the current investigation because of its importance from both a theoretical and an applied perspective. The present results provide some practical implications concerning intervention efforts that might be undertaken to increase condom use among sexually-active people. It is no surprise to find that people hold specific beliefs that tend to support or undermine condom use. As Fishbein and colleagues have suggested in their application of TRA to AIDS-related behaviours (e.g., Fishbein & Middlestadt, 1989), specific populations and cultures may adhere more strongly to certain behavioural and normative beliefs than to others with respect to specific health behaviours. The present finding that a person's single most important behavioural belief or single most important normative belief reliably predicts condom use intentions argues for the promotion of public health campaigns that emphasise these specific beliefs (see Table 6.1). The current findings underscore the importance of conducting extensive pilot research in order to determine the most important beliefs within a given population or culture prior to developing media messages, educational programs, community interventions, or one-on-one counselling strategies. In this way, the belief underpinnings of TRA may be applied effectively to develop interventions aimed at increasing condom use.

The current findings also provide insight regarding concerns about the presence or absence of cognitive activity within the physical, hormone-driven context in which condom use occurs (cf. Loewenstein & Furstenberg, 1991). The current detailed examination of condom use beliefs indicates that people's intentions *are* related to their beliefs. Given the massive social psychological literature demonstrating the robust linkage between intentions and subsequent behaviour, it is clear that possessing specific behavioural and/or normative beliefs plays a role in the enactment (or lack of enactment) of this important health behaviour. Thus, attempts to strengthen specific pro-condom use beliefs (such as those in Table 6.1) are likely to ultimately reduce both the number of unintended pregnancies and cases of sexually-transmitted disease.

Limitations and Future Research Directions

Several limitations of the current study should be noted. First, this study was cross-sectional and, therefore, did not allow for an examination of the intention-behaviour relationship. It would be insightful to see the degree to which subject-generated beliefs predict actual behaviour, either directly or indirectly. Second, the subjects in this study were all involved in a romantic relationship at the time of their participation, a requirement imposed to increase the possibility that participants would have experience with condom use. However, as a result, the underlying behavioural and normative beliefs concerning condom use reported here may be qualitatively different from those that might be generated by individuals not involved in such close relationships. Future research might explore the extent to which subject-generated condom beliefs predict the relevant theoretical constructs with a sample of subjects whose sexual behaviour occurs within a more casual context.

Beliefs clearly play an important role in the development and maintenance of a number of important health behaviours, including condom use. The theory of reasoned action provides a tremendously useful heuristic framework for isolating and examining the effects of specific cognitive determinants of behaviour. While a variety of measurement strategies can be adopted by researchers who utilise the theory, the present study demonstrates that it continues to provide social and health science researchers with useful information for understanding the manner in which beliefs support or undermine healthy behaviour.

NOTES

1. Although a bit odd, this last question is suggested by Ajzen and Fishbein (1980) to ensure that respondents have the opportunity to list all possible beliefs relevant to the behavior under investigation.
2. As noted in Table 1, there were some beliefs that were listed by over 20% of one sex but not the other. Beliefs were retained if they were listed by a minimum of 20% of the *overall* preliminary sample, irrespective of sex differences.
3. Nine spaces were included because of the assumption that any beliefs listed beyond that number would not be salient (cf. Fishbein & Ajzen, 1975).
4. Subjects' own beliefs were collected prior to the assessment of the modal beliefs to ensure that subjects would not be influenced by having seen the list of modal beliefs.

5. The reduction in sample size was due to the failure of some subjects to circle their 'most important' beliefs ($n = 5$ for behavioral beliefs, $n = 11$ for normative beliefs) or to list more than two behavioral ($n = 5$) and/or normative beliefs ($n = 12$). For purposes of direct comparison among the various measurement approaches, subjects with incomplete data were not included in the reported analyses. Results from analyses conducted using all possible subjects in each correlational pairing did not differ markedly from those reported here.

6. To determine whether the most accessible behavioral belief (i.e., the first belief listed) also tended to be rated by subjects as among the 'most important', the correlation between these two variables was computed. The two variables were found to be moderately correlated ($r = .40$, $p < .001$) indicating that participants tended to begin their own belief listings with subjectively more important beliefs.

7. To determine whether the most accessible normative belief (i.e., the first referent listed) also tended to be rated by subjects as among the 'most important', the correlation between these two variables was calculated and found to be very high ($r = .64$, $p < .001$), indicating that participants tended to begin their own normative belief listings with subjectively more important referents.

8. The median percentage of idiosyncratic behavioral beliefs was also 20%; the maximum percentage of idiosyncratic behavioral beliefs held by a subject was 55%. Similarly, the median percentage of idiosyncratic normative beliefs was 17%; the maximum percentage of idiosyncratic normative beliefs held by a subject was 60%.

9. Subject's partners figured prominently in the subject-generated normative belief listings. More than two-thirds of subjects (67.1%) included their current partner in their listing. Of these subjects, nearly all of them (94.5%) marked their subject as 'most important' in determining whether they used a condom.

10. Subjects' partners figured prominently in the subject-generated normative belief listings. More than two-thirds of subjects (67.1%) included their current partner in their listing. Of these subjects, nearly all of them (94.5%) marked their subject as 'most important' in determining whether they used a condom.

REFERENCES

Agnew, C. R. (1999). Power over interdependent behavior within the dyad: Who decides what a couple does? In L. J. Severy & W. B. Miller (eds.), *Advances in Population: Psychosocial Perspectives, Volume 3* (pp. 163–188). London: Jessica Kingsley Publishers.

Agnew, C. R. & Loving, T. J. (1998). The role of social desirability in self-reported condom use attitudes and intentions. *AIDS and Behavior, 2*, 229–239.

Ajzen, I. & Fishbein, M. (1980). *Understanding Attitudes and Predicting Social Behavior*. Englewood Cliffs, NJ: Prentice Hall.

Aral, S. O. & Holmes, K. K. (1991). Sexually transmitted diseases in the AIDS era. *Scientific American, 264*, 62–69.

Bentler, P. M. & Speckart, G. (1979). Models of attitude-behavior relations. *Psychological Review, 86*, 452–464.

Budd, R. J. (1986). Predicting cigarette use: The need to incorporate measures of salience in the theory of reasoned action. *Journal of Applied Social Psychology, 16*, 663–685.

Budd, R. J., North, D., & Spencer, C. (1984). Understanding seat-belt use: A test of Bentler and Speckart's extension of the 'theory of reasoned action'. *European Journal of Social Psychology, 14*, 69–78.

Conner, M. T. (1993). Individualized measurement of attitudes towards foods. *Appetite, 20*, 235–238.

Crawford, T. J. & Boyer, R. (1985). Salient consequences, cultural values, and childbearing intentions. *Journal of Applied Social Psychology, 15*, 16–30.

Davidson, A. R. & Morrison, D. M. (1983). Predicting contraceptive behavior from attitudes: A comparison of within- versus across-subjects procedures. *Journal of Personality and Social Psychology, 45*, 997–1009.

Eiser, J. R. & Van der Pligt, J. (1988). *Attitudes and Decisions*. London: Routledge.

Fazio, R. H. & Williams, C. J. (1986). Attitude accessibility as a moderator of the attitude-perception and attitude-behavior relations: An investigation of the 1984 presidential election. *Journal of Personality and Social Psychology, 51*, 505–514.

Feather, N. T. (1982). *Expectations and Actions: Expectancy-Value Models in Psychology*. Hillsdale, NJ: Erlbaum.

Fishbein, M. (1963). An investigation of the relationships between beliefs about an object and the attitude toward that object. *Human Relations, 16*, 233–240.

Fishbein, M. (1993). Introduction. In D. J. Terry, C. Gallois, & M. McCamish (eds.), *The Theory of Reasoned Action: Its Application to AIDS-Preventive Behaviour* (pp. xv-xxv). Oxford: Pergamon Press.

Fishbein, M. & Ajzen, I. (1975). *Belief, Attitude, Intention, and Behavior: An Introduction to Theory and Research*. Reading, MA: Addison-Wesley.

Fishbein, M. & Middlestadt, S. E. (1989). Using the theory of reasoned action as a framework for understanding and changing AIDS-related behaviors. In V. M. Mays, G. W. Albee and S. F. Schneider (eds.), *Primary Prevention of AIDS: Psychological Approaches* (pp. 93–110). Newbury Park, CA, Sage.

Fisher, J. D. & Fisher, W. A. (1992). Changing AIDS-risk behavior. *Psychological Bulletin, 111*, 455–474.

Hewstone, M. & Young, L. (1988). Expectancy-value models of attitude: Measurement and combination of evaluations and beliefs. *Journal of Applied Social Psychology, 18*, 958–971.

Jaccard, J. J. & Davidson, A. R. (1972). Toward an understanding of family planning behaviours: An initial investigation. *Journal of Applied Social Psychology, 2*, 228–235.

Jaccard, J. J. & Wood, G. (1985). An idiothetic analysis of attitude-behavior models. *Advances in Consumer Research, 13*, 600–605.

Janz, N. K. & Becker, M. H. (1984). The Health Belief Model: A decade later. *Health Education Quarterly, 11*, 1–47.

Jemmott, J. B. & Jones, J. M. (1993). Social psychology and AIDS among ethnic minority individuals: Risk behaviors and strategies for changing them. In J. B. Pryor & G. D. Reeder (Eds.), *The Social Psychology of HIV Infection* (pp. 183–224). Hillsdale, NJ: Erlbaum.

Kaplan, D. (1978). To have or not to have another child: Family planning attitudes, intentions, and behavior. *Journal of Applied Social Psychology, 8*, 29–46.

Kaplan, K. J. & Fishbein, M. (1969). The source of beliefs, their saliency, and prediction of attitude. *Journal of Social Psychology, 78*, 63–74.

Liska, A. E. (1984). A critical examination of the causal structure of the Fishbein/Ajzen attitude-behavior model. *Social Psychology Quarterly, 47*, 61–74.

Loewenstein, G. & Furstenberg, F. F. (1991). Is teenage sexual behavior rational? *Journal of Applied Social Psychology, 21*, 957–986.

Mandler, G. (1967). Verbal learning. In T. M. Newcomb (ed.), *New Directions in Psychology* (Vol. 3, pp. 1–50). New York: Holt.

Miller, G. A. (1956). The magic number seven, plus or minus two: Some limits on our capacity for processing information. *Psychological Review, 63*, 81–97.

Miller, W. B. & Pasta, D. J. (1995). Behavioral intentions: Which ones predict fertility behavior in married couples? *Journal of Applied Social Psychology, 25,* 530–555.

O'Keefe, D. J. (1990). *Persuasion: Theory and Research.* Newbury Park, CA: Sage.

Oliver, R. L. & Berger, P. K. (1979). A path analysis of preventive health care decision models. *Journal of Consumer Research, 6,* 113–122.

Peak, H. (1955). Attitude and motivation. In M. R. Jones (ed.), *Nebraska Symposium on Motivation* (Vol. 3, pp. 149–188). Lincoln, NE: University of Nebraska Press.

Pomazal, R. J. & Brown, J. D. (1977). Understanding drug use motivation: A new look at a current problem. *Journal of Health and Social Behavior, 18,* 212–222.

Poppen, P. J. & Reisen, C. A. (1994). Heterosexual behaviors and risk of exposure to HIV: Current status and prospects for change. *Applied and Preventive Psychology, 3,* 75–90.

Prentice-Dunn, S. & Rogers, R. W. (1986). Protection Motivation Theory and preventive health: Beyond the Health Belief Model. *Health Education Research, 1,* 153–161.

Prochaska, J. O., DiClemente, C. C., & Norcross, J. C. (1992). In search of how people change: Applications to addictive behaviors. *American Psychologist, 47,* 1102–1114.

Pryor, J. B. & Reeder, G. D. (Eds.). (1993). *The Social Psychology of HIV Infection.* Hillsdale, NJ: Erlbaum.

Rippetoe, P. A. & Rogers, R. W. (1987). Effects of components of protection-motivation theory on adaptive and maladaptive coping with a health threat. *Journal of Personality and Social Psychology, 52,* 596–604.

Rosenberg, M. (1956). Cognitive structure and attitudinal affect. *Journal of Abnormal and Social Psychology, 53,* 367–372.

Rosenstock, I. M. (1990). The Health Belief Model: Explaining health behavior through expectancies. In K. Glanz, F. M. Lewis, & B. K. Rimer (eds.), *Health Behavior and Education: Theory, Research, and Practice* (pp. 39–62). San Francisco: Jossey-Bass.

Rutter, D. R., & Bunce, D. J. (1989). The theory of reasoned action of Fishbein and Ajzen: A test of Towriss's amended procedure for measuring beliefs. *British Journal of Social Psychology, 28,* 39–46.

Sheppard, B. H., Hartwick, J., & Warshaw, P. R. (1988). The theory of reasoned action: A meta-analysis of past research with recommendations for modifications and future research. *Journal of Consumer Research, 15,* 325–343.

Terry, D. J., Gallois, C., & McCamish, M. (eds.). (1993). *The Theory of Reasoned Action: Its Application to AIDS-Preventive Behaviour.* Oxford: Pergamon Press.

Towriss, J. G. (1984). A new approach to the use of expectancy value models. *Journal of the Market Research Society, 26,* 63–75.

van den Putte, B. (1993). *On the Theory of Reasoned Action.* Unpublished doctoral dissertation, University of Amsterdam, Amsterdam, The Netherlands.

van der Plight, J. & Eiser, J. R. (1984). Dimensional salience, judgment, and attitudes. In J. R. Eiser (Ed.), *Attitudinal Judgement* (pp. 161–177). New York: Springer-Verlag Vinokur

Warshaw, P. R. & Davis, F. D. (1984). Self-understanding and the accuracy of behavioral expectations. *Personality and Social Psychology Bulletin, 10,* 111–118.

Zuckerman, M. & Reis, H. T. (1978). Comparison of three models for predicting altruistic behavior. *Journal of Personality and Social Psychology, 36,* 498–510.

CHAPTER SEVEN

Discriminating Between Behavioural Intention and Behavioural Willingness: Cognitive Antecedents to Adolescent Health Risk

Frederick X. GIBBONS, Meg GERRARD, Judith A. OUELLETTE and Rebecca BURZETTE

INTRODUCTION

Is human social behaviour always 'reasoned' action? Most models of attitude/behaviour consistency, such as Fishbein and Ajzen's (1975; 1980) Theory of Reasoned Action and Ajzen's (1985; 1991) Theory of Planned Behaviour, are based on some version of that premise. According to these 'rational' models, behaviour is a direct result of behavioural intentions (BI). Intentions, in turn, reflect consideration of relevant attitudes and beliefs about the behaviour and its outcomes. This deliberative approach has been quite successful at predicting a number of rational or reasoned behaviours (see Conner & Sparks, 1996; van den Putte, 1993, for reviews). In the domain of health, for example, these models have been used to predict health-protective behaviours, such as exercise (Godin, Valois & Lepage, 1993) and food choice (Sparks & Shepherd, 1992). They have been less successful, however, at predicting behaviours that, by their nature, are less rational, but also exciting or enticing (Johnson, 1988; Stacy, Bentler & Flay, 1994; cf. Conner and Sparks, 1996). A prime example of this – one that has both intrigued and puzzled behavioural scientists for years – is behaviour that jeopardizes one's health, such as unprotected sex or smoking (Stacy et al., 1994), especially among young people.

These behaviours do not appear to be attributable to ignorance about risk. In fact, in many countries, health education begins as early as age 7 or 8, so that by the time a child is a pre-teen, she or he is well aware of the dangers inherent in such activities as drinking or drug use. When asked, young people frequently point to these dangers as reasons why they do not intend to engage in the behaviour, even though they often mistakenly believe that their friends and peers are heavily involved (Prentice & Miller, 1993; Sussman et al., 1988). From this perspective, their reasoning appears quite rational. Good intentions notwithstanding, however, health risk behaviours are quite common (Brooks-Gunn & Furstenberg, 1989). In a number of countries (including the U.S.), the incidence of some of these behaviours is actually increasing (Centers for Disease Control, 1992; 1993; University of Michigan, 1995). Why that is the case is not clear.

A Prototype/Willingness Model of Adolescent Health Risk

Pathways to risk. In an effort to further explain and predict these risky actions, we have developed a model of adolescent health risk, called the Prototype/Willingness (P/W) model, that is described in detail elsewhere (Gibbons & Gerrard, 1995, 1997; Gibbons, Gerrard & Love, in press). We will present a summary here. The model is consistent with other health models in its emphasis on the social nature of adolescent risk behaviour (Graham, Marks & Hansen, 1991; Kandel, 1980; Stein, Newcomb & Bentler, 1987); but it diverges from most theories of attitude/behaviour consistency by claiming that some adolescent risk behaviour is not intentional. Instead, we argue that there are two 'pathways; to risk.[1] One, labelled the 'reasoned path,' represents more or less rational decision making, as outlined by the various deliberative or expectancy-value models. The second route to behaviour, which we have labelled the 'social reaction' path, involves that element of behaviour that is less 'reasoned' or deliberate and often less rational. This path includes some of the same influential factors as the earlier models (i.e., subjective norms and attitudes toward the behaviour, plus previous behaviour, cf. Bagozzi & Warshaw, 1992; Sutton, 1994), but it has two important distinctions. First, it includes an additional antecedent, which reflects its emphasis on social factors, and that is the social image or *prototype* associated with the behaviour – the adolescent's perception of the *type* of person who does it (e.g., the 'typical smoker' or 'typical drinker'). The second difference is that this path proceeds through a construct, which is distinct from BI, that we have called behavioural 'willingness' (BW). This construct reflects an adolescent's willingness to engage in a particular behaviour given the opportunity to do so.

Prototypes and willingness. One result of the health education that most young people receive is that their perceptions of risk behaviours and of the type of people who engage in them tend to be fairly negative. They include some positive characteristics (e.g., independence, toughness), and quite a few negative ones (unhealthy, unwise). This is true even among those who are actually doing the behaviours. Nonetheless, as numerous studies have demonstrated (see Gibbons & Gerrard, 1997, for a review), these images are influential in adolescents' decisions to engage or not engage in these activities. The reason, according to the P/W model, is that young people realize that if they engage in the behaviour in public settings, they will be identified as members of the group that the image represents – they will be seen as a (typical) smoker or drinker. This means the images are actually social *consequences* of engaging in the behaviour rather than goal states. It also means that many young people engage in risk behaviour not because they want to acquire the characteristics associated with the image (cf. Leventhal and

Cleary, 1980) – this would reflect intentional behaviour – but rather in spite of these characteristics. They don't find the image attractive, but they do find it acceptable (i.e., reflecting reactive behaviour); and therefore are willing to engage in the behaviour given the opportunity. Thus, for most young people the impact of images or prototypes on behaviour is mediated more by BW than by BI. This distinction between deliberate and reactive behaviour, and between BI and BW, is central to the P/W model; it is also the focus of the current paper.

Willingness vs. Intention

The belief that cognitive processing varies in terms of amount and extent of deliberation is not a new one in psychology; in fact, the idea is central to a number of 'dual-processing' models in the social cognition literature. For example, Petty and Cacioppo's Elaboration Likelihood Model (Petty & Cacioppo, 1986) describes two routes to attitude change and persuasion, one of which involves careful and detailed consideration of relevant information (the 'central' route), the other a more cursory type of processing (the 'peripheral' route). The former route requires some minimum level of motivation, as well as the ability or opportunity to process, and it typically results in behaviour that is more closely aligned with attitudes. Similarly, Fazio's MODE model (Fazio, 1990) also draws a distinction between spontaneous and deliberative types of information processing, claiming that opportunity (to think about one's attitudes) and (high) level of motivation are necessary for attitudes to affect behaviour in a reasoned fashion (see also Thaler's, 1980, discussion of planned vs. impulsive consumer behaviour). More generally, these models suggest that the link between attitudes, intentions, and behaviour will be stronger when individuals take the time and have the inclination to consider the behaviour and their own attitudes before acting (Dovidio & Fazio, 1992; cf. Bagozzi, 1992; Norman & Conner, 1996).

Deliberation. A similar dichotomy exists between intentions and willingness in the P/W model.[2] According to the model, intentions are plans that have been formulated in order to achieve a particular goal state through certain, instrumental actions. They involve contemplation of the behaviour and, usually, of its consequences (as Ajzen and Fishbein, 1980, suggested in discussing BI, 'People consider the implications of their actions before they decide to engage or not to engage in a particular behaviour ...' p. 5). Willingness, on the other hand, does not involve goal states, plans, or instrumental actions. Compared to intentions, BW involves relatively little forethought, which means less consideration of outcomes or consequences. As a result, it also means less acceptance of responsibility for the behaviour and its outcomes (cf. Kruglanski, 1975; Wells, 1980).

Consider excessive drinking on college campuses as an example. The student who states that he intends to get drunk this coming Friday night has made some commitment to the behaviour and has spent some time considering its requirements and sequelae; the same would be true for the student who says he intends *not* to get drunk. Some students fall into a middle-ground category, however; they would be willing to drink, even to excess, *if* the opportunity is afforded, but getting drunk is not a goal for them. They have not given much thought to the prospect and have no specific plans as to how they might get drunk. Unlike the intending (or 'willful") student, who creates risk opportunities, the willing student responds to them. Of course, risk opportunities are common, and in fact, BW has been shown to predict a number of risk behaviours among adolescents and young adults including substance use (Blanton, Gibbons, Gerrard, Conger and Smith, 1997; Gerrard, Gibbons, Zhao, Russell & Reis-Bergan, 1999; Gibbons, Gerrard Blanton & Russell, 1998), and unprotected sexual behaviour (Gibbons et al., 1998). In these prospective studies, BW and BI were shown to predict changes in risk behaviour independent of one another.

Acceptance of responsibility. This type of thinking, which may appear to adults as some form of self-deception (adults' actions are more likely to be both rational and deliberate), appears to be common among young people, especially with regard to risky behaviours. They may spend some time considering the type of social situation in which the risk behaviour might occur, as well as the type of person who does it. But they spend relatively little time thinking about the potential negative impact the behaviour might have on themselves or others (we would expect that compared with the student who intended to get drunk, the willing student would be less likely to accept responsibility for the hangover he experiences the next morning). Indeed, they may actively *avoid* such consideration. More specifically, relative to those who have expressed a commitment to a particular risky behaviour, i.e., an intention to engage, those who are only willing to engage are less likely to accept responsibility for their behaviour or its consequences, and to have considered the potential risks associated with the behaviour – they are not intending to do it, so they don't see the need to seriously consider the consequences (cf. Gerrard, 1982). Those who are only willing should also be less likely to acknowledge their *personal vulnerability* (PV) to those risks, i.e., likelihood that they will experience the negative consequences associated with the behaviours. In fact, they may even deny personal vulnerability. These last two hypotheses were tested in the studies reported here.

Personal Vulnerability

Some evidence of the relation between perceptions of personal vulnerability and intention comes from research indicating that people who engage in risk behaviours acknowledge more PV than those who do not (Gerrard, Gibbons and Bushman, 1996). Research with adolescents, for example, has shown that as their use of substances such as alcohol and tobacco increases, so do their intentions to use in the future *and* their estimates of the likelihood that they themselves will experience the illnesses and accidents associated with these behaviours (Gerrard, Gibbons, Benthin & Hessling, 1996). Research with adults has indicated that smokers are less likely than nonsmokers to accept the validity of scientific research linking cancer and smoking (Dawley, Fleischer & Dawley, 1985), but they do admit that their own risk (PV) of contracting lung cancer is higher than that of nonsmokers (Chapman, Wong & Smith, 1993). Moreover, perceptions of PV are positively correlated with plans to quit smoking (Gibbons, McGovern & Lando, 1991; Klesges et al., 1988). Those who quit and then relapse report a marked decline in their PV after relapsing, however, as well as a decline in their commitment to quitting (Gibbons, Eggleston & Benthin, 1997). In sum, the fact that PV to illness is positively associated with health risk behaviour, even among adolescents, *and* with intentions to stop vs. continue engaging in these behaviours is consistent with the belief that unlike BW, BI is associated with some acknowledgment of risk. This is one important way in which BI and BW differ.

Measuring BW and BI

Willingness. BW is assessed by asking respondents to imagine being in a situation that is risk-conducive. Some of these situations are fairly common (being at a party where cigarettes are available), some less so (an attractive person of the opposite sex offers you another drink after you've already decided you've had enough). In fact, the particular risk-conducive circumstances are not that important. The items are not designed to measure situation-specific intentions (intentions are not mentioned explicitly or implicitly); instead, what is being assessed is a general openness to risk opportunity independent of the specific circumstances. After being assured that no assumptions are being made that they would ever be in such a situation, respondents are asked to indicate how willing they would be to act in several different ways, each varying in level of risk (e.g., say no, try some, 'get high').[3] Combining these responses provides an index of BW.

Intentions vs. expectations. A distinction has been drawn in the deliberative-model literature between the concept of BI and that of behavioural expectation (BE) (Sheppard, Hartwick & Warshaw, 1988; Warshaw & Davis, 1985). The latter, which is an individual's assessment of the likelihood that she/he will actually engage in a particular behaviour, includes acknowledgment of relevant past behaviour, as well as estimations of opportunity. BE measures are frequently used in studies of substance use (Morojele & Stephenson, 1994) and other behaviours that are low in social desirability (Beck & Ajzen, 1991), such as drunk driving (Aberg, 1994), and reckless driving (Parker, Manstead, Stradling, Reason & Baxter, 1992). We have used BE measures in our studies of health risk primarily because they predict better – adolescents are more likely to acknowledge some likelihood of risk behaviour than to admit that they intend to engage in this behaviour (e.g., 'I intend to drive drunk' vs. 'I expect that I will drive drunk'). Conceptually, BI and BE are very similar and, in fact, some have suggested they can be used interchangeably (Ajzen & Fishbein, 1980, p. 42), especially for volitional behaviours (Fishbein & Stasson, 1990). In the current two studies we again use BE measures to predict behaviour. Because BE includes some consideration of opportunity as well as intention, however, it is clearly more similar to BW than is BI. Thus, using BE measures actually provides a conservative test of the distinction between planned and reactive behaviour, or between intentions and willingness. Presumably, the differences uncovered in these studies would be more pronounced if 'traditional' BI measures were used.

The Current Studies

Previous research with the BW construct has provided evidence of its construct validity and its predictive validity (net BE) *vis-à-vis* adolescent risk behaviours, such as smoking and drinking. The primary purpose of the current studies was to provide some evidence of its discriminant validity by comparing the relations of BW and BE with another health-relevant cognition, PV. The following specific hypotheses were tested in the first study: (a) BW and BE will both relate prospectively to adolescent health risk behaviour, independent of one another, as they have in previous studies; and (b) because it involves greater consideration of behaviour and its consequences than does BW, BE will be more closely associated with acknowledgment of PV to the risks associated with those behaviour than will BW. This first study included new analyses of adolescent smoking behaviour from the sample used in Gibbons et al. (1998, Study 1).

STUDY 1

METHOD

Participants and Procedure

The original sample began with 245 males and 255 females from small towns in Iowa, USA, who had been recruited, along with their families, to participate in a study of social psychological factors related to health behaviour. Half of the sample was age 13 at T1 and half was age 15. From that group, 470 completed all of the measures at Tl, 464 at T2, and 447 at T3. Data collection occurred in the families' homes at intervals of approximately one year. Families were paid $50 at T1 and T2, and $55 at T3 (for additional description of the samples and measures, see Gibbons, Gerrard & Boney-McCoy, 1995; Gerrard, Gibbons, Benthin & Hessling, 1996).

Measures

Behaviour. There were two measures of smoking behaviour, one lifetime and the other current: 'What is the most that you have ever smoked cigarettes?' followed by a 6-pt. scale with anchors 'never' to 'I have smoked every day.' and 'How often do you smoke now?' followed by a 4-pt. scale with anchors 'not at all' to 'every day.' The two were standardized, and then their average was used as the behavioural measure (α at all three waves > 0.83).

Behavioural Expectation. BE was assessed with a single item: 'Do you think that you will smoke cigarettes in the future?' followed by a 7-pt. scale with anchors 'I definitely will not' to 'I definitely will.'

Behavioural Willingness. BW was assessed by asking subjects to imagine themselves in the following situation, and then think about how they might respond if they were in that situation: 'Suppose you were with some friends and one of them offered you a cigarette. How likely is it that you would do *each* of the following?' This was followed by three responses: 'Take it and try it,' 'Tell them 'no thanks,''' and 'Leave the situation,' each with a 7-pt. scale with anchors 'not at all likely' to 'very likely.[4] The last two items were reversed, and the three were averaged together at each wave (αs > 0.78).

Personal Vulnerability. Finally, there were two PV items; one was absolute: 'How likely is it that you will have a smoking-related illness (for example, lung cancer) at some time in the future?'; the other was comparative: 'Compared to others your age, how likely is it …' Each was accompanied by a 7-pt. scale, with anchors 'no chance' to 'definitely will happen,' for the first item, and then 'much less likely than others' to 'much more likely than others,' for the second. These pairs also were averaged together at each wave (αs > 0.78).

RESULTS

Behaviour

Table 7.1 presents the means, SDs and correlations among all of the relevant variables. As can be seen in the table, BW and BE were correlated with each

Table 7.1 Means, standard deviations and correlations among smoking behaviour, BE, BW, and PV across three waves (Study 1)

	Time 1 (N = 470)				Time 2 (N = 464)				Time 3 (N = 447)			
	B	BE	BW	PV	B	BE	BW	PV	B	BE	BW	PV
Time 1												
Behaviour					0.67	0.43	0.43	0.34	0.50	0.29	0.36	0.27
BE	0.62				0.50	0.55	0.47	0.38	0.44	0.41	0.36	0.32
BW	0.65	0.64			0.52	0.48	0.58	0.30	0.43	0.30	0.45	0.23
PV	0.25	0.31	0.24		0.15	0.19	0.14	0.41	0.12	0.10	0.12	0.39
Time 2												
Behaviour									0.67	0.49	0.51	0.46
BE					0.63				0.56	0.61	0.54	0.44
BW					0.66	0.70			0.61	0.54	0.68	0.45
PV					0.43	0.50	0.40		0.34	0.38	0.29	0.55
Time 3												
Behaviour												
BE									0.69			
BW									0.74	0.68		
PV									0.56	0.54	0.45	
MEAN	1.59	1.62	2.51	2.04	1.79	1.87	2.99	1.95	2.02	1.89	3.15	2.02
SD	0.79	1.20	1.50	1.23	1.00	1.40	1.71	1.13	1.25	1.54	1.74	1.16

Note: B = Behaviour, BE = Behavioural Expectation, BW = Behavioural Willingness, PV = Personal Vulnerability. *N*s for correlations across time periods (e.g., T1 with T3) range from 419 to 435. All *p*s < 0.05.

Table 7.2   Hierarchical regressions of smoking behaviour (Part A), and PV to smoking-related disease (Part B) on previous behaviour, BE and BW (Study 1)

	Criterion	Predictors	β	t	R^2
Part A: Predicting Subsequent Behaviour	T2 Behaviour	T1 Behaviour	0.53 (0.67)	11.18**	0.45
		T1 BE	0.13 (0.17)	2.84**	0.47
		T1 BW	0.11	2.21*	0.48
	T3 Behaviour	T2 Behaviour	0.46 (0.67)	9.84**	0.46
		T2 BE	0.10 (0.22)	2.02*	0.48
		T2 BW	0.24	4.74**	0.51
Part B: Predicting Concurrent PV	T1 PV	T1 Behaviour	0.09 (0.25)	1.41	0.06
		T1 BE	0.23 (0.24)	3.70**	0.10
		T1 BW	0.04	0.65	0.10
	T2 PV	T2 Behaviour	0.09 (0.43)	3.34**	0.19
		T2 BE	0.37 (0.38)	6.26**	0.27
		T2 BW	0.02	0.41	0.27
	T3 PV	T3 Behaviour	0.34 (0.56)	5.63**	0.32
		T3 BE	0.27 (0.28)	4.79**	0.36
		T3 BW	0.05	0.83	0.36

Note: Betas at entry are in parentheses. $*p < 0.05$ $**p < 0.001$.

other, sharing about 40–45% of their variance ($M\ r = 0.67$), and they were both correlated with smoking behaviour ($M\ r = 0.65$ and 0.68). In addition, the mean of BW exceeded BE, and both increased along with behaviour over time. Table 7.2 presents results of two hierarchical regression analyses. In the first analysis (Part A), using some data reported in a previous study (i.e., waves 2 and 3 in Gibbons et al., 1998), smoking behaviour was predicted by the following measures, entered in this order: previous behaviour, BE, and, finally, BW. Because previous behaviour is included, these prospective analyses actually are predicting change in behaviour over tine. Results from the final step are displayed in the table along with the βs in parentheses for previous behaviour and BE at their entry (steps 1 and 2, respectively). The coefficient for previous behaviour, i.e., behavioural stability, was quite high (both βs > 0.45, $p < 0.001$). Nonetheless, BE did predict above and beyond previous behaviour, and then BW predicted net both behaviour and BE. These results remained essentially unchanged when the adolescents who were regular smokers were excluded from the analyses, and when the criterion was switched to just current smoking behaviour.

Personal Vulnerability

Part B of the table presents results of the analyses in which PV was regressed on the same variables in the same order as was behaviour in Part A, but this time the criterion and the predictors were all assessed concurrently. Previous behaviour was strongly related to PV at the time it entered the equation (all $p < 0.001$), and remained significant at T2 and T3, after BE was entered. In addition, BE was also strongly related to PV to smoking risk (all $ps < 0.001$). The more these adolescents expected to smoke in the future, taking into account their current smoking, the more PV to smoking-related illnesses they acknowledged. In contrast, there was no relation between BW and PV at all (this was the case for both absolute and comparative PV, and for non-regular smokers as well as the entire sample). Comparison of the βs for BW vs. BE indicated that the BE βs were significantly stronger than the BW βs in each instance (all $ps < 0.001$). In short, even though BW predicted behaviour it was not (independently) related to PV.

Given the zero-order correlation between BW and PV ($M\ r = 0.37$), the lack of any relation between them in the regression is surprising. When the regressions were re-run, reversing the order of entry of BW and BE, however, BW did relate significantly to PV (net behaviour) at all three waves, when it was first entered (βs $= 0.13$, 0.21 and 0.15; $ps < 0.03$, 0.001 and 0.01); it became nonsignificant only when BE was entered. What this suggests is that the variance in BW that does relate to PV is the variance that it shares with BE. To test this directly, we conducted a commonality analysis (Pedhazur, 1982), which assessed the contributions of the unique and shared variance of the two constructs. This analysis indicated that the unique variance of BE (R^2 increments: T1 = 3%; T2 = 6%; T3 = 3%), but not BW (all R^2 increments < 0.1%), related significantly to PV. An additional amount of variance in PV, albeit small (1% or 2% increments in R^2), was explained by the variance shared by BW and BE.

DISCUSSION

As in previous studies, both expectations and willingness to engage in risky behaviour predicted subsequent involvement in that behaviour, taking into account previous behaviour, and they did so independent of one another (Gibbons et al., 1998). Only expectations of behaviour were independently associated with a recognition of risk, however. The lack of relation between BW and PV was not attributable to the fact that those who were 'only' willing but not intending to smoke actually smoked less, because we had accounted for amount of behaviour in the regression equation. One possible interpretation of the lack of independent relation between BW and PV is that those adolescents who were willing, but not intending, did not believe they would be able to smoke in the future. If they can't smoke they aren't at risk. This seems unlikely given the availability of substances such as tobacco among young people; but it is the case that a belief that one is not personally vulnerable to negative consequences because one will not have the opportunity to engage does reflect rational, and perhaps even deliberative, reasoning. Yet another possibility is that BW is associated with avoidance of risk consideration, and a denial of personal vulnerability. That is, adolescents rationalize their willingness to engage in an unhealthy behaviour by denying or minimizing their PV to its associated risk. This type of dissonance reduction – the idea being 'If I were to try it, I could get away with it' – is similar to the logic demonstrated by smokers who reduce their PV to smoking risk after they have quit and then relapsed (Gibbons et al., 1997).

One way to assess these two possibilities would be to eliminate likelihood or opportunity to engage as a variable; in other words, ask subjects what their personal risk would be *if* they were to engage in the behaviour, a form of conditional personal vulnerability (ConPV). If BW involves some denial of risk, then a negative relation between it and ConPV would be expected. In other words, the more willing they are to engage in a risk behaviour, the more likely they would be to think they could 'get away with it,' *if* they were to do it. If the lack of relation between BW and absolute risk, noted in Study 1, simply reflects a belief by the willing subjects that they will not have an opportunity to engage, however, then eliminating opportunity as a variable should again result in no relation between ConPV and BW – high as well as low willing subjects would be equally likely to acknowledge some risk *if* they were to smoke.

BE and PV. A different type of reasoning applies to BE. On one hand, those who engage and those who expect to engage in risky behaviours do not completely delude themselves; they are more likely than those who do not engage to acknowledge the personal risks associated with the behaviour (Gerrard, Gibbons & Bushman, 1996). Smokers, for example, report higher personal risk of lung cancer than do nonsmokers (Chapman et al., 1993). The same is true among those who intend to smoke (as in Study 1), presumably because they expect to do the behaviour. On the other hand, risk participants do show some signs of defensiveness; smokers are less convinced of the relation between smoking and lung cancer than are nonsmokers (Dawley et al., 1985). This being the case, we would expect that eliminating the differences in anticipated risk behaviour, by using a conditional measure, should result in more denial among regular participants than occasional or nonparticipants. Assume, for example, that three individuals: a nonsmoker, someone who smokes half a pack a day, and someone who smokes three packs a day, were asked 'What is the likelihood you will develop lung cancer if you were to smoke two packs a day,' the nonsmoker should report the greatest risk, and the heavy smoker the least. Hence, a negative relation between BE and ConPV was expected.

STUDY 2

In order to test these assumptions, a second series of analyses was conducted that examined a different type of risk behaviour, drunk driving, within a sample of college students. Once again, there were two parts to the analyses. First, a prospective analysis tested the extent to which BE and BW predicted drunk driving, as before, taking into account prior behaviour. Second, the concurrent relations among drunk driving behaviour, its associated BE and BW, and ConPV were assessed. Our hypotheses were the following: (a) taking into account previous behaviour, BE and BW would both predict risky behaviour independent of one another; (b) the concurrent relation between ConPV and BE will be negative; i.e., the more subjects intend to do it, the more they will think they can get away with it (even deliberative decision-making, as reflected in stated intentions, is accompanied by some defensiveness when it applies to risky behaviour (Gerrard, Gibbons, Smith & Ouellette, 1997); (c) because BW is thought to reflect more denial of risk we anticipated that its relation with ConPV would be stronger (more negative) than would the relation of BE with ConPV.

METHOD

Participants and Procedures

The first full wave of data collection (T1) was obtained from 229 male and 290 female American college students who were recruited to participate in a different ongoing study of health attitudes and health behaviours. T1 occurred during spring semester of their second year on campus. In addition, baseline data for the prospective analyses of behaviour (i.e., previous behaviour, BW and BE) were obtained 6 months earlier. Successive waves (T2 and T3) occurred 6 months later and then again 18 months after that.[5] Participants answered the questionnaires individually in our laboratory and were paid $25 each time (see Gibbons & Gerrard, 1995, for further description).

Measures

Behaviour. There were two drunk driving behaviour items at T1 and T2, and then four such items at T3. At T1 and T2, students were asked how often they had 'driven while under the influence of alcohol or drugs,' followed by a 7-pt. scale with anchors 'never' to 'frequently.' The second item was: 'Approximately how many times have you driven after drinking alcohol (more than two drinks) in the last 6 months? Please indicate a number: _____ times.'[6] These two were averaged (α at T1 and T2 = 0.71 and 0.61). Two items were added to the behaviour index at T3, which improved the α (0.89), and produced the same pattern of results as T1 and T2 (the overall α for all measures of the behaviour across the three waves, plus the baseline, was 0.91). The two new items were: 'How often in the past 12 months have you... (a) gotten drunk on alcohol at a party and then driven home; (b) driven home shortly after having several drinks of alcohol?' These were followed by scales from 1 = 'never' to 7 = 'frequently.'

Behavioural Expectations. The BE item at T1 and T2 was: 'If you were to drive in the next year, what is the likelihood that you would drive while under the influence of alcohol or drugs?' followed by a 7-pt scale with anchors 'No chance' to 'Definitely would happen.' At T3, a second BE item was added ('Do you think that you will drive under the influence of alcohol in the next year?' from 1 = 'Definitely will not' to 7 = 'Definitely will'; α = 0.95). This addition increased the predictive power of the BE measure somewhat (see Table 7.4).

Behavioural Willingness. The BW items were preceded by the same instructions as in Study 1, followed by: 'Suppose you had been drinking alcohol (several drinks) and it was time for you to go home. Under these circumstances, how likely is it that you would do *each* of the following? (a) go ahead and drive yourself home; (b) ask someone else to drive you home.' The two options were each accompanied by a 7-pt. scale with anchors 'not at all likely' to 'very likely.' The second item was reversed and then the two items were averaged (αs = 0.74, 0.60 and 0.70).

Conditional Personal Vulnerability. Finally, ConPV was assessed with a single item: 'If you were to have several drinks of alcohol and then drive, what do you think the chances are that you would be involved in an accident?' followed by a 7-pt. scale with anchors 'no chance' to 'definitely would happen.'

RESULTS

Behaviour

The means, SDs and correlations of the relevant variables are presented in Table 3. Once again, BW and BE both increased over time, and the BW means were generally greater. Part A of Table 7.4 presents results of the same type of hierarchical regression analyses (predicting behaviour change) reported in Study 1 for the three waves of data. As can be seen in the table, stability of drunk driving behaviour was very high for the first two waves (βs > 0.53), and then was lower for the third wave, which had an 18-month time lag. More important, BE predicted change in drunk driving behaviour at all three waves (all $ps < 0.001$), and BW predicted significantly at two of the three waves (both $ps < 0.05$), and did so net BE, as expected.

Personal Vulnerability

Part B of Table 7.4 presents results of the final step of the hierarchical regression in which ConPV was regressed first on behaviour, then BW, and then BE, for all three waves of data. As in Study 1, all measures in the PV analyses were assessed concurrently. The βs for both behaviour and BE in the blocks at which they were first entered are presented in parentheses. As can be seen, behaviour was negatively related to ConPV at the time it entered the equation, although in each case it became nonsignificant when BE, or BE and BW entered. Similarly, BE was a predictor of ConPV at each wave at the time it was entered (the more they expected to do it, the less ConPV they acknowledged), but became nonsignificant when BW was entered – a pattern essentially opposite to that seen in Study 1. More important, BW was strongly related to ConPV: the more willing they were to drink and drive, taking into account both prior behaviour and BE, the less likely they thought it was that they would have an accident if they did (all $|\beta s| > 0.34$, $p < 0.0001$). In each case, the β for BW was significantly stronger than that for BE (all $ps < 0.001$). These results remained essentially the same when conducted separately for only those who reported they had engaged in the behaviour. Finally, a commonality analysis was again conducted examining the contributions of BW

Table 7.3 Means, SDs, correlations among drunk driving behaviour, BE, BW, and ConPV across three waves of data (Study 2)

	Time 1 (N = 519)				Time 2 (N = 475)				Time 3 (N = 408)			
	B	BE	BW	ConPV	B	BE	BW	ConPV	B	BE	BW	ConPV
Time 1												
Behaviour					0.70	0.54	0.36	-0.21	0.56	0.48	0.31	-0.15
BE	0.67				0.60	0.75	0.55	-0.39	0.67	0.65	0.53	-0.29
BW	0.52	0.66			0.45	0.57	0.69	-0.48	0.52	0.51	0.61	-0.37
ConPV	-0.25	-0.35	-0.49		-0.20	-0.34	-0.39	0.65	-0.32	-0.32	-0.44	0.60
Time 2												
Behaviour									0.52	0.49	0.34	-0.18
BE					0.65	0.63			0.64	0.67	0.56	-0.33
BW					0.45				0.49	0.51	0.61	-0.38
ConPV					-0.27	-0.38	-0.50		-0.29	-0.34	-0.48	0.61
Time 3												
Behaviour												
BE									0.79	0.68		
BW									0.58			
ConPV									-0.35	-0.43	-0.48	
MEAN	1.54	2.15	2.34	4.98	1.86	2.27	2.44	4.73	1.92	2.46	2.67	4.50
SD	2.15	1.59	1.41	1.28	3.00	1.63	1.36	1.27	1.12	1.65	1.47	1.27

Note: B = Behaviour, BE = Behavioural Expectation, BW = Behavioural Willingness, ConPV = Conditional Personal Vulnerability. Prospective correlations for T1 behaviour with *baseline* variables (not reported here) are: $r = 0.74$ for behaviour, $r = 0.60$ for BE, and $r = 0.44$ for BW. Ns for correlations across time periods (e.g., T1 with T3) range from 399 to 464. All $ps < 0.01$.

Table 7.4 Hierarchical regressions of drunk driving behaviour (Part A), and ConPV to alcohol-related accidents (Part B) on previous behaviour, BE and BW (Study 2)

	Criterion	Predictors	β	t	R^2
Part A: Predicting Subsequent Behaviour	T1 Behaviour	Baseline Beh	0.59 (0.74)	18.96**	0.55
		Baseline BE	0.24 (0.31)	6.32**	0.62
		Baseline BW	0.12	3.43**	0.63
	T2 Behaviour	T1 Behaviour	0.54 (0.70)	12.57**	0.49
		T1 BE	0.23 (0.24)	4.54**	0.53
		T1 BW	0.03	0.53	0.53
	T3 Behaviour	T2 Behaviour	0.17 (0.51)	3.53**	0.26
		T2 BE	0.45 (0.52)	7.85**	0.42
		T2 BW	0.11	2.17*	0.43
Part B: Predicting Concurrent PV	T1 PV	T1 Behaviour	0.03 (−0.25)	0.66	0.06
		T1 BE	−0.07 (−0.33)	−1.23	0.12
		T1 BW	−0.46	−8.90**	0.24
	T2 PV	T2 Behaviour	−0.01 (−0.27)	−0.21	0.07
		T2 BE	−0.10 (−0.36)	−1.71	0.15
		T2 BW	−0.43	−8.49**	0.26
	T3 PV	T3 Behaviour	−0.05 (−0.38)	−0.75	0.14
		T3 BE	−0.15 (−0.35)	−1.91	0.19
		T3 BW	−0.35	−5.89**	0.25

Note: Betas at entry are in parentheses. *$p < 0.05$ **$p < 0.001$.

and BE to the prediction of ConPV. This analysis indicated that the unique variance of BW (R^2 increments: T1 = 12%; T2 = 11%, and T3 = 6%), and the variance it shared with BE (R^2 increments: T1 = 6%; T2 = 7%; and T3 = 4%) both related to ConPV, but there was no unique relation between BE and ConPV (all R^2 increments < 1%).

DISCUSSION

As in previous studies of drunk driving, those who had done it before were more likely to report that they could do it in the future without negative consequences (Agostinelli & Miller, 1994; Guppy, 1993). In addition, both expectations and willingness to drink and drive were also related to perceived immunity. However, BE became nonsignificant at each wave when BW was added into the equation. Thus, the only variance within BE that was related to ConPV (i.e., defensiveness) was the variance that it shared with BW. In contrast, the relation between BW and ConPV existed independent of BE; and it existed independent of previous behaviour, which means, once again, it was not simply the result of some of the students having engaged in the behaviour in the past without consequence (Martens, Ross & Mundt, 1991). It also was not related to other 'logical' factors, such as ethanol tolerance, weight, or gender.[7] In short, there was little evidence of what could be considered 'reasoned action' associated with subjects' BW, even though it was related to their behaviour. Instead, their willingness appeared to reflect some defensiveness on their part.

Given the concurrent nature of the assessment of BW and ConPV, an alternative causal path must be considered, which is that conditional risk judgments precede BW. In other words, it is possible that adolescents are willing to engage in a risk behaviour because they believe they are immune to its negative consequences. In fact, some risk consideration probably does precede BE, and even BW, among adolescents. However, the idea that perceptions of low risk lead to either BW or BE appears to us to be a less plausible cognitive sequence. First, it seems unlikely that adolescents give a lot of serious consideration to the consequences of a particular behaviour before they consider engaging in it (cf. Brown, DiClemente & Reynolds, 1991). That type of reasoning may be more common among adults (however, Gibbons et al., 1997, reported that adult smokers' change in smoking PV *followed* their behaviour – i.e., relapse – rather than preceded it). Second, the interpretation that perceptions of PV $\rightarrow$ BE would suggest a parallel, but somewhat illogical interpretation of the data from Study 1, which is that the positive correlation between PV and BE in that study was due to the fact that recognition of PV to smoking risk led to greater intention or expectation of smoking (prior behaviour being held constant). Although the causal direction of the relation is not crucial to the central focus of the paper (i.e., the difference between BW and BE), we recognize the causal ambiguity inherent in our correlational data; that ambiguity may be resolved in future studies. In the meantime, we would suggest that the relation between ConPV and both BW and BE is most likely nonrecursive. The most accurate interpretation of the current analysis, however, appears to be that willingness to engage in a behaviour promotes defensiveness regarding the likelihood of experiencing its negative consequences.

GENERAL DISCUSSION

The overall results of these two studies present a picture of the constructs of BW and BE that appears to be congruent with the reasoning of the P/W model. First, the means of the two measures were as expected: willingness to engage in health risk behaviour was greater than intention (more so for the younger sample), and both tended to increase over time along with behaviour. Second, the two constructs were correlated with one another, but, as was evident in the regressions, were not redundant; each one predicted change in behaviour and did so net the other (cf. Gibbons et al., 1998). Those regression (commonality) analyses also indicated that the variance shared by BW and BE related directly to the two types of PV. In Study 1, the variance that BW shared with BE was related to perceived risk, but there was no independent relation between BW and risk. In Study 2, the variance that BE shared with BW related to ConPV (and that relation was negative, indicating defensiveness), but this time there was no independent relation between BE and ConPV.

What this shared variance suggests is that BW does include an element of planning and forethought, just as BE includes an element of defensiveness. It is the variance that they do *not* share, however, that provides evidence of discriminant validity between the two constructs. Moreover, their independence is consistent with two basic contentions of the P/W model: (a) that there are two paths to adolescent risk behaviour, one deliberate, the other reactive; and (b) that these paths share some influential factors, such as attitudes toward the behaviour and perceptions of norms, but ultimately influence behaviour through distinct proximal antecedents and through processes that are distinguishable.

Decision-making

Although there was some evidence of defensiveness associated with BE in Study 2, generally speaking, it would appear that consideration of risk followed a process quite similar to that outlined by the Theories of Reasoned Action and Planned Behaviour, and by other rational models as well. The relation between PV and smoking expectations was strong at each wave for the adolescents (all $\beta s > 0.23$, $ps < 0.002$), suggesting that those who were expecting to smoke had given at least some thought to the negative outcomes associated with the behaviour. In contrast, there was relatively little evidence of 'reasoned' thought associated with subjects' willingness to engage in the behaviour – i.e., evidence that either the adolescents who were willing to smoke (a number of whom did) or the young adults who were willing to drink and drive had contemplated the behaviours and of their outcomes in a rational manner. In fact, the opposite appeared to be the case for drunk driving: the more willing they were to imbibe and drive, the more defensive they were, which means the less likely they were to acknowledge personal risk.

This defensiveness is consistent with the reactive nature of willingness. Placing some of the responsibility for the behaviour within its social context, as is the case with willingness to act, obviates a need for serious contemplation and much of the deliberative effort that rational models of behaviour suggest accompany a decision to perform a particular behaviour. Moreover, we suspect this applies both prospectively and retrospectively. On one hand, willing adolescents may assume that whether or not they engage in risk behaviours in the future will be determined by factors that are external to themselves and perhaps not entirely within their control. On the other hand, 'willing' adolescents who have engaged in 'unintended' risk behaviour in the past may also conclude that these previous incidents were largely attributable to external factors. In both cases, there is little acceptance of responsibility.

Consideration of Risk

Although BW involves less deliberation than does intention, we do not believe that it (BW) is simply the result of cursory or 'top of the head' (Langer, 1989) responding. The fact that some cognitive elements relate to it, apparently in a causal fashion (Blanton et al., 1997), suggests that some consideration of the behaviour has occurred. For example, a belief that others are doing the behaviour or that they are favorably predisposed toward it is associated with greater willingness to do it (Gibbons et al., 1998). That consideration appears to involve primarily social factors, however, and has not carried through to the point of a logical deliberation of possible negative outcomes.

Another contextual factor that is associated with a willingness to engage in behaviour is the social image that one has of the type of person who does it. This image includes a number of characteristics that young people associate with the behaviour, such as independence; but, for those who are doing the behaviour, vulnerability is apparently not one of those characteristics. Once again, this reflects the social or external perspective associated with the construct; the consequences of the behaviour are more external – What will others think of me? What will I look like? – than internal – What will happen to me? Will I be injured? Consistent with this thinking, other analyses we have conducted have demonstrated that willingness to drink excessively, for example, is more closely related to the social expectancies (Brown, Christiansen & Goldman, 1987) associated with alcohol consumption (e.g., its impact on sociability) than to expectancies associated with its *physiological* effects (e.g., relaxation).

The Relation between BW and BE

Defining acceptable behaviour. Although the current results indicate that BE and BW have independent relations with behaviour, it is also clearly the case that the two constructs are related to one another. In fact, for many young people, BW and BE are congruent – they are either intending and willing to engage or they're not. These individuals have identified a latitude of acceptance (Sherif & Hovland, 1961) regarding certain activities, and their willingness most likely defines the limits or risky boundary of the behaviours included within this range (seldom would one's behavioural intentions be riskier than one's behavioural willingness). These individuals are likely to have given some thought to the behaviour and its consequences and to have a plan of action that they could implement. Results of the current and previous studies, however, indicate that there is another significant subset of adolescents who are not intending to engage in risk, but are willing to do so. It may very well be the case that what these young people are willing to do, under certain circumstances, actually falls outside of their latitudes of acceptance. In other words, they realize the behaviour (e.g., drunk driving) is inappropriate and do not plan on doing it; but they are nonetheless open to the possibility should the opportunity afford itself. Not only is this hypothesis interesting, it also has implications for risk interventions (see below) and therefore seems worthy of future investigation.

A behavioural sequence: BW → BE. The P/W model also proposes a temporal or maturational link between BW and BE. For example, although relatively few adolescents intend to smoke cigarettes, drink heavily, or have unprotected sex (fewer than actually do it; Gibbons et al., 1996; Brooks-Gunn & Furstenberg, 1989), some are willing. Thus, the manifestation of these behaviours among adolescents is usually a result of BW rather than BE (cf. Blanton et al., 1997).

If this manifestation continues, many of them will come to realize that their willingness to behave does, sometimes, result in the behaviour. Assuming these experiences have not been aversive, their willingness most likely will progress into intention. Thus, for some behaviours (such as substance use), the BW and BE curves will tend to converge. Eventually, BE will become dominant, at which point awareness and acknowledgment of PV and risk are likely to increase.

Not all willingness develops into intention, however. For some individuals, certain risk behaviours are always thought to be (and may very well be) reactions to circumstances that they did not create or consciously promote. This is analogous to the dieter who claims (facetiously, of course) that the chocolate soufflé she consumed after dinner really had very few calories because it was proffered by a friend and not actually ordered. For these people, full acknowledgment of risk may never happen. The behaviour may only occur on certain occasions that are unexpected and perhaps rare; but it will happen. In short, for some people and some behaviours, BW is a developmental antecedent to BE; for others and other behaviours (e.g., adultery, recreational drug use; cf. Buunk & Gibbons, 1996), willingness may remain a social reaction and never develop into a reasoned or even intended action.

Which is Worse?

The adolescent who intends to smoke or take drugs can certainly find the resources to do so, and most of them eventually will. Moreover, the fact that BE is usually more closely linked with behaviour than is BW might lead one to conclude that BE is more of a concern for health educators and counselors. The relation of both constructs with PV suggests that may not necessarily be the case, however. PV has been linked with a number of risk behaviours, both prospectively and retrospectively (Harrison, Mullen & Green, 1992; Janz & Becker, 1984; see Footnote 7) and, in fact, it is a central element in most models of health behaviour (Weinstein, 1993). For example, Weinstein (1988) has suggested that acknowledgment of risk is an important step in the sequence leading up to the adoption of health precaution. What the current data suggest is that some of the adolescents who are willing, but not intending, to engage in risk have not yet reached that stage; in fact, the ConPV results suggest they may actually be avoiding or denying it. As a result, the 'willing adolescent' may be less likely than an 'intending adolescent' to take precautionary actions, such as carrying a condom or arranging ahead of time for a 'designated driver.' In this sense, the social reaction path may be more dangerous.

Premeditation and pregnancy protection. A similar dynamic has been demonstrated in regard to the relation between the disposition of sex guilt (Mosher, 1973) and another type of risky behaviour, unprotected sex. Although adolescents with high sex guilt typically do not intend to have intercourse, a number of them eventually do (Gerrard, 1987). In this sense, they are similar to the adolescents in the current studies who did not intend to drink and drive or smoke, but were willing to, and then did. Because their sexual behaviour is not planned, and because effective contraception requires planning, high-guilt, sexually-active adolescents often fail to protect themselves from unplanned pregnancy and sexually transmitted diseases (Gerrard, 1982; Mosher, 1973). In short, there is some benefit to acknowledging an intention to engage in behaviour that is risky (drunk driving), or potentially risky (sex).

Practical Implications. At the same time, there are reasons for optimism with regard to the prospects for altering BW as opposed to BE. The first and simplest reason has to do with the issue of perceived 'ownership' of the behaviour. It would be safe to assume that those who are 'only' willing and not intending to do it are less committed to the behaviour; presumably, they will be more open to efforts to dissuade them from doing it. A second, related reason is that because BW represents a more socially-oriented perspective, it should be more amenable to attempts to modify (its) social antecedents. Along these lines, there are several aspects of the BW construct that lead us to expect that efforts to lower willingness and/or bring it more in line with intentions may be successful. First, results of the current analyses suggest that encouraging young people to seriously consider the potential negative consequences of various risk behaviours would be effective. Many of them have not given much thought to these consequences. This would be the case for all young people, of course, but especially those who are willing but not intending – a group that has apparently avoided considering these consequences, and may be denying them.

Another characteristic of BW that suggests it may be amenable to change has to do with its relation with perceived culpability. According to the P/W model, willingness is a reaction (openness) to risk opportunity – opportunity that is often not sought nor created by the individual. As such, it involves relatively little acceptance of responsibility for the behaviour or its consequences (the idea being, 'I never intended to do it, so I can't really be blamed for what happened'). In fact, we find that self-reports of BW tend to be higher when the hypothetical risk scenario is described in such a way that responsibility can be externally attributed. In contrast, because intended behaviour is planned and premeditated, it is more difficult to deny responsibility for it and the harm it may produce. Thus, interventions that encourage young people to accept responsibility for their risk behaviour and its potential consequences should help reduce levels of BW. Once again, that should be particularly true for those whose BW exceeds their intentions.

Finally, the social images or prototypes that are precursors to BW (but not to intention; see Gibbons & Gerrard, 1997; Gibbons et al., 1998) are often based on misperceptions of others' attitudes and opinions toward the behaviour – a type of 'pluralistic ignorance' (Prentice & Miller, 1993; Gibbons & Gerrard, 1997). More specifically, young people typically overestimate the extent to which their friends and peers maintain favourable opinions of risk behaviours and people who engage in them (i.e., risk images), much as they tend to overestimate the extent to which their friends are engaging in the behaviours (Marks, Graham & Hansen, 1992). Thus efforts to educate an adolescent as to the actual opinions of his/her peers about the type of person who engages in these behaviours – opinions that are often considerably more negative than she/he realises – should result in less willingness to engage in the behaviour, and that alteration should be mediated by a change in the associated social image.

Limitations

Before concluding, some limitations to these data and our interpretations of them should be mentioned. First, we chose to use a BE measure and not a BI measure. As indicated previously, we believe this provides a conservative test of the distinction between reactive and deliberative behaviour, but it does mean that we were not directly assessing students' stated intentions to engage. Second, BE in Study 1 and ConPV in Study 2 were assessed with single items and that raises some questions about their reliabilities. Third, we did not assess both ConPV and PV for the two behaviours in the two studies, which means we cannot determine for sure if the different pattern of results was due to the type of cognition being assessed or the type of behaviour with which it was associated. These last two issues are being addressed in current studies. Finally, it is worth noting that the constructs that correlated most highly in Study 2 also were most similar in wording. BE and behaviour both included timeframes whereas BW and ConPV did not. In addition, BW and ConPV were both worded in the subjunctive, whereas BE and (of course) behaviour were not. This measurement difference could have contributed to the magnitude of the relations between the two pairs of variables. We do not believe that any of these points argues against the interpretations of the results presented here, or suggests alternative interpretations that are more viable. Nonetheless, taken together, they do indicate that some caution is warranted in evaluating our interpretations.

CONCLUSIONS

As the P/W model would predict, BW and BE are related constructs, but they involve different cognitive processes and, therefore, are conceptually and empirically distinguishable. In particular, those who are intending to engage in risky behaviour acknowledge their personal risk; those who are only willing to engage do not. In contrast, those who are willing are more likely to deny the relation between the risk behaviour and its personal consequences than are those who are intending to engage. We believe these distinctions reflect differences in degrees of 'ownership,' and consideration of consequences, of future risk behaviours.

Acknowledgements:

This research was supported by NIMH grant MH 48165-01 and NIAAA grant AA 10208-02. The authors thank Dan Russell for his comments on the manuscript.

NOTES

1. The Theory of Planned Behaviour (Ajzen, 1985) adds the construct of perceived behavioural control to the elements of the Theory of Reasoned Action. Ajzen (1991)

has shown that for behaviours that are difficult to perform (e.g., dieting), perceived behavioural control can have a direct influence on behaviour, independent of BI. With this exception, however, *all* 'pathways' to behaviour proceed through BI in both theories.

2. The P/W model is somewhat more circumscribed in its perspective than these other models – it concerns cognitive processes that are associated with decision making primarily relevant to health and health risk, and that are much more common among adolescents.

3. When we ask adolescents if they could obtain substances such as tobacco or alcohol, or find a sexual partner, the vast majority say they could. That is the case whether they are willing or not. Thus, BW is not a proxy for perceived behavioural control. Moreover, confirmatory factor analyses (Gibbons et al., 1998) have demonstrated statistical independence among the constructs of BW, BI, and perceived behavioural control, including refusal efficacy (ability to 'say no').

4. We have also used two items (see Study 2) or three items to assess the BE construct, but have found that a single, face-valid item ('How likely it is …') usually works just as well. Willingness is typically assessed with either 3 or 4 items, depending on the behaviour involved. It makes little difference, in terms of prediction, if the willingness scenario involves some social influence (e.g., a friend offers a cigarette, as was the case in this study) or not (e.g., alcohol is simply available; you want to have sex, but no contraception is available).

5. In fact, our first contact with this sample occurred during the fall of their first year on campus, a year earlier. Thus, the baseline reported here was actually the third wave of data collection. However, one of the two earlier waves did not include all of the drunk driving measures necessary for the current analyses, and the other had very little drunk driving behavior reported. Nonetheless, the pattern across these first two waves was essentially the same as that reported here, but with less variance in the behaviour to predict. For brevity, only waves 3–5, plus the baseline for the prospective analysis, are presented here.

6. Three or more (or 'several') drinks is a common cut-off for signifying 'influence' (Guppy, 1993; Stacy et al., 1994), even though it may not produce a BAC above the legal limit (which varies in the U.S. according to state, but is usually around 0.08 – noticeably higher than in most European countries). We chose a lower level because these is significant impairment (especially at this age) in driving ability at three drinks. Also, although the behavioural and BE items did include mention of drug influence, very few of these students reported using drugs (e.g., only 6% reported using marijuana more than once or twice); thus, we believe it is accurate to interpret these drunk driving items as measures of alcohol influence.

7. Gerrard et al.'s (1997) study of the relation between ConPV and actual risk behaviour (substance use and abuse) found that ConPV (e.g., the alcohol consumption-accident vulnerability measure reported here) did predict changes in risk behaviour. For example, those who thought they could drive while under the influence and not become involved in an accident were more likely to increase their drunk driving behaviour over time. This adds some significance to the ConPV measure. In addition, Gerrard et al.'s analyses indicated that alternative factors, such as ethanol tolerance, weight, and gender, were related to ConPV, as would be expected (cf. Agostinelli & Miller, 1994), but did not explain the relation between ConPV and BW or between ConPV and behaviour. In short, there was no obvious 'rational' explanation for subjects' perceived immunity to the negative consequences of drunk driving behaviour.

REFERENCES

Aberg, L. (1994). Relations among variable influencing drivers' intentions to drive after drinking. In D. R. Rutter and L. Quine (eds.), *Social Psychology and Health: European Perspectives* (pp. 89–100). Aldershot, England: Avebury.

Agostinelli, G. & Miller, W. R. (1994). Drinking and thinking: How does personal drinking affect judgments of prevalence and risk? *Journal of Studies on Alcohol*, **55**, 327–337.

Ajzen, I. (1985). From intentions to actions: A theory of planned behavior. In J. Kuhl and J. Beckman (eds.), *Action Control: From Cognition to Behavior* (pp. 11–39). Berlin: Springer.

Ajzen, I. (1988). *Attitudes, Personality, and Behavior*. Chicago: Dorsey.

Ajzen, I. (1991). The theory of planned behavior. *Organizational Behaviour and Human Decision Processes*, **50**, 179–211.

Ajzen, I. & Fishbein, M. (1980). *Understanding attitudes and predicting social behaviour*. Englewood Cliffs, NJ: Prentice Hall.

Bagozzi, R. P. (1992). The self-regulation of attitudes, intentions and behaviour. *Social Psychology Quarterly*, **55**, 178–204.

Bagozzi, R. P. & Warshaw, P. R. (1992). An examination of the etiology of the attitude-behaviour relation for goal-directed behavior. *Multivariate Behavioural Research*, **27**, 601–634.

Beck, L. & Ajzen, I. (1991). Predicting dishonest actions using the theory of planned behavior. *Journal of Research in Personality*, **25**, 285–301.

Blanton, H., Gibbons, F. X., Gerrard, M., Conger, K. J. & Smith, G. E. (1997). Development of health risk prototypes during adolescence: Family and peer influences. *Journal of Family Psychology*, **11**, 1–18.

Brooks-Gunn, J. & Furstenberg, F. F., Jr. (1989). Adolescent sexual behavior. *American Psychologist*, **44**, 249–257.

Brown, S. A., Christiansen, B. A. & Goldman, M. S. (1987). The alcohol expectancy questionnaire: An instrument for the assessment of adolescent and adult alcohol expectancies. *Journal of Studies on Alcohol*, **48**, 483–491.

Brown, L. K., DiClemente, R. J. & Reynolds, L. A. (1991). HIV prevention for adolescents: Utility of the health belief model. *AIDS Education and Prevention*, **3**, 50–59.

Buunk, B. & Gibbons, F. X. (1996). *Temptations: Can prototypes predict adultery?* Research in progress.

Centers for Disease Control (1992). Recent trends in adolescent smoking, smoking-uptake correlates, and expectations about the future. *Advance Data*, No. 221.

Centers for Disease Control (1993). Teenage pregnancy and birth rates – United States 1990. *Morbidity and Mortality Weekly Report*, **42**, 39.

Chapman, S., Wong, W. L. & Smith, W. (1993). Self-exempting belief about smoking and health: Differences between smokers and ex-smokers. *American Journal of Public Health*, **83**, 215–219.

Conner, M. & Sparks, P. (1996). The theory of planned behaviour and health behaviours. In M. Conner and P. Norman (eds.), *Predicting Health Behaviour: Research and Practice with Social Cognition Models* (pp. 121–162). Buckingham, U.K.: Open University Press.

Dawley, H. H., Fleischer, B. J. & Dawley, L. T. (1985). The discouragement of smoking in a hospital setting. *International Journal of the Addictions*, **20**, 783–793.

Dovidio, J. F. & Fazio, R. H. (1992). New technologies for the direct and indirect assessment of attitudes. In J. M. Tanur (ed.), *Questions About Questions* (pp. 204–237). New York: Russell Sage Foundation.

Fazio, R. H. (1990). Multiple processes by which attitudes guide a behavior: The MODE model as an integrative framework. In M. P. Zanna (ed.), *Advances in Experimental Social Psychology*. (Vol. 23, pp. 75–109). San Diego, CA: Academic Press.

Fishbein, M. & Ajzen, I. (1975). *Belief, Attitude, Intention, and Behaviour: An Introduction to Theory and Research*. Reading, MA: Addison-Wesley.

Fishbein, M. & Ajzen, I. (1980). Predicting and understanding consumer behavior: Attitudes-behavior correspondence. In I. Ajzen and M. Fishbein (eds.), *Understanding Attitudes and Predicting Social Behavior* (pp. 148–172). Englewood Cliffs, NJ: Prentice-Hall.

Fishbein, M. & Stasson, M. (1990). The role of desires, self-predictions, and perceived control in the prediction of training session attendance. *Journal of Applied Social Psychology*, **20**, 173–198.

Gerrard, M. (1982). Sex, sex guilt, and contraceptive use. *Journal of Personality and Social Psychology*, **42**, 153–158.

Gerrard, M. (1987). Sex, sex guilt, and contraceptive use revisited: Trends in the 1980's. *Journal of Personality and Social Psychology*, **52**, 975–980.

Gerrard, M., Gibbons, F. X., Benthin, A. C. & Hessling, R. M. (1996). The reciprocal nature of risk behaviors and cognitions: What you think shapes what you do and vice versa. *Health Psychology*, **15**, 344–354.

Gerrard, M., Gibbons, F. X., Love, D. J. &. Ouellette, J. (1997). *Does optimistic bias promote risk behavior?* Research in progress.

Gerrard, M., Gibbons, F. X. & Bushman, B. J. (1996). The relation between perceived vulnerability to HIV and precautionary sexual behavior. *Psychological Bulletin*, **119**, 390–409.

Gerrard, M., Gibbons, F. X., Zhao, L., Russell, D. W., & Reis-Bergan, M. (1999). The effect of peers' alcohol consumption on parental influence: A cognitive mediational model. *Journal of Studies on Alcohol*, 13, 32–44.

Gibbons, F. X., Eggleston, T. J. & Benthin, A. (1997). Cognitive reactions to smoking relapse: The reciprocal relation between dissonance and self-esteem. *Journal of Personality and Social Psychology*, **72**, 184–195.

Gibbons, F. X. & Gerrard, M. (1995). Predicting young adults' health risk behaviour. *Journal of Personality and Social Psychology*, **69**, 505–517.

Gibbons, F. X. & Gerrard, M. (1997). Health images and their effects on health behaviour. In B. P. Buunk and F. X. Gibbons (eds.), *Health, Coping, and Well-Being: Perspectives from Social Comparison Theory*. (pp. 63–94) Hillsdale, NJ: Erlbaum.

Gibbons, F. X., Gerrard, M., Blanton, H. & Russell, D. W. (1998). Reasoned action and social reaction: Willingness and intention as independent predictors of health risk. *Journal of Personality and Social Psychology*, **74**, 1164–1181.

Gibbons, F. X., Gerrard, M. & Boney-McCoy, S. (1995). Prototype perception predicts (lack of) pregnancy prevention. *Personality and Social Psychology Bulletin*, **21**, 85–93.

Gibbons, F. X., Gerrard, M. & Love, D. J. (in press). A social reaction model of adolescent health risk. In J. M. Suls and K. Wallston (eds.), Social Psychological Foundations of Health and Illness. Oxford: Blackwell.

Gibbons, F. X., McGovern, P. G. & Lando, H. A. (1991). Relapse and risk perception among members of a smoking cessation clinic. *Health Psychology*, **10**, 42–45.

Godin, G., Valois, P. & Lepage, L. (1993). The pattern of influence of perceived behavioral control upon exercising behavior. An application of Ajzen's theory of planned behavior. *Journal of Behavioral Medicine*, **16**, 81–102.

Graham, J. W., Marks, G. & Hansen, W. B. (1991). Social influence processes affecting adolescent substance use. *Journal of Applied Psychology*, **76**, 291–298.

Guppy, A. (1993). Subjective probability of accident and apprehension in relation to self-other bias, age, and reported behavior. *Accident Analysis and Prevention*, **25**, 375–382.

Hanison, J. A., Mullen, P. D. & Green, L. W. (1992). A meta-analysis of studies of the health belief model with adults. *Health Education Research*, **7**, 107–116.

Janz, N. K. & Becker, M. H. (1984). The health belief model: A decade later. *Health Education Quarterly*, **11**, 1–47.

Johnson, V. (1988). Adolescent alcohol and marijuana use: A longitudinal assessment of a social learning perspective. *American Journal of Drug and Alcohol Abuse*, **14**, 419–439.

Kandel, D. B. (1980). Drug and drinking behavior among youth. *Annual Review of Sociology*, **6**, 235–285.

Klesges, R. C., Somes, G., Pascale, R. W., Klesges, L. M., et al. (1988). Knowledge of beliefs regarding the consequences of cigarette smoking and their relationships to smoking status in a biracial sample. *Health Psychology*, **7**, 387–401.

Kruglanski, A. W. (1975). The endogenous-exogenous partition in attribution theory. *Psychological Review*, **82**, 387–406.

Langer E. J. (1989). *Mindfulness*. Reading, MA: Addison-Wesley.

Marks, G., Graham, J. W. & Hansen, W. B. (1992). Social projection and social conformity in adolescent substance use: A longitudinal analysis. *Personality and Social Psychology Bulletin*, **18**, 96–101.

Martens, C. H., Ross, L. E. & Mundt, J. C. (1991). Young drivers' evaluation of driving impairment due to alcohol. *Accident Analysis and Prevention*, **23**, 67–76.

Morojele, N. K. & Stephenson, G. M. (1994). Addictive behaviours: Predictors of abstinence intentions and expectations in the Theory of Planned Behaviour. In D. R. Rutter & L. Quine (eds.), *Social Psychology and Health: European Perspectives*. Aldershot, England: Avebury.

Mosher, D. L. (1973). Sex differences, sex experience, sex guilt and explicitly sexual films. *Journal of Social Issues*, 29, 95–112.

Norman, P. & Conner, M. (1996). The role of social cognition models in predicting health behaviours: Future directions. In M. Conner & P. Norman (eds.), *Predicting Health Behaviour: Research and Practice with Social Cognition Models* (pp. 197–225). Buckingham, U.K.: Open University Press.

Parker, D., Manstead, S. R., Stradling, S. G., Reason, J. T. & Baxter, J. S. (1992). Intention to commit driving violations: An application of the theory of planned behaviour. *Journal of Applied Psychology*, **77**, 94–101.

Pedhazur, E. J. (1982). *Multiple Regression in Behavioral Research: Explanation and Prediction*. New York: Holt, Rinehart and Winston.

Petty, R. E. & Cacioppo, J. T. (1986). The elaboration likelihood model of persuasion. In L. Berkowitz (ed.), *Advances in Experiment Social Psychology* (Vol. 19, pp. 123–205). San Diego, CA: Academic Press.

Prentice, D. A. & Miller, D. T. (1993) Pluralistic ignorance and alcohol use on campus: Some consequences of misperceiving the social norm. *Journal of Personality and Social Psychology*, 64, 243–256.

Rogers, R. W. (1975). A protection motivation theory of fear appeals and attitude change. *Journal of Psychology*, **91**, 93–114.

Sheppard, B. H., Hartwick, J. & Warshaw, P. R. (1988). The theory of reasoned action: A meta-analysis of past research with recommendations for modifications and future research. *Journal of Consumer Research*, **15**, 325–343.

Sherif, M. & Hovland, C. I. (1961). *Social judgment: Assimilation and Contrast Effects in Communication and Attitude Change*. New Haven: Yale Univ. Press.

Sparks, P. & Shepherd, R. (1992). Self-identity and the theory of planned behavior: Assessing the role of identification with 'green consumerism.' *Social Psychology Quarterly*, **55**, 388–399.

Stacy, A. W., Bentler, P. M. & Flay, B. R. (1994). Attitudes and health behavior in diverse populations: Drunk driving, alcohol use, binge eating, marijuana use, and cigarette use. *Health Psychology*, **13**, 73–85.

Stein, J. A., Newcomb, M. D. & Bentler, P. M. (1987). An 8-year study of multiple influences on drug use and drug use consequences. *Journal of Personality and Social Psychology*, **53**, 1094–1105.

Sussman, S., Dent, C. W., Rauch, J. M., Johnson, C. A., Hansen, W. B. & Flay, B. R. (1988). Adolescent nonsmokers, triers, and regular smokers' estimates of cigarette smoking prevalence: When do over estimations occur and by whom? *Journal of Applied Social Psychology*, **18**, 537–555.

Sutton, S. (1994). The past predicts the future: Interpreting behaviour-behaviour relationships in social psychological model of health behaviour. In D. R. Rutter and L. Quine (eds.), *Social psychology and health: European perspectives* (pp. 71–88). Aldershot, England: Avebury.

Thaler, R. (1980). Toward a positive theory of consumer choice. *Journal of Economic Behaviour and Organization*, **1**, 39–60.

University of Michigan, Survey Research Center. (1995) *Monitoring the Future*. Ann Arbor, MI: Author.

Van den Putte, B. (1993). *On the theory of reasoned action.* Unpublished doctoral dissertation. University of Amsterdam.

Warshaw, P. R. & Davis, F. O. (1985). Disentangling behavioral intention and behavioral expectation. *Journal of Experimental Social Psychology*, **21**, 213–228.

Weinstein, N. D. (1988). The precaution adoption process. *Health Psychology*, **7**, 355–386.

Weinstein, N. D. (1993). Testing four competing theories of health-protective behavior. *Health Psychology*, **12**, 324–333.

Wells, K. (1980). Adolescents' attributions for delinquent behavior. *Personality and Social Psychology Bulletin*, **6**, 63–67.

Section 4 –
Stages of Change

CHAPTER EIGHT

The Attitude–Social Influence– Efficacy Model Applied to the Prediction of Motivational Transitions in the Process of Smoking Cessation

Hein DE VRIES, Aart MUDDE and Arie DIJKSTRA

This chapter presents the Attitude – Social influence – Efficacy Model (ASE model) (De Vries & Mudde, 1998). Moreover, two longitudinal studies are reported in which the validity of the ASE-model was tested.

The ASE model originated in the Theory of Reasoned Action (TRA) (Ajzen & Fishbein, 1980; Fishbein & Ajzen, 1975), but has evolved in several areas since Bandura's concept of self-efficacy was added to it (Bandura, 1986). Moreover, the model integrated insights of the Trans-theoretical Model (TM) (Prochaska & DiClemente, 1983), by incorporating the concept of motivational and behavioural phases. The ASE model is aimed at understanding the motives people have to engage in a particular behaviour. A variety of models are available in health psychology. A basic distinction can be made between planning models, explanatory models and change models.

Planning models focus on the description and explanation of the planning process. Well known examples of this type include the community change model developed by Bracht (1990) and the PRECEDE model (Green & Kreuter, 1991), which is probably the best known health promotion planning model. A later variant of this model is the ABC-planning model, which indicates that three basic planning phases can be distinguished in the planning, evaluation and implementation of health psychology interventions. The first, preparatory phase is the Analysis phase, which focuses for instance on analysing the motives behind health behaviours in a particular group. The second phase involves the development and testing of Behavioural interventions. The third phase is the Continuation of successful programmes by diffusing and implementing them on a regional or national scale (De Vries, 1998). Within each phase, various models can be chosen. In the first phase, for instance, a variety of explanatory models can be used to analyse people's motives to perform a particular behaviour; the ASE model is one of them. In the second phase, for example, McGuire's model of attitude change can be used to change attitudes and behaviour, while, for instance, Rogers' theory of diffusion of innovation (Rogers, E. M., 1983) can be used in the third phase.

Explanatory models focus on understanding the factors that determine a behaviour. A variety of motivational models focus on understanding peoples' motivations by analysing their cognitions, i.e., the ideas that people have about a particular (health) behaviour. The ASE model is one of a range of health psychology models that can be used (De Vries, Backbier, Kok & Dijkstra, 1995; De Vries, Dijkstra & Kuhlman, 1988; De Vries & Mudde, 1998). Other available models include the Health Belief Model (Janz & Becker, 1984), the Protection Motivation Theory (Rogers, R., 1983), and the Transtheoretical Model (TM) (Prochaska & DiClemente, 1983; Prochaska, Norcross & DiClemente, 1994). These models focus explicitly on health behaviours. Other, more general psychological models have also been applied to health behaviours, such as the Social Learning Theory (SLT) (Bandura, 1986), the Theory of Reasoned Action (TRA) (Ajzen & Fishbein, 1980; Fishbein & Ajzen, 1975) and its revised version, as described by Ajzen (1991), the Theory of Planned Behaviour (TPB), the Self-Perception Theory (Bem, 1972), and the Attribution Theory (AT) (Weiner, 1986). Some of these explanatory models and theories focus on behaviour change as well, as the TM, the SLT and the AT, and can be considered as change models. We will briefly discuss the TRA, the TM, the ASE model and the integration of the latter two.

THE THEORY OF REASONED ACTION

The TRA developed by Fishbein and Ajzen (1975) is one of the models that has often been used to explain health behaviours. The model assumes that behaviour can be predicted by the behavioural intention, which is determined by the individual's attitude and the perceived, subjective norms imposed by other people.

The theory states that behaviour is a function of a person's intention, which in turn is determined by attitudes and social norms. An attitude represents a person's general feeling of favourableness or unfavourableness regarding a behaviour (e.g. smoking is bad). Attitudes can be assessed directly by asking subjects to indicate on an evaluation scale whether a particular behaviour is, for instance, good or bad, pleasant or unpleasant, etc.. Attitudes can also be determined indirectly by assessing relevant (or salient) beliefs (b) whether the behaviour will result in specific consequences (e.g. smoking causes breathing problems) and corresponding evaluations (e) of these consequences (e.g. having breathing problems is bad). A measure for attitude can be obtained by multiplying the beliefs by the evaluations, and then adding up the products ($\Sigma b*e$).

Social norms are the perceptions that a person has about what others in the social environment expects him or her to do. The social norm, or subjective norm, can be measured directly by asking more generally whether other people who are important to the respondent think that he/she should perform a particular behaviour. Social norms can also be determined indirectly by assessing normative beliefs (nb) of important referent persons about a behaviour, and the motivations to comply (mc) with important referent persons on, e.g., smoking. A measure for social norms can be obtained by multiplying the normative beliefs by the corresponding motivation to comply, and then adding up the products: Σnb*mc.

Several recommendations to improve or adapt the Theory of Reasoned Action have been suggested (see e.g Ajzen, 1991; Bagozzi, 1992; Bentler & Speckart, 1981; Grube, Morgan, & McGee 1986). It was found, for instance, that attitudes sometimes influenced behaviour directly (see also Bagozzi, Blaumgartner, & Yi, 1989) and that the effects of past behaviour were sometimes not fully mediated by the model (Ajzen, 1991; Bagozzi, 1981; Bentler & Speckart, 1981; Fredricks & Dosset, 1983). It has therefore been suggested to include past behaviour as a factor in the model (De Vries et al., 1995). Another comment was that the model did not address self-efficacy expectations. This factor, however, has been added to the model by Ajzen and Madden (1986) and is also referred to as perceived behavioural control. The revised model is referred to as the Theory of Planned Behaviour (TPB) (Ajzen, 1991). Others have mentioned the incomplete measurement of perceived social influences and have suggested the inclusion of other concepts such as perceived behaviour and perceived social pressure against the health behaviour or the social support in favour of the health behaviour (De Vries et al., 1995; Grube et al., 1986; Urberg, Shyu, & Liang, 1990).

The use of multiplicative functions has also been criticised. In the first place, scaling effects may form a serious threat to reliability of additive product terms, meaning that researchers decisions about coding of answering options are crucial (Evans, 1991). In the second place, from a statistical point of view, the multiplicative concept is a combined concept of several interaction terms between for instance the beliefs and the evaluations of these beliefs, implying that the separate concepts (beliefs and evaluations) should be entered in the regression analyses too (Evans, 1991).

THE TRANSTHEORETICAL MODEL

The TM states that the behavioural change process should be regarded as a process consisting of five different motivational stages (Prochaska, 1994; Prochaska & DiClemente, 1983; Velicer, Fava, Prochaska, Abrams, Emmonds & Pierce, 1995). The TM proposes that two interrelated dimensions are needed to adequately assess the behavioural change process. The first dimension is labelled the stages of change. People can move from precontemplation via contemplation and preparation to action, and then to maintenance or relapse. Moreover, movement through the stages involves a cycling and recycling process. Applied to smoking cessation, this implies that smokers in precontemplation do not consider quitting. In contemplation, smokers consider cessation within six months. Preparation implies that cessation within a month is considered. In action, smokers are trying to quit which may lead to maintenance of non-smoking, or to a relapse to smoking, which in turn leads to either precontemplation, contemplation or preparation.

The second dimension is called the processes of change, focussing on ten different styles of coping activities, five of which have a more experiential nature and five a more behavioural nature (Prochaska, Redding, Harlow, Rossi & Velicer, 1994; Prochaska, Velicer, DiClemente & Fava, 1988). Recently a Dutch study tried to replicate the impact of the ten processes (De Vries, Mudde & Peters, 1997). In a cross-sectional sample of 321 smokers and ex-smokers, the processes were assessed by means of a 36-item written questionnaire. In only a minority of the processes was statistical verification for the hypotheses found, although roughly the same patterns emerged as in previous studies. An important difference was that behavioural processes were already frequently used in the contemplation stage. It is concluded that more research is needed to study the potential impact of these processes, and to analyse whether all ten processes play an important role in the explanation of health behaviour.

A third dimension concerns two sets of dependent variables that mediate stage movement (Prochaska et al., 1994). The first set is referred to as the decisional balance, which measures the pros and cons of behaviour change (Velicer, DiClemente, Prochaska & Brandenburg, 1985). Although this concept is not assumed to assess attitude, it does measure the sum of perceived beliefs regarding a particular behaviour and thus provides an estimation of the attitudes which is somewhat comparable to that obtained when measuring the sum of the beliefs (without, however, multiplying them by evaluations) according to the TRA. The second set assesses self-efficacy by measuring two related constructs: 1) a person's situation-dependent confidence in his ability to change, and 2) the situational temptations to engage in the problem behaviour (Velicer, DiClemente, Rossi & Prochaska, 1990).

Research by Prochaska and colleagues suggests that smokers moving from precontemplation to action become more convinced of the advantages of quitting and the disadvantages of smoking, while also experiencing higher levels of self-efficacy (DiClemente, Prochaska, Fairhurst, Velicer, Velasquez & Rossi, 1991; Fava, Velicer & Prochaska, 1995; Velicer et al., 1985). Furthermore, their research suggests that the five experiential processes of change are more important in precontemplation and contemplation, while the behavioural processes are more important in the action and maintenance phases (Prochaska, Norcross et al., 1994).

The Transtheoretical Model has been applied to explain a variety of health behaviours, such as smoking, nutrition, exercise (Prochaska & Di Clemente, 1998). The theory has also been subject to criticism. One criticism concerns the fact that Prochaska and colleagues use the concept of stages, while in developmental psychology this concept refers to irreversible developments (Bandura, 1997; De Vries, Mudde, Dijkstra & Willemsen, 1998). Since the TM stages seem to refer to consecutive motivational and behavioural echelons through which both forward and backward transitions are possible, we have suggested that it might be better to replace the word phase (Bolman & De Vries, 1998; De Vries et al., 1998). Another criticism concerns the utilisation of an algorithm to measure stages that may be useful for smokers, but may be less applicable to other behaviours. As regards nutrition, for instance, researchers have shown that the classic utilisation of the algorithm may result in substantial mis-classifications by placing subjects in maintenance because they think that they have changed their behaviour, while in-depth analysis showed that they did not perform the recommended behaviour and thus should have been labelled as precontemplators (Lechner, Brug & De Vries, 1997). Despite caution about the application of the stage algorithm, the concept of stages or motivational phases has caused an important paradigm shift in health psychology by indicating that behaviour change should not be regarded as a dichotomy but as a process. The Precaution Adoption Model by Weinstein (1988) also elaborates this idea, but then mainly for people in the earlier motivational phases.

The distinction between motivational phases also implies that the importance of motivational determinants such as attitudes might differ per motivational phase. This is also the main reason why the present study analysed the impact of integrating the concept of motivational phases into the ASE model, which is the main subject of this chapter.

THE ASE MODEL

The ASE model originated in the TRA, but has evolved in several areas since Bandura's concept of self-efficacy was added to it (see also: De Vries & Backbier, 1994; De Vries et al., 1988, 1995). In accordance with the TRA (Ajzen & Fishbein, 1980) and its successor the TPB (Ajzen, 1988, 1991; Ajzen & Madden, 1986), the ASE model states that behaviour is a function of a person's intention. Intention and behaviour are assumed to be most directly determined by three types of proximal cognitive factors: attitudes, social influences, and self-efficacy expectations. The ASE model has been used to explain various health behaviours, such as nutrition (Brug, Lechner & De Vries, 1995), exercise (Lechner & De Vries, 1995a, 1995b), alcohol consumption (Oostveen, Knibbe & De Vries, 1996), child safety (Wortel, De Vries, & De Geus, 1995) and smoking (Bolman & De Vries, 1998; De Vries & Backbier, 1994; De Vries et al., 1998; Willemsen, De Vries, Van Breukelen & Genders, 1998). However, in spite of their similarities, the ASE model differs from the TPB on seven points, which are discussed briefly below.

First, the ASE does not use multiplicative functions, since it is believed that multiplicative functions should be entered separately into regression equations (Evans, 1991; Hosmer & Lemeshow, 1989). In addition, research by Lechner, De Vries & Kok (submitted) showed that the inclusion of evaluations for the measurement of attitudes did not contribute to the explanation of participation in exercise programmes.

Second, the ASE model assesses attitude by measuring the outcome expectations of a behaviour using two dimensions. The first involves assessing both the advantages and disadvantages of a particular behaviour (Janis & Mann, 1977; Velicer, DiClemente, Prochaska & Brandenburg, 1985). The second aims at measuring both cognitive and emotional outcome beliefs. Current research is focussing on the identification of further useful subfactors predicting behaviour (see e.g., De Vries, Backbier, Dijkstra, Van Breukelen, Parcel & Kok, 1994; Dijkstra, Bakker & De Vries, 1997).

Third, the ASE model distinguishes three types of social influences: social norms, perceived behaviours of others, and direct pressure or support to perform a particular behaviour, since each of the three constructs has been found to make a unique contribution towards explaining behaviour. Inspired by the work of Friedman, Lichtenstein and Biglan (1985) and Grube et al. (1986), a longitudinal study was set up among 495 adolescents to test the impact of three different constructs for measuring social influence. Social influence was assessed by measuring the social norms, perceived smoking behaviour and direct pressure. The three constructs showed modest inter-correlations, indicating that they were measuring different aspects of the social influence process. Both perceived smoking behaviour and direct pressure were found to have significant unique contributions in addition to social norms. When attitudes and self-efficacy were added to the model, social norms hardly made a unique contribution, while perceived behaviour and pressure did have significant unique contributions (De Vries et al., 1995).

Fourth, self-efficacy expectations are measured instead of perceived control by measuring the level of difficulty in performing the desired behaviour (see e.g., De Vries et al., 1988; Dijkstra, De Vries & Bakker, 1996; Van Assema, Pieterse, Kok, Eriksen & De Vries, 1993), and/or by measuring the confidence a person has in his ability to perform this behaviour (Lechner & De Vries, 1995ab; Mudde, De Vries & Dolders, 1995; Mudde, Kok & Strecher, 1995; Schaalma, Kok & Peters, 1993).

Fifth, the ASE model has adopted the notion of the Transtheoretical Model, indicating that behavioural change should be regarded as a process (Prochaska, Norcross, et al., 1994). Therefore, apart from measurements of intention and behaviour, the principles underlying the motivational stages suggested by the transtheoretical theory were integrated into the ASE model (see Figure 8.1).

Sixth, the impact of the three proximal factors is assumed to be moderated by four types of distal factor (see also Flay & Petraitis, 1994): behavioural

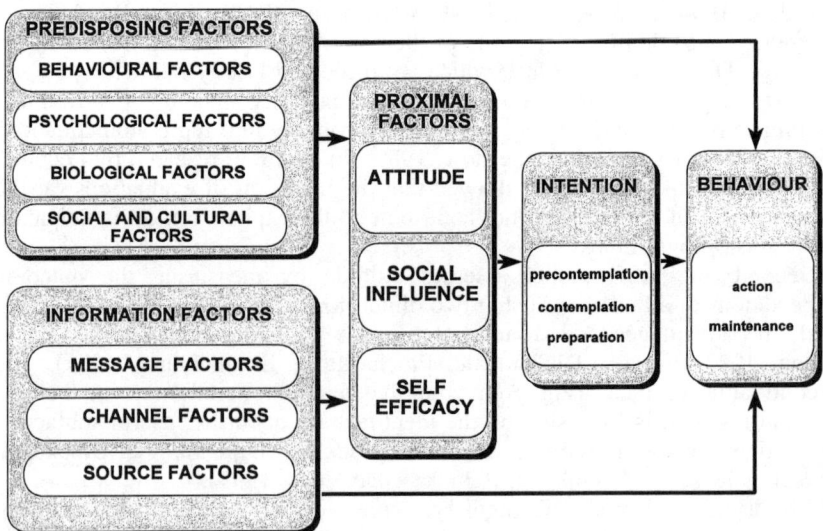

Figure 8.1   The ASE model for motivational changes.

factors (e.g. acquisition of skills, previous experiences with the behaviour, previous experiences with related behaviours), psychological factors (e.g. attributions, vicarious learning processes), biological factors (e.g. gender, age, hereditary variables), and social and cultural factors (e.g. social climate, socio-economic status) (De Vries, 1995). It has furthermore been acknowledged that behaviours that have become habitual may have a direct effect of past behaviour on future behaviour as well (Ajzen, 1991; Bagozzi, 1992; Bentler & Speckart, 1981; De Vries et al., 1995; Fredericks & Dosset, 1983; Grube et al., 1986) and may thus prompt the individual to a less elaborate processing of information (Petty & Cacioppo, 1986).

Seventh, the proximal cognitions of an individual about the behaviour are assumed to be influenced by predisposing factors, but can also be changed by interventions, which may be elaborate but can also be a simple 'cue to action' (Janz & Becker, 1984). The effectiveness of a behavioural intervention in motivating an individual to change is assumed to be influenced by four types of information factors (McGuire, 1985): receiver factors, which refer to the characteristics of the target group (e.g. age, level of education, motivation) and which influence the effectiveness of the intervention; message factors (e.g. level of discrepancy between the message and the opinions of the target group); channel variables (e.g. mass media strategies); and source variables (e.g. reliability of the source). In accordance with the notions developed by Petty and Cacioppo (1986) described above, it is acknowledged that interventions may also have a direct influence on behaviour.

The ASE model is therefore in line with other social cognitive change theories and could be described as a theory of motivational change, since the assumption of the ASE model is that behavioural change can be realised by motivating individuals to change unhealthy behaviour and to reinforce healthy behaviour.

INTEGRATION OF THE CONCEPT OF MOTIVATIONAL PHASES INTO THE ASE MODEL

Earlier Dutch smoking cessation research integrating the ASE model with the motivational phases concepts of the TM model showed that precontemplators could be distinguished from contemplators by their less positive perception of the outcomes of quitting, while contemplators could be distinguished from smokers in preparation and actors by their lower levels of self-efficacy (De Vries & Backbier, 1994; Dijkstra, et al., 1996). The studies demonstrated that subjects in precontemplation had a negative attitude towards quitting and perceived few advantages of the healthy behaviour, while those in contemplation were significantly more convinced of the advantages. Moreover, the latter group also reported more social support to engage in the healthy behaviour. Subjects in preparation were somewhat more convinced of the advantages of the healthy behaviour and reported more support than those in contemplation. However, the greatest difference occurred with regard to self-efficacy. Subjects in preparation reported higher levels of self-efficacy than those in contemplation or in precontemplation. The resulting Ø-pattern, as

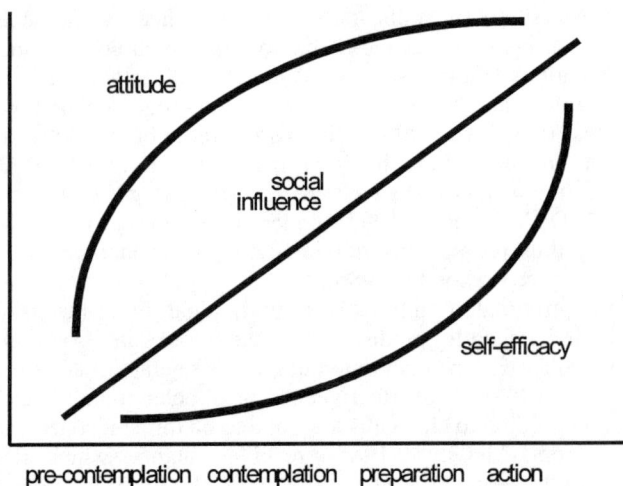

Figure 8.2   The ø-pattern.

depicted in Figure 8.2 (De Vries & Backbier, 1994), was replicated in several other Dutch studies on smoking cessation (Bolman & De Vries, 1998; De Vries et al., 1988; De Vries & Mudde, 1998) and fat intake (Brug & Van Assema, 1995). However, these Dutch studies had a cross-sectional nature and could therefore not demonstrate which factors would predict transition from one motivational phase to another

The two longitudinal studies that are described in the present chapter aspire to test the ASE model and the related Ø-pattern. In the first study, the Ø-pattern is applied to predict changes through the motivational phases. It was expected that forward movement among smokers who are not motivated to quit (precontemplators) could be predicted by perception of higher levels of the pros of quitting (hypothesis 1). Secondly, it was expected that forward movement among smokers who are motivated to quit (smokers in preparation) could be predicted by perceptions of higher levels of self-efficacy to quit (hypothesis 2). Since the Ø-pattern hypothesises that perceptions of social support increase gradually over the subsequent phases and were relatively modest, it was difficult to foretell whether the transitions from one stage to another could be predicted by this factor. Finally, although the occurrence of backward movements through the stages had been described earlier (Martin, Velicer & Fava, 1996; Mudde, 1994; Velicer et al., 1995), no evidence had been reported concerning the relation with cognitions. Therefore, no specific hypotheses were formulated regarding these transitions either. In the second study it was tested whether interventions aimed at changing different cognitions lead to the hypothesised transitions over the motivational phases. The interventions consisted of computer tailored feedback letters, which were based on the answers of participating smokers to a questionnaire. It was expected that contemplators would be more likely to proceed over the phases when they received messages containing attitudinal information that dealt with describing the advantages and disadvantages of smoking cessation (hypothesis 3), while providing messages containing information about how to cope with various barriers (self-efficacy enhancing information) would stimulate smokers in preparation to proceed over the phases (hypothesis 4).

METHOD

Study 1: A Longitudinal Study on Smoking Cessation

Goal

The goal of this study was to replicate the Ø-pattern and to analyse which motivational determinants would predict changes in motivation to quit smoking.

Sample and Design

The study was carried out in 1991, and focussed on assessing the determinants of smoking cessation in the general public. It was part of a prospective evaluation study of a three-month national mass-media smoking cessation campaign (Mudde, 1994). At base-line, smokers aged 15 or older were selected by means of telephone screening of a random sample drawn from all Dutch private telephone numbers. This group (n = 1338) was subjected to three computer-assisted telephone interviews: a baseline interview before the start of the campaign (December 1990), a post campaign interview (April 1991) and a follow-up interview after a 10-months follow-up (February 1992). Data of 918 participants who took part in both the post-campaign interview (referred to as time 1) and the 10-months follow-up interview (referred to as time 2) were analysed for the purpose of the present study. The sample at time 1 consisted of smokers and ex-smokers who had stopped smoking during the campaign. This sample included subjects in the phases of precontemplation, contemplation, preparation and action. Ex-smokers in the maintenance stage were not yet available, since the period between base-line and time 1 was only three months.

Questionnaire

The items of the questionnaire were based on a earlier study of the effectiveness of a community-based smoking cessation programme (Mudde, De Vries & Dolders, 1995). Attitudes were assessed by means of five advantages of quitting (pros: will smoking cessation reduce your cancer risk and cardiovascular risk, will it improve the health of others, will it improve your physical condition, and will it reduce the inconvenience for others; these were scored on 4-point scales ranging from no (0) to very much (3); Cronbach's alpha = .66) and four disadvantages of quitting using 4 items (cons: will smoking cessation cause weight gain, will it reduce your relaxation opportunities, will it make you nervous, and will it cause yearning for the sociable feeling of smoking; these were scored on 4-point scales ranging from no (0) to very much (–3); Cronbach's alpha = .55).

Social support from partner, friends and colleagues was measured on 4-point scales, ranging from no support (0) to much support (3). For smokers, the perceived support for quitting was assessed, while for ex-smokers the support for remaining a non-smoker was measured. These items were not intended to measure one construct, since the intensity of the support may vary among important others. Therefore, the three items were described separately.

Self-efficacy was assessed by means of the subjects' confidence in succeeding to refrain from smoking in six specific social, emotional and habitual situations (when feeling stressed, after dinner, when seeing others smoke, when drinking alcoholic beverages, when drinking coffee or tea, and when offered a cigarette) scored on 5-point scales, ranging from very certain (2) to very uncertain (−2); Cronbach's alpha = .80).

With regard to behaviour, smokers and ex-smokers were categorised using the algorithm developed by Prochaska and colleagues (Prochaska & DiClemente, 1983; Velicer et al., 1985). Smokers in precontemplation were defined as those who did not intend to quit smoking within six months; those in contemplation intended to quit smoking within six months but not within a month. Smokers in preparation indicated their intention to quit within one month. Actors were subjects who were non-smokers (not having smoked during the last seven days before measurement) and had quit smoking within the 6 last months, while those in the maintenance stage were non-smokers who had quit smoking more than 6 months ago.

Finally, a number of background variables were measured. Exposure to elements of the preceding campaign was measured by means of correct recall of at least one campaign element, and the number of campaign TV elements watched. Demographic variables (age, gender, and educational level) were assessed, as well as smoking variables: average daily cigarette consumption, addiction (defined by: 1. smoking at least 25 cigarettes a day, or 2. smoking between 16 and 25 cigarettes a day and either smoking within 30 minutes after awakening, or smoking when sick and in bed, or finding it hard to refrain from smoking for 24 hours), type of tobacco use (manufactured cigarettes, hand-rolled cigarettes or combinations of tobacco products), and attempts at quitting lasting at least 24 hours during the previous year.

Analyses

The means of pros, cons, and self-efficacy and the scores on social pressure items were transformed into z-scores. Contrasts with respect to ASE variables between phases at time 1 were assessed by means of multiple variance analysis (MANOVA), comparing subjects in each stage with subjects in the subsequent stage. Logistic regression analyses were used to compare subjects who had moved forward with those who had not (i.e. those who had remained at the same stage plus those who had moved backward). The same procedure was followed for backward transitions from each stage: subjects who had moved backward were compared with those who had not (i.e. those who had remained in the same stage plus those who had moved forward). Background variables related to forward and backward transitions were included as co-variates (see for more details: De Vries & Mudde (1998)).

Characteristics of the Sample

The sample was almost equally distributed between men (51%) and women (49%). The mean age in the sample as measured at time 1 was 38.9 years (sd. 13.9). One quarter (26%) had only attended primary school or lower vocational training, while 39% had completed intermediate vocational training. Moreover, 8% had completed highschool without any subsequent training, and 27% had higher vocational training or had graduated from university. Analysis of attrition showed that there was no selective drop-out between time 1 and time 2. A majority of the subjects (69%) had tried to quit in the previous year. At baseline, 48% of the subjects smoked manufactured cigarettes and 40% smoked hand-rolled cigarettes, while 40% were addicted. Of the total sample of 918 subjects, 852 were smokers at time 1 (93%), with a mean daily consumption of 16.6 cigarettes (sd 10.1). The distribution of smokers over the phases showed that 604 smokers were in precontemplation (66%), 188 were in contemplation (20%), 60 were in preparation (7%), while 66 (7%) were in action.

Replication of the Ø-Hypothesis

As regards the differences between the groups at time 1 (see Figure 8.3), the results reveal the following pattern. Precontemplators scored significantly lower on the pros of quitting ($F(1,788) = -5.23$, $p < 0.001$) and on support from the partner ($F(1,788) = -3.56$, $p < 0.001$), friends ($F(1,788) = -3.95$, $p < 0.001$), and colleagues ($F(1,788) = -2.63$ $p < 0.01$), and higher on self-efficacy ($F(1,788) = 2.79$, $p < 0.01$) than did contemplators. Contemplators, in turn, reported less support from their partners than did those in preparation ($F(1,788) = 2.16$, $p < 0.05$). Preparers perceived more cons of quitting ($F(1,788) = 2.98$, $p < .01$), and more support from their partner ($F(1,788) = 5.95$, $p < 0.001$), friends ($F(1,788) = 4.00$, $p < 0.001$) and colleagues ($F(1,788) = 2.45$, $p < 0.05$), but had lower self-efficacy expectations ($F(1,788) = 10.13$, $p < 0.001$) than did actors. These results indicate that the Ø-hypothesis that emerged from earlier studies was replicated in the present study, although the finding that precontemplators having stronger self-efficacy expectations than contemplators was not expected.

Predicting Factors for Stage Transition

At time 2, a majority of the subjects was found in the same phase as at time 1. Forward movement over the phases was seen in 28% of the subjects, while 15% of the subjects moved backward (for details, see Table 8.1).

Those who progressed from precontemplation perceived significantly more pros of quitting than those who stayed in precontemplation (confirm hypothesis 1). Moreover, trends indicated that perceiving fewer cons and more support from partners and colleagues may also influence forward transition from precontemplation. Only a trend indicated that forward movement from contemplation may be connected with the perception of more pros. Subjects moving forward from preparation had stronger self-efficacy expectations than those who did not progress (confirm hypothesis 2). Because of a lack of power, a relatively small group of subjects was in the action phase at time 1, no significant time 1 predictors could be found for forward transitions from the action stage.

Regressing contemplators had significantly lower scores on pros, and may have perceived less support from their friends (trend), than contemplators who did not regress. Time 1 preparers who moved backward over the phases may have had weaker self-efficacy expectations at time 1 than those who did not regress, although this was also only indicated by a trend. No predictors could be found for backward transitions from action, again because of lack of power.

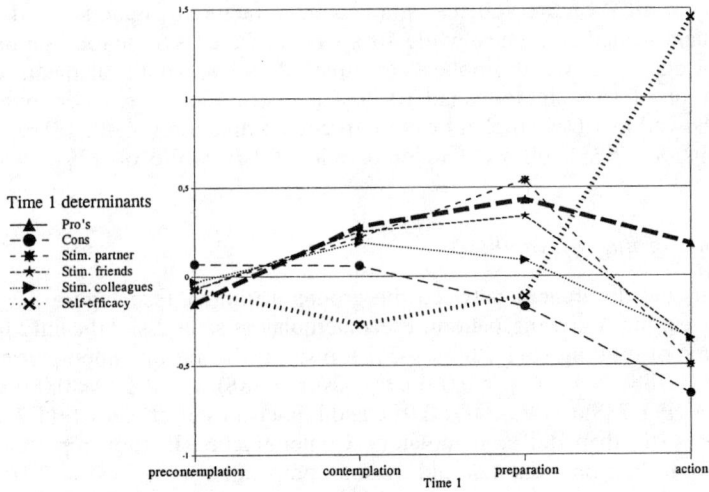

	time 1 precontemplation	time 1 contemplation	time 1 preparation	time 1 action
Pro's (−2.07 = no pro's, 2.17 = many pro's)	−0.15[1]	0.28	0.43	0.18
Con's (−2.31 = no pro's, 1.82 = many pro's)	0.07	0.06	−0.17	−0.66
Support from Partner (−0.58 = low, 2.30 = high)	−0.07	0.22	0.54	−0.50
Support from friends (−0.45 = low, 3.98 = high)	−0.07	0.25	0.34	−0.36
Support from Colleagues (−0.42 = low, 3.69 = high)	−0.03	0.19	0.09	−0.35
Self-efficacy (−2.03 = low, 1.62 = high)	−0.07	-0.27	−0.11	1.45

[1] Means adjusted for related demographic variables (gender), smoking behaviour (quit attempt in previous year, addiction, type of tobacco use), and exposure (correct recall of at least one campaign element, number of TV-clinic broadcasts watched).

Figure 8.3 Distribution of ASE variables over stages at time 1.

Table 8.1 Transition over the motivational phases between time 1 and time 2, and factors predicting forward and backward transitions (n = 918)

	Forward (backward)	*Backward (1) versus same phase or forward (0)*	*Forward versus (1) same phase or backward (0)*
Overall n = 918	28% (15%)		
T1 precontemplation	26%	–	pros OR = 1.34 ** cons OR = 0.82• support partner OR = 1.21• support colleagues OR = 1.20•
T1 contemplation	27% (38%)	pros OR = 0.58 ** support friends OR = 0.76•	pros OR = 1.43•
T1 preparation	15% (70%)	self-efficacy OR = 0.49•	self-efficacy OR = 7.85 *
T1 action	59% (32%)		

Results adjusted for gender, smoking behaviour (quit-attempt in previous year, addition, type of tobacco use), and exposure to previous campaign.

* p < 0.05 ** p < 0.01 • trend: 0.05 < p < 0.10

Study 2: Computerised Tailoring to Stimulate Smokers to Quit

Goal

The goal of this study was to analyse the impact on forward transition over the motivational phases of four intervention conditions offering: 1) attitudinal information 2) self-efficacy enhancing information; 3) both types of information; 4) no information. Four groups of smokers were distinguished: immotives (very much unmotivated), precontemplators (unmotivated), contemplators (moderately motivated), preparators (motivated to quit). This distinction was based on the results of an earlier study showing that 70% of the smoking population in the Netherlands were in the precontemplation phase (Mudde, Dolders & De Vries, 1994). Further analyses showed that this group of precontemplative smokers could be divided into immotives and precontemplators (Dijkstra et al., 1997)

Sample and design

Smokers were recruited by advertisements in local newspapers throughout the Netherlands in 1994. Smokers were invited to participate in this study regardless of their motivation to quit in the next six months. They were asked to volunteer for a research project on minimal interventions for smoking cessation including the possibility of being a control group member. Participants completing all three questionnaires had a chance to win one of the 10 bonus prizes amounting to $100. After participants had phoned the

..rsity to register (N = 1733), they were sent the pre-test questionnaire ..nich could be returned in a pre-paid envelope. After two weeks, 1540 pretest questionnaires (89%) had been returned.

Smokers were randomly assigned to one of the four conditions providing 1) information about the positive and negative outcomes of quitting (OC; N = 384); 2) information about self-efficacy expectations towards quitting (SE; N = 385); 3) information about both outcomes and self-efficacy expectations (BO; N = 386) or 4) no information (the control condition (CO; N = 385). Four weeks (T2) and twelve weeks (T3) after the pretests (T1), follow-up assessments were obtained (Dijkstra, De Vries & Roijackers, 1998).

Intervention

The respondents of the experimental conditions received computer generated letters of four to five pages, which tailored the information using the questionnaire responses of the participants. Hence, respondents in the OC condition only received information that was tailored to their responses about perceived advantages and disadvantages of quitting, respondents in the SE condition received information that was tailored to their responses about self-efficacy expectations with respect to quitting, and respondents in the BO condition received both types of tailored feedback. The participants in the control condition received no information.

Questionnaire

The questionnaires were based on the questionnaire used in a previous study (De Vries & Backbier, 1994), but was more elaborate since the goal of this study was to provide detailed feedback on outcome expectations and self-efficacy expectations. As a result, the questionnaire included 15 questions about the advantages of quitting (measured on 4-point scales, Cronbach's alpha = 0.87), 6 questions about the disadvantages of quitting (measured on 4-point scales, Cronbach's alpha = 0.57), 4 questions about situational self-efficacy (measured on 7-point scales, Cronbach's alpha = .81) and 3 questions about emotional self-efficacy (measured on 7-point scales, Cronbach's alpha = .86). Smokers who indicated a desire to quit but not within the next five years, or who planned to remain smokers were defined as immotives (N = 502). Smokers who indicated a desire to quit within the next five years were defined as precontemplators (N = 409). Smokers who indicated to quit within the next year were defined as contemplators (N = 374), while smokers who indicated a desire to quit within the next month were defined as preparers (N = 255). This adapted version of the stage algorithm appeared to discriminate better between the groups of smokers in the Netherlands, and the distinctions were also based on the smokers' scores on cognitive determinants discriminating the various groups (see Dijkstra et al., 1997 for more details). The questionnaire measured smoking habits by assessing (among others): 1) Severity of smoking habit by using the Fagerström Test for Nicotine Dependence (FTND) (Heatherton, Kozlowski, Frecker & Fagerström, 1991; Cronbach's alpha = 0.71); 2) smoking behaviour by asking, how many cigarettes they smoked on average.

Demographics measured were gender, age and educational level (low, medium, high).

Analyses

Logistic regression analyses were used to compare subjects who had moved forward with those who had not (i.e. those who had remained at the same stage plus those who had moved backward).The factor condition was dummy-coded. Background variables gender, age and educational level were included as covariates.

Participant Characteristics

Of the 1540 respondents, 59% were female; the average age was 39.7. With respect to the level of education, 22% were classified as 'low', 43% as 'medium', and 35% as 'high'. The respondents smoked an average of 20.3 cigarettes a day, the average FTND score was 4.6. The results showed that the randomisation was successful, and that attrition from pretest to post test 3 was 28.8% (N = 440). More men dropped out from the study than women did. Furthermore, the drop-out rates were significantly higher in the CO condition compared to the OC and the BO conditions, and among base-line contemplators and smokers in preparation compared to immotives and precontemplators. The analyses were rerun, including dropouts and replacing their missing value (T3) by their last recording. These analyses did not result in different findings.

Results

As regards stage transition, the conditions involving outcome information (OC and BO conditions) led to significant more forward movements compared to the control group (see Table 8.2). Smokers in precontemplation benefited most from information about self-efficacy. Both conditions involving self-efficacy information (SE and BO conditions) led to significant more motivational progress than in the control condition (resp. 40.7% in the SE condition and 34.5% in the BO condition versus 17.1% in the CO condition). Outcome information alone did not lead to a significant difference with the control condition. Smokers in contemplation benefited most from the condition containing both sorts of information (39.3% forward movement in the BO condition versus 20% in the CO condition).

The self-efficacy enhancing condition was most beneficial for smokers in preparation: 54.3% motivational progress in the SE condition compared to 25.7% in the control group.

CONCLUSIONS

Both studies support earlier findings that the process of change with respect to smoking cessation can be characterised as a dynamic process (Prochaska &

Table 8.2   Transition over the motivational phases between time 1 and time 3 by phase and information condition predicting forward and backward transitions (n = 1100)

	OC Forward (backward)	OC vs CO Forward vs same phase or backward (OR)	SE Forward (backward)	SE vs CO Forward vs same phase or backward (OR)	BO Forward (backward)	BO vs OC Forward vs same phase or backward (OR)	OC Forward (backward)
Overall n = 1100	31% (12%)	1.89 **	37% (10%)	2.42 ***	36% (8%)	2.34 ***	19% (17%)
T1 immotives	32%	2.11 *	28%	1.85	31%	2.09 *	17%
T1 precontemplation	29% (6%)	1.90	41% (5%)	3.23 **	35% (2%)	2.50 *	17% (16%)
T1 contemplatinon	29% (15%)	1.71	32% (19%)	1.91	39% (16%)	2.64 *	20% (29%)
T1 preparation	38% (49%)	1.10	54% (31%)	3.49 *	46% (31%)	2.60	26% (49%)

OC = outcome information; SE = self-efficacy information; BO = both sorts of information; OC = no information.
OR's adjusted for gender, age and education.

* p<0.05   ** p<0.01   *** p<0.001

DiClemente, 1983; Velicer et al., 1995). Between measurements, smokers in various motivational phases moved forward in this process and may have engaged in an attempt to change. A significant number of smokers, however, became less motivated to quit, resulting in a backward transition.

The concept of motivational and behavioural stages, developed by Prochaska and colleagues, was integrated in the ASE model, which is itself an integration of the model of Ajzen and Fishbein (1980) with concepts from Bandura's Social Cognitive Theory (1986). The distribution of the scores on attitudes, social pressure and self-efficacy measured in study 1 at time 1 demonstrated a pattern, referred to as the Ø-pattern, which had also been found before in various populations (Bolman & De Vries, 1998; De Vries & Backbier, 1994; De Vries et al., 1988; De Vries & Mudde, 1998). This pattern implies that the perceived advantages of quitting discriminate stronger between the earlier phases, whereas the self-efficacy expectations differentiate better between the later phases.

Study 1 analysed also the longitudinal impact of perceptions of pros, cons, social influences and self-efficacy on transitions over the motivational and behavioural phases. It was expected that forward movement among smokers in precontemplation would be predicted by a perception of higher levels of the pros of quitting (hypothesis 1). The results of the logistic regression analysis indeed demonstrated that forward movement of time 1 precontemplators was predicted only by a greater perception of the pros of quitting. It was furthermore expected that forward movement among smokers in preparation could be predicted by a perception of higher levels of self-efficacy to quit at time 1 (hypothesis 2). The results confirmed hypothesis 2 by showing that forward movement for smokers in preparation was predicted by a greater perception of their self-efficacy to quit measured at T1. Although no specific hypotheses were formulated regarding the prediction of backward transitions, backward transition at time 2 was found to be predicted among contemplators by a lower score on the perceived pros of quitting. Finally, the data of study 1 provided some indications that perceptions of lower levels of the cons of quitting and higher levels of social support from the partner and colleagues could stimulate precontemplators to progress, while a perception of higher levels of the pros of quitting may also contribute to forward transition from contemplation. Furthermore, the support from friends may have a preventive impact on backward transitions for those in contemplation, while greater self-efficacy expectations may prevent backward transitions from preparation. However, more research on the roles of these factors is needed, since only trends were found for these relationships.

A longitudinal study of the predictors of stage transition has also been performed by Prochaska, DiClemente, Velicer, Ginpil and Norcross (1985), who analysed which cognitive factors could predict stage transition. In their study, the predictive effects of the ten processes of change, the pros and cons, and self-efficacy were analysed using discriminant analysis for predicting changes among precontemplators, contemplators, recent quitters and relapsers. They found that precontemplators who moved forward scored lower on the pros of smoking and higher on the cons of smoking, and experienced less temptation to smoke. They also found that precontemplators who moved forward emphasised self-reevaluation more and social liberation less than precontemplators who remained in the precontemplation stage. Furthermore, they found that contemplators who were more likely to take action were less tempted to smoke (a factor similar to self-efficacy). However, it is difficult to compare their results with those of our study 1 because of the differences regarding the analytic procedures and the measurement of the constructs.

Study 2 investigated whether different types of information induced forward movement over the motivational and behavioural phases in smokers in the subsequent phases. Smokers who differed in their motivation to quit were randomly assigned to four groups, who received different types of messages. One group received information about the advantages of quitting, the second group received self-efficacy enhancing information, the third group received both types of information and a control group did not get any information. Smokers who were unmotivated to quit at base-line benefited most from messages that contained information about the advantages of quitting (attitudinal information). The combination of information about the advantages and self-efficacy enhancing information had a similar effect, but self-efficacy information alone did not result in significant differences with the control group. Precontemplators and contemplators profited from the combination of both types of information, although the results for precontemplators were not conclusive: they also benefited from uniquely self-efficacy information. Moreover, it was found that preparers benefited most from messages that contained self-efficacy enhancing information.

As regards the implications for the development of behavioural interventions for smoking cessation, the results confirm the suggestions that have been formulated in earlier studies (De Vries & Backbier, 1994; De Vries et al., 1998). Smokers who are very unmotivated to quit may profit most from information concerning the advantages of quitting, since a higher score is associated with an increased motivation to quit. Similarly, smokers who are prepared to quit may profit most from information enhancing their self-efficacy. This result may also help counsellors when selecting priorities in their process of counselling. If a person is not motivated to quit, this suggests that the counsellor needs at least to discuss the advantages of quitting and disadvantages of smoking. If the smoker is motivated to quit, the counsellor can probably skip this step, but needs to explore barriers to quit and ways of coping with these barriers.

Furthermore, the results of the computerised tailoring study 2, and the results of other studies involving computerised tailoring, suggest that tailored health information may significantly improve the credibility, relevance and effectiveness of the information (Brug, Steenhuis, Van Assema & De Vries, 1996; Dijkstra, De Vries & Royackers, 1998; Dijkstra, De Vries, Roijackers & Van Breukelen, 1998). Similar findings on the impact of computerised tailoring have been found for other behaviours, such as nutrition (Brug et al., 1995) and exercise (Bull, Jamrozik & Blanksby, 1999). These results suggest that further fine-tuning of messages to very specific characteristics of the target group may have an additional benefit.

Although the present studies provided support for the Ø-pattern and the predictions that can be derived from this pattern, one cannot conclude that a similar pattern will be found for all health behaviours. It is conceivable that this pattern can be replicated for behaviours where the subjects can make a fair estimation of the pros and cons, the social support and the self-efficacy expectations. For behaviours where such an estimation cannot be made (e.g. new behaviours), it is conceivable that individuals may overestimate or underestimate the advantages, or overestimate their levels of self-efficacy to perform the behaviour. The latter has been found for subjects at work sites engaging in new behaviours, such as avoiding exposure to carcinogenic substances (De Vries & Lechner, submitted) or participation in exercise programmes (Lechner & De Vries, 1995a).

It is recommended to further explore how to measure motivational progress. Although the TM stage algorithm provides an easy way to discriminate groups, it can also be argued that this algorithm may not be the best way to assess various motivational groups, for several reasons. Firstly, a distinction in time does not provide a conceptual base to discriminate groups. For this reason, Dijkstra et al. (1997) proposed an alternative method of assessing motivational phases and suggested four groups in the process of quitting: immotives, precontemplators, contemplators, preparers. Secondly, the distinction in time does not always make sense. For instance, in studying the process of quitting among pregnant women, a time-frame of one year or six months does not make sense for those women who are in their fourth month of pregnancy. De Vries and Backbier (1994) therefore used the traditional intention scale to group the respondents. Thirdly, the algorithm may lead to mis-classifications when complex behaviours are studied, such as nutrition (Lechner et al., 1997) or exercise (Lechner & De Vries, 1995ab).

ACKNOWLEDGEMENT

The contributions by De Vries and Dijkstra were made possible by grants from the Dutch Cancer Society. The contribution by Mudde was made possible by a grant from the Dutch Smoking and Health Foundation.

REFERENCES

Ajzen, I. (1988). *Attitudes, Personality and Behavior*. Milton Keynes: Open University Press.
Ajzen, I. (1991). The theory of planned behavior. *Organizational Behavior and Human Decision Processes, 50*, 179–211.
Ajzen, I. & Fishbein, M. (1980). *Understanding Attitudes and Predicting Social Behaviour*. Englewood Cliffs: Prentice Hall.
Ajzen, I. & Madden, J. T. (1986). Prediction of goal-directed behavior: Attitudes, intentions, and perceived behavioral control. *Journal of Experimental Social Psychology, 22*, 453–474.
Bagozzi, R. P. (1981). Attitudes, intentions, and behavior: A test of some key hypotheses. *Journal of Personality and Social Psychology, 41*, 607–627.
Bagozzi, R. P. (1992). The self-regulation of attitudes, intentions, and behavior. *Social Psychology Quarterly, 55*, 178–204

Bagozzi, R. P., Baumgartner, J. & Yi, Y. (1989). An investigation into the role of intentions as mediators of the attitude-behavior relationship. *Journal of Economic Psychology, 10*, 35–63.

Bandura, A. (1986). *Social Foundations of Thought and Action: A Social Cognitive Theory.* New York: Prentice-Hall.

Bandura, A. (1997). *The Exercise of Control.* New York: Freeman.

Bem, D. J. (1972). Self-perception theory. In: L. Berkowitz (Ed.), *Advances in Experimental Social Psychology, 6*, 2–57.

Bentler, P. M. & Speckart, G. (1981). Attitudes cause behaviors: A structural equation analysis. *Journal of Personality and Social Psychology, 40*, 225–238.

Bolman, C. & De Vries, H. (1998). Psycho-social determinants and motivational phases in smoking behavior of cardiac inpatients. *Preventive Medicine, 27*, 738–747.

Bracht, N. (1990). *Health Promotion at the Community Level.* Newbury Park: Sage.

Brug, J., Lechner, L. & De Vries, H. (1995). Psychosocial determinants of fruit and vegetable consumption. *Appetite, 25*, 285–296.

Brug, J., Steenhuis, I., Van Assema, De Vries, H. (1996). The impact of a computer tailored nutrition intervention. *Preventive Medicine, 25*, 236–242.

Brug, J. & Van Assema, P. (1995). Factors differentiating between stages of change for fat reduction. *Appetite, 24*, p. 296.

Bull, F. C., Jamrozik, K. & Blanksby, B. A. (1999). Tailored advice on exercise: Does it make difference? *American Journal of Preventive Medicine, 16*, 230–239.

De Vries, H. (1995). Socio-economical differences in smoking: Dutch Adolescents' beliefs and behavior. *Social Science & Medicine, 41*, 419–424.

De Vries, H. (1998) Planning health promotion. In: R. Weson & D. Scott. *Evaluation of Health Promotion* (pp. 92–108). Cheltenham: Stanley Thornes.

De Vries, H. & Backbier, M. P. H. (1994). Self-efficacy as an important determinant of Quitting among smoking pregnant women: the Ø-phenomenon. *Preventive Medicine, 23*, 167–164.

De Vries, H., Backbier, E., Dijkstra, M., van Breukelen, G., Parcel, G. & Kok, G. (1994). A Dutch social influence smoking prevention approach for vocational school students. *Health Education Research, 9*, 365–374.

De Vries, H., Backbier, E., Kok, G., & Dijkstra, M. (1995). The impact of social influences in the context of attitude, self-efficacy, intention and previous behavior as predictors of smoking onset. *Journal of Applied Social Psychology, 25*, 237–257.

De Vries, H., Dijkstra, M. & Kuhlman, P. (1988). Self-efficacy: The third factor besides attitude and subjective norm as a predictor of behavioral intentions. *Health Education Research, 3*, 273–282.

De Vries, H. & Lechner, L. Motives for protection against carcinogenic substances at the workplace: A pilot study among Dutch workers. Submitted.

De Vries, H. & Mudde, A. N. (1998). Predicting stage transitions for smoking cessation applying the attitude-social influence-efficacy model. *Psychology and Health, 13*, 369–385.

De Vries, H., Mudde, A., Dijkstra, A. & Willemsen, M. (1998). Differential beliefs, perceived social influences and self-efficacy expectations among smokers in various motivational phases. *Preventive Medicine, 27*, 681–689.

De Vries, H., Mudde, A. N. & Peters, L. (1997). Stadia and processen van stoppen met roken [Stages and processes of smoking cessation]. *Gedrag & Gezondheid, 26*, 230–240.

DiClemente, C. C., Prochaska, J. O., Fairhurst, S. K., Velicer, W. F., Velasquez, M. M. & Rossi, J. (1991). The process of smoking cessation; an analysis of precontemplation, contemplation and preparation stages of change. *Journal of Consulting and Clinical Psychology, 59*, 295–304.

Dijkstra, A., Bakker, M. & De Vries. (1997). Subtypes within a sample of precontemplating smokers: A preliminary extension of the stages of change. *Addicitive Behaviours, 22,* 327–337.

Dijkstra, A., De Vries, H., Bakker, M. (1996). Pros and cons of quitting, self-efficacy and the stages of change in smoking cessation. *Journal of Consulting and Clinical Psychology, 64,* 758–776.

Dijkstra, A., De Vries, H., & Roijackers, J. (1998). Long-term effectiveness of computer-generated tailored feed-back in smoking cessation. *Health Education Research, 13,* 207–214.

Dijkstra, A., De Vries, H., Roijackers, J. & Breukelen, van, G. (1998). Tailoring information to enhance quitting in smokers with low motivation to quit: Three basic efficacy questions. *Health Psychology, 17,* 513–519

Evans, M. G. (1991). The problem of analysing multiplicative composites. *American Psychologist, 46,* 6–15.

Fava, J. L., Velicer, W. F. & Prochaska, J. O. (1995). Applying the transtheoretical model to a representative sample of smokers. *Addictive Behaviours, 20,* 189–203.

Fishbein, M., & Ajzen, I. (1975). *Belief, Attitude, Intention and Behavior: An Introduction to Theory and Research.* Reading, MA: Addison-Wesley.

Flay, B. R. & Petraitis, J. (1994). The theory of triadic influence: A new theory of health behaviour with implications for preventive interventions. *Advances in Medical Sociology, 4,* 19–44.

Fredericks, A. R. & Dossett, D. L. (1983). Attitude-behavior relations: A comparison of the Fishbein-Ajzen and Bentler-Speckart models. *Journal of Personality and Social Psychology, 40,* 226–238.

Friedman, L. S., Lichtenstein, E. & Biglan, A. (1985) Smoking onset among teens: An empirical analysis of initial situations. *Addictive Behaviors, 10,* 1–3.

Green, L. W. & Kreuter, M. W. (1991). *Health Promotion Planning; An Educational and Environmental Approach.* Palo Alto: Mayfield Publishing Company.

Grube, J. W., Morgan, M. & McGee, S. T. (1986). Attitudes and normative beliefs as predictors of smoking intentions and behaviours: A test of three models. *British Journal of Social Psychology, 25,* 81–93.

Heatherton, T. F., Kozlowski, L. T., Frecker, R. C. & Fagerström, K. O. (1991). The Fagerström Test for Nicotine Dependence: A revision of the Fagerström Tolerance Questionnaire. *British Journal of Addiction, 86,* 1119–127.

Hosmer, D. W., Lemeshow, S. (1989). *Applied Logistic Regression.* New York: John Wiley & Sons, pp. 34–35.

Janz, N. K. & Becker, M. H. (1984). The Health Belief Model: A decade later. *Health Education Quarterly, 11,* 1–47.

Janis, I. L. & Mann, L. (1977). *Decision Making: A Psychological Analysis of Conflict, Choice Commitment.* New York: Free Press.

Lechner, L, Brug, J. & De Vries, H. (1997). Misconception of fruit and vegetable consumption: Interpretation and consequences. *Journal of Nutrition Education, 29,* 313–320.

Lechner, L. & De Vries, H. (1995a). Participation in an employee fitness program: Determinants of high adherence, low adherence and drop-out. *Journal of Occupational and Environmental Medicine, 37,* 429–436.

Lechner, L. & De Vries, H. (1995b). Starting participation in an employee fitness program: Attitudes, self-efficacy and social influence. *Preventive Medicine, 24,* 633–637.

Lechner, L., De Vries, H. & Kok, G. J. *Attitudes according to the Theory of Reasoned Action: Do we need to include evaluations?* Manuscript submitted for publication.

Martin, R. A., Velicer, W. F. & Fava, F. L. (1996). Latent transition analysis to the stages of change for smoking cessation. *Addictive Behaviors, 21,* 67–80.

McGuire, W. J., (1985) Attitudes and attitude change. In: G. Lindzey & E. Aronson (Eds.) *Handbook of Social Psychology*, Volume II, New York: Lawrence Erlbaum Associates, pp. 233–246.

Mudde, A. N. (1994). *The development and evaluation of a community and a mass media approach to smoking cessation.* Unpublished doctoral dissertation, University of Limburg, The Netherlands.

Mudde, A. N., De Vries, H. & Dolders, M. G. T. (1995). Evaluation of a Dutch community-based smoking cessation intervention. *Preventive Medicine, 24,* 61–70.

Mudde, A. N., Dolders, M. & De Vries, H. (1994). Publieksevaluatie van de actie: Volwassen bevolking. [Evaluation of the action: The adult population]. In: B. Baan, M. H. M. Breteler & G. A. J. van der Rijt (Eds.): *Samen Stoppen Met Roken* [Quitting smoking together]. The Hague, The Netherlands, Stichting Volksgezondheid en Roken, p. 22–44.

Mudde, A. N., Kok, G. J. & Strecher, V. J. (1995). Self-efficacy as predictor for the cessation of smoking: Methodological issues and implications for smoking cessation programs. *Psychology and Health, 10,* 353–67.

Oostveen, T., Knibbe, R. A., & De Vries, H. (1996). Social influences on young adults' alcohol consumption: Norms, modelling, pressure, socializing and conformity. *Addictive Behaviors, 21,* 187–197.

Petty, R. E. & Cacioppo, J. T. (1986). The elaboration likelihood model of persuasion. In: Berkowitz, L. (Ed.), *Advances in Experimental Social Psychology*, Vol. 19. London: Academic Press.

Prochaska, J. O. (1994). Strong and weak principles for progressing from precontemplatin to action on the base of twelve problem behaviors. *Health Psychology, 13,* 1–5.

Prochaska, J. O. & DiClemente, C. C. (1983). Stages and processes of self-change of smoking: Toward an integrative model of change. *Journal of Consulting and Clinical Psychology, 51,* 390–395.

Prochaska, J. O. & DiClemente, C. C. (1998). Comments, criteria, and creating better models: In response to Davidson. In: Miller, W. R. & Heather, N. (Eds) *Treating Addictive Behaviors* (2nd ed.). New York: Plenum Press, pp. 39–45.

Prochaska, J. O., DiClemente, C. C., Velicer, W. F., Ginpil, S. & Norcross, J. C. (1985). Predicting change in smoking status for self-changers. *Addictive Behaviors, 10,* 395–406.

Prochaska, J. O., Norcross, J. C., & DiClemente, C. C. (1994). *Changing for Good.* New York: William Morrow and Company, Inc.

Prochaska, J. O., Redding, C. A., Harlow, L. L., Rossi, J. S. & Velicer, W. F. (1994). The transtheoretical model of change and HIV prevention: A review. *Health Education Quarterly, 21,* 471–486

Prochaska, J. O., Velicer, W. F., DiClemente, C. C., & Fava, J. (1988) Measuring processes of change: Applications to the cessation of smoking. *Journal of Consulting and Clinical Psychology, 56,* 520–528.

Rogers, E. M. (1983). *Diffusion of Innovations.* New York: Free Press.

Rogers, R. (1983). Cognitive and physiological processes in fear appeals and attitude change: A revised theory of protection motivation. In: J. T. Cacioppo, J. T & Petty, R. E. (Eds.) *Social Psychophysiology–A Source Book.* New York: Guilford Press, p. 153–176.

Schaalma, H., Kok, G. J. & Peters, L. (1993). Determinants of consistent condom use by adolescents: The impact of experience with sexual intercourse. *Health Education Research, 8,* 255–269.

Urberg, K. A., Shyu, S. & Liang, J. (1990). Peer influence in adolescent cigarette smoking. *Addictive Behaviors, 15,* 247–255.

Van Assema, P., Pieters, M., Kok, G., Eriksen, M. & De Vries, H. (1993). The determinants of four cancer-related risk behaviours. *Health Education Research, 8,* 461–472.

Velicer, W. F., DiClemente, C. C., Prochaska, J. O., & Brandenburg, N. (1985). A decisional balance measure for predicting smoking cessation. *Journal of Personality and Social Psychology, 48,* 1279–1289.

Velicer, W. F., DiClemente, C. C., Rossi, J. S. & Prochaska, J. O. (1990). Relapse situations and self-efficacy: An integrative model. *Addictive Behaviors, 15,* 271–283.

Velicer, W. F., Fava, J. L., Prochaska, J. O., Abrams, D. B., Emmonds, K. M. & Pierce, J. P. (1995). Distribution of smokers by stage in three representative samples. *Preventive Medicine, 24,* 401–411.

Weiner, B. (1986). *An Attributional Theory of Motivation and Emotion.* New York: Springer-Verlag Inc..

Weinstein, N. D. (1988). The precaution adoption process. *Health Psychology, 7,* 355–386.

Willemsen, M. C. & De Vries, H. (1996). The evaluation of the PTT-telecom smoking cessation program. *Tobacco Control, 4,* 351–354.

Willemsen, M. C., De Vries, H., Van Breukelen, G. & Genders, R. (1998). Long-term effectiveness of two Dutch work site smoking cessation programs. *Health Education and Behavior, 25,* 418–435.

Wortel, E., De Vries, H. & De Geus, G. H. (1995). Lessons learned from a community campaign on child safety in The Netherlands. *Family & Community Health, 18,* 60–77.

CHAPTER NINE

Relationships Among The Theory of Planned Behaviour, Stages of Change, and Exercise Behaviour in Older Persons Over a Three Year Period

Kerry S. COURNEYA, Claudio R. NIGG, and Paul A. ESTABROOKS

Much of the previous research applying theoretical models to exercise behaviour has attempted to predict which individuals are, or will be, inactive or active at a given point in time (Courneya, 1995a, b). Such an approach implies a two stage model of exercise behaviour change (i.e., from inactive to active) and has led to a search for determinants and interventions to facilitate such a change. Recent theorising, however, has suggested that individuals may progress through multiple discrete stages when changing their exercise behaviour and that each stage transition may have different determinants and require different intervention strategies (e.g., Dishman, 1991; Sallis & Hovell, 1990; Sonstroem, 1988). Although a number of stage models have been proposed and applied to the exercise domain (e.g., Booth, Macaskill, Owen, Oldenburg, Marcus & Bauman, 1993; Dishman, 1990; Godin, Desharnais, Valois & Bradet, 1995; Sallis & Hovell, 1990; Weinstein, 1988), the most popular and validated has been Prochaska's stages of change model (SCM; DiClemente, Prochaska, Fairhurst, Velicer, Velasquez & Rossi, 1991; Prochaska & DiClemente 1983, 1985; Prochaska & Velicer, 1997).

Overview of the Stages Of Change Model

The SCM was originally developed for application in the area of smoking cessation but has recently been applied to a wide variety of health behaviours including exercise (Prochaska et al., 1994). The stage construct was developed to reflect the temporal dimension of health behaviour change (Prochaska & Velicer, 1997). That is, the SCM highlights the dynamic nature of health behaviour change and attempts to demarcate 'when' meaningful (i.e., clinically significant) health behaviour change has occurred. Six stages of change have been proposed for the SCM.

In the first stage, precontemplation, the person is not engaged in the appropriate health behaviour and has no intention of changing in the foreseeable future. In the contemplation stage, the person has formed an intention to change in the near future but still has not attempted the behaviour change. The third stage, preparation, is reached when the person intends to take action in the immediate future, has a detailed plan for taking action, and may have taken some small steps toward behaviour change. The action stage is achieved when behaviour has been changed to the target level that is recommended for that behaviour (e.g., exercising 3 times per week for 30 minutes at moderate to vigorous intensity). Once this level of behaviour has been maintained for six months, the person enters the maintenance stage which lasts until about 5 years. The sixth and final stage, termination, is reached when the risk of returning to the previous unhealthy behaviour has been completely eliminated (i.e., the risk is zero) which is usually defined as zero temptation to engage in the old behaviour and 100% self-efficacy in all previously tempting situations.

The SCM is part of a larger theoretical framework called the transtheoretical model (TTM) developed by Prochaska and DiClemente (1983; 1985; 1986). The TTM incorporates variables from other theories to help understand health behaviour change. The processes of change were combined with the SCM to explain 'how' people change their health behaviours (DiClemente et al., 1991). These processes include overt and covert activities that individuals use to modify their experiences and environments in order to modify their behaviour (Prochaska & Velicer, 1997). The TTM has highlighted 10 processes of change which can be divided into two higher order factors labelled cognitive/experiential (i.e., consciousness raising, dramatic relief, environmental reevaluation, self-reevaluation, and social liberation) and behavioural/environmental (i.e., counterconditioning, helping relationships, contingency management, self-liberation, and stimulus control).

Moreover, self-efficacy, decisional balance (i.e., pros and cons), and temptation have been incorporated into the TTM (DiClemente, Prochaska, Fairhurst, Velicer, Valasquez, & Rossi, 1991; Prochaska & Velicer, 1997; Velicer, DiClemente, Prochaska, et al., 1985). These integrations appear to be an attempt to help explain 'why' health behaviour change occurs. Self-efficacy was taken from Bandura's (1986) social cognitive theory and reflects a person's confidence in completing the health behaviour change. The pros and cons were borrowed from Janis and Mann's (1977) decisional balance theory and reflect the costs and benefits of health behaviour change. Temptation reflects the intensity of urges to engage in the problem behaviour when faced with difficult situations (Prochaska & Velicer, 1997).

Approximately 40 studies have examined the TTM in the exercise domain (see Buxton, Wyse, & Mercer, 1996; Cardinal, 1995; Prochaska & Marcus, 1994 for partial reviews). The vast majority of these studies have been cross-sectional although studies employing longitudinal and experimental designs are beginning to emerge (e.g., Calfas, Sallis, Oldenburg, & French, 1997; Cardinal & Sachs, 1995; Marcus, Banspach, Lefebvre, Rossi, Carleton, & Abrams, 1992; Marcus et al., 1998). These studies have supported the TTM across a wide range of populations including different worksite groups (e.g., medical, industrial, retail, government), age groups (e.g., children, adolescents, older adults), places of residence (e.g., rural, urban), medical conditions (e.g., cardiac patients), and countries (e.g., United States, Canada, Britain, Australia). Thus, considerable empirical evidence is available to confirm that the first five stages of the SCM are applicable to exercise behaviour and that the TTM constructs are capable of discriminating across the stages of change. Preliminary evidence concerning the termination stage, however, indicates that this stage may not be relevant for exercise behaviour change (Courneya & Bobick, in press).

Overview of the Theory of Planned Behaviour

Other researchers in the exercise domain have applied constructs from the theory of planned behaviour (TPB; Ajzen, 1991) to aid in understanding 'why' stage change has occurred (e.g., Courneya, 1995a; Lee, 1993; Murphy, 1993; Nguyen, Potvin, & Otis, 1997; Sonstroem, 1988). Although the TPB was originally developed to predict intention and behaviour, it may also be relevant for understanding stage change. The TPB proposes that a person's intention to perform a behaviour is the central determinant of behaviour because it captures certain motivational factors such as how hard one is willing to try. Intention is in turn determined by three conceptually independent variables. One variable, termed attitude, focuses on a positive or negative evaluation of performing the behaviour. A second variable, termed subjective norm, is intended to reflect the perceived social pressure that individuals may feel to perform or not perform the behaviour. The third conceptually independent variable indicates the perceived ease or difficulty of performing the behaviour and is labelled perceived behavioural control. Perceived behavioural control may also be an immediate determinant of behaviour if the behaviour is not completely volitional (i.e., not free of practical constraints). The summary proposition of the TPB is that people will intend to perform a behaviour when they evaluate it positively, believe that important others think they should perform it, and perceive it to be under their own control (Ajzen, 1988).

Integration of the Theory of Planned Behaviour and the Stages of Change

Courneya (1995a) has argued that the TPB is the most validated model for understanding 'why' people exercise. The TPB shares many conceptual similarities with the 'why' constructs from the TTM but may possess certain advantages over them. First, the pros from the TTM are similar to the behavioural beliefs from the TPB which form the basis of attitude toward the behaviour. The TPB has the added advantage, however, of including a global assessment of attitude which is arguably the most fundamental construct in social psychology. Second, the cons from the TTM may be partially reflected in the control beliefs of the TPB which underlie perceived behavioural control. These control beliefs are conceptually similar to self-efficacy beliefs and perceived barriers (Ajzen, 1991). Once again, however, the TPB includes a global indicator of perceived behavioural control. Third, the TPB also includes a social influence construct, subjective norm, which is neglected by the TTM. While this construct has been criticised in the exercise domain (Courneya & McAuley, 1995), it is at least an attempt to account cognitively for social influence in exercise behaviour change. Finally, intention from the TPB appears to be relevant for defining the early stages of change whereas behavioural criteria come into play in the later stages. Thus, the TPB's two major dependent variables are key elements in most conceptions of stage models (e.g., Godin et al., 1995; Prochaska & Velicer, 1997; Weinstein, 1988). Research has confirmed that TPB constructs are useful for discriminating the stages of change in the exercise domain (Courneya, 1995a; Lee, 1993; Murphy, 1993; Sonstroem, 1988) and preliminary evidence suggests that they may actually outperform their TTM counterparts (Courneya, 1995a).

Purpose of the Study

Marcus et al. (1994) have used the 'why' and 'when' constructs from TTM to predict and explain exercise behaviour in an employee sample over a six month period. Their study is one of the few longitudinal designs in the exercise domain. Structural equation modelling was used to examine a model that hypothesised that exercise stage would mediate the effects of self-efficacy, pros, and cons on physical activity six months later. Although the stage construct was not originally proposed to predict behaviour, it certainly makes sense that it should demonstrate predictive validity with behaviour. Moreover, its early stages are precursors to behaviour change. Results were consistent with the hypothesis showing the important mediational role of exercise stage and its predictive validity with exercise behaviour.

The purpose of the present study was to complement and extend the Marcus et al. (1994) research in a number of important ways. The first and most important extension was to test a model that combined the TPB with the SCM rather than the 'why' constructs from the TTM. This approach allows for a comparison of the relative utility of a combined TPB/SCM model compared to a TTM/SCM model for understanding 'why' people exercise over time. A second extension was the inclusion of a measure of current exercise stage to allow for an examination of the mediational role of the stage construct measured at two time points, baseline and follow-up. Third, the present study used a more appropriate self-report measure of exercise behaviour, namely, the Godin Leisure Time Exercise Questionnaire (GLTEQ; Godin, Jobin & Bouillon, 1986; Godin & Shephard, 1985). The GLTEQ has two major advantages in the present context over the Seven Day Physical Activity Recall (7DPAR) questionnaire (Blair, 1984) used by Marcus et al. (1994). One advantage is that the GLTEQ focuses on an *average* week without a specified time period whereas the 7DPAR measures the last seven days of physical activity which may not be typical of normal activity patterns. A second advantage is that the GLTEQ assesses only leisure time exercise which is consistent with how exercise stage is typically defined whereas the 7DPAR includes occupational and household activity. Finally, the follow-up time period was extended from six months to 3 years to provide an even stronger test of predictive validity and to eliminate any potential confound that may have resulted from seasonal changes in exercise levels.

The main hypotheses for the present study were drawn from the TPB and the longitudinal study of Marcus et al. (1994). The hypotheses were as follows:

(a) baseline TPB constructs would be significant predictors of current exercise stage, (b) baseline intention would mediate the effects of baseline TPB constructs on both baseline and current exercise stage, and (c) baseline and current exercise stage would mediate the effects of baseline intention on current exercise behaviour.

METHOD

Participants

Participants in the study were recruited from a baseline sample of volunteers who participated in a previous study (Courneya, 1995a, b). Participants were members of the Kerby Center, which is a multi-purpose social service, recreational, and educational facility operated by and for persons aged 60 years and over. The original sample consisted of 288 participants. The only identifying information provided by the original participants was their name. A search of the local telephone book identified telephone numbers for 191 of the original participants. Ten telephone call attempts to each person resulted in contact with 140 of the original participants. Five persons were deceased and four refused to participate which resulted in 131 participants. This number represents 45% of the original 288 participants and 94% of the 140 participants who could be contacted. The demographic profile of the 131 participants at baseline was as follows: age (M = 71.5, SD = 6.0); 56% females, 45% married, 71% completed at least high school, and 86% had a family income of less than $40,000.

Design and Procedure

The study was a three year follow-up of a cohort sample with baseline data collected in February/March of 1993 (Courneya, 1995a, b) and the current data collected in February, 1996. The baseline assessment was made using mail survey methodology (Courneya, 1995a, b) and the current three year follow-up assessment was made using a telephone protocol. Data collected at baseline included demographics, subjective norm, attitude, perceived behavioural control, intention, and exercise stage. The follow-up assessment included exercise stage and exercise behaviour.

Measures

This section details the measures for the 131 participants who completed both the baseline and follow-up assessments. Physical activity was defined for participants as 'any planned physical exertion aimed at improving or maintaining physical fitness and health'. The term 'regular' physical activity was defined for subjects as at least 3 times per week for at least 20–30 minutes each session at a moderate intensity (e.g., at least very brisk walking).

Subjective norm was measured by a single item 'Most people who are important to me think I should engage in regular physical activity' and scored on a 7 point scale that ranged from strongly disagree (−3) to strongly agree (+ 3). A single item to represent subjective norm is quite common and consistent with TPB (Ajzen, 1991). The traditional 'motivation to comply' assessment was not used because previous research had shown that it is not necessary and may in fact attenuate the correlation between subjective norm and intention (Ajzen 1991; Ajzen & Driver, 1992).

Attitude was measured using 7 point (−3 to + 3) bipolar adjective scales as suggested by Fishbein and Ajzen (1975; Ajzen & Fishbein, 1980). The statement that preceded the adjectives was 'My participating in regular physical activity is/would be...'. Four items tapped the evaluative or instrumental aspect of attitude (useful-useless, harmful-beneficial, wise-foolish, bad-good) and four items tapped the affective aspect of attitude (enjoyable-unenjoyable, boring-interesting, pleasant-unpleasant, stressful-relaxing). Alpha for the eight item scale was 0.84.

Perceived behavioural control was measured by three questions as suggested by Ajzen and Madden (1986): (1) 'How much control do you have over whether or not you engage in regular physical activity?' (− 3 = no control at all; + 3 = complete control), (2) 'For me to engage in regular physical activity is...' (+ 3 = extremely easy; −3 = extremely difficult), and (3) 'If I wanted to I could easily engage in regular physical activity.' (−3 = strongly disagree; + 3 = strongly agree). Alpha for this three item scale was 0.60.

Intention was assessed using four different scales (Courneya, 1994; Courneya & McAuley, 1993a). The individual items were (1) 'I intend to engage in physical activity at least _____ times in the next 4 weeks'', (2) 'I intend to engage in physical activity the following number of times in the next 4 weeks' with responses of 0–4, 5–8, 9–12, 13–16, 17–20, 21–24, and 25 + scored from 1 to 7 respectively, (3) 'I intend to engage in physical activity with the following regularity in the next 4 weeks' with responses on a 7 point scale anchored by (1) not at all and (7) everyday, and (4) 'I intend to engage in physical activity at least 12 times in the next 4 weeks' and scored on a 7 point scale that ranged from (1) definitely not to (7) definitely. Each scale was transformed into a z score and summed to provide the intention scale (a = 0.95). It should be pointed out that the four week time frame for intention does not correspond to the exercise behaviour assessment three years later. This lack of correspondence was due to the fact that the study was not originally conceived as longitudinal.

Exercise stage at baseline was measured using a questionnaire adapted from Marcus, Selby et al. (1992) who adapted theirs from the original stages of change measure developed by Prochaska and DiClemente (1983). The specific statements were 'I currently do not engage in physical activity and I am not thinking about starting' (precontemplation), 'I currently do not engage in physical activity but I am thinking about starting' (contemplation), 'I currently engage in some physical activity but not on a regular basis' (preparation), 'I currently engage in regular physical activity but I have only begun to do so within the last six months' (action), and 'I currently engage in regular physical activity and I have done so for longer than six months' (maintenance). Participants were required to select only one stage that best described their current physical activity pattern. Courneya (1995a) reported a two week test-retest reliability of 0.79 for this measure (*n* = 148) and Marcus, Selby et al.

(1992) reported a Kappa index of reliability over a two week period of 0.78 (n = 20). Concurrent validity has been demonstrated by Marcus and Simkin (1993) using the Seven Day Physical Activity Recall questionnaire (Blair, 1984). The participant by stage breakdown at baseline was as follows: precontemplation –15 (11%), contemplation –12 (9%), preparation –18 (14%), action –4 (3%), and maintenance –82 (63%).

Exercise stage at follow-up was measured using the same statements as at baseline but in a sequential or algorithmic format. Participants were first asked if they currently engaged in physical exercise. If no, participants were then asked if they were thinking about starting in the near future. If no, they were placed in the precontemplation stage, if yes, they were placed in the contemplation stage. If participants answered yes to the first question concerning physical exercise, they were then asked if it was regular physical exercise. If no, they were placed in the preparation stage. If yes, participants were asked if they had done so for longer than six months. If no, they were placed in the action stage, if yes, they were placed in the maintenance stage. The participant by stage breakdown at follow-up was as follows: precontemplation – 15 (11%), contemplation – 15 (11%), preparation – 29 (22%), action – 10 (8%), and maintenance – 62 (47%).

Exercise behaviour at follow-up was assessed using the leisure score index (LSI) of the Godin Leisure Time Exercise Questionnaire (GLTEQ; Godin et al., 1986; Godin & Shephard, 1985). The LSI of the GLTEQ contains three questions covering the frequency of mild, moderate, and strenuous exercise done during free time for at least 20 minutes duration in a typical, week. A LSI is calculated by weighting each frequency by intensity and summing for a total score using the following formula: 3 x mild + 5 x moderate + 9 x strenuous. An independent evaluation of this instrument found it to be easily administered, brief, reliable, and possess concurrent validity based on various criteria including objective activity monitors and fitness indices (Jacobs, Ainsworth, Hartman & Leon, 1993).

RESULTS

Table 9.1 provides means, standard deviations, and Pearson correlations for each of the constructs. These results show moderate to strong correlations among baseline TPB constructs, baseline and current exercise stage, and current exercise behaviour.

A oneway multivariate analysis of variance (MANOVA) was conducted to determine the relationships between TPB constructs (intention, attitude, subjective norm, and perceived behavioural control), current exercise behaviour (moderate and total), and current exercise stage. The MANOVA used current exercise stage as the independent variable. Moderate and total exercise were selected as the measures of exercise behaviour because participants were asked to focus on moderate exercise when answering stage questions. Evidence for this focus was found in the correlations between exercise stage and exercise behaviour which showed the highest correlations were with moderate exercise (see Table 9.1).

Table 9.1   Means, standard deviations, and Pearson correlations among variables

	2	3	4	5	6	7	8	9	10	M	SD
Current											
1. Total Exercise	0.56	0.67	0.46	0.72	0.35	0.49	0.18	0.34	0.08	22.2	17.99
2. Strenuous Exercise		-0.08	-0.09	0.25	0.11	0.10	-0.03	0.15	-0.07	0.44	1.29
3. Moderate Exercise			0.13	0.64	0.31	0.48	0.22	0.22	0.17	2.24	2.37
4. Mild Exercise				0.30	0.16	0.25	0.14	0.23	0.03	2.60	2.62
5. Stage					0.35	0.43	0.21	0.28	0.10	3.68	1.45
Baseline											
6. Stage						0.78	0.56	0.55	0.53	3.96	1.47
7. Intention							0.49	0.51	0.47	0.07	0.93
8. Attitude								0.49	0.48	1.71	0.91
9. Perceived Control									0.43	1.59	1.19
10. Subjective Norm										1.82	1.35

Note: The intention scale was converted to a standard score. Attitude, perceived control, and subjective norm range from > 3 to + 3. Correlations > 0.14 are significant ($p < 0.05$).

Table 9.2 **Descriptive statistics, ANOVA results, and effect sizes for TOPB constructs by current stage**

Construct		Stage of Exercise Change[a]					$F(4, 126)$[b]	Omega[2c]
		PC	C	P	A	M		
Intention	M	–0.67	–0.57	0.03	0.00	0.43	7.81	0.17
	SD	0.85	0.64	1.02	0.63	0.83		
Attitude	M	1.28	1.28	1.77	2.21	1.80	2.80	0.05
	SD	1.12	1.16	0.71	0.37	0.87		
Perceived Control	M	0.82	1.13	1.62	1.90	1.82	3.08	0.06
	SD	1.49	1.28	0.99	0.75	1.15		
Subjective Norm	M	1.53	1.33	2.00	2.30	1.86	1.12	0.00
	SD	1.41	1.63	1.44	0.82	1.28		
Moderate Exercise	M	0.27	0.00	1.03	2.50	3.79	25.34	0.43
	SD	1.03	0.00	0.91	1.58	2.38		
Total Exercise	M	4.53	3.40	14.28	28.40	35.26	36.84	0.52
	SD	10.17	5.99	7.35	12.77	15.41		

Note: The intention scale was converted to a standard score. Attitude, perceived control, and subjective norm range from –3 to +3.
[a] PC = precontemplation, C = contemplation, P = preparation, A = action, M = maintenance.
[b] All F tests are significant ($p < 0.05$) except for subjective norm.
[c] Effect size based on formula provided by Tolson (1980).

The MANOVA revealed a main effect for current exercise stage (Wilks' lambda = 0.36, approximate F(24, 423) = 6.01, $p < 0.00$ 1) and follow-up univariate ANOVAs showed significant differences for all constructs except subjective norm (Table 9.2). These findings support the first hypothesis that baseline TPB constructs would be significantly related to current exercise stage in a linear fashion.

Path analysis (Pedhauzer, 1982) was undertaken to determine if the theoretical relationships among the constructs were as hypothesised. The approach taken in this study is referred to as 'theory trimming' whereby all possible paths are tested and nonsignificant ones are deleted (Pedhauzer, 1982). This approach involved three multiple regression analyses beginning with total current exercise being regressed on exercise stage and the four TPB constructs (intention, perceived control, attitude, and subjective norm). Constructs that emerged with significant standardized betas ($p < 0.01$) are shown with direct paths to exercise behaviour. Exercise stage was then regressed on the four TPB constructs and those that emerged with significant standardized betas ($P < 0.01$) are shown with direct paths to exercise stage. Intention was then regressed on perceived control, attitude, and subjective norm as hypothesised by TPB. Constructs that emerged with significant standardized betas ($p < 0.0$ 1) are shown with a direct path to intention.

Two path models were tested. The first model included the baseline TPB constructs, baseline exercise stage, and current exercise behaviour (Figure 9.1). The second path model included the baseline TPB constructs, current exercise

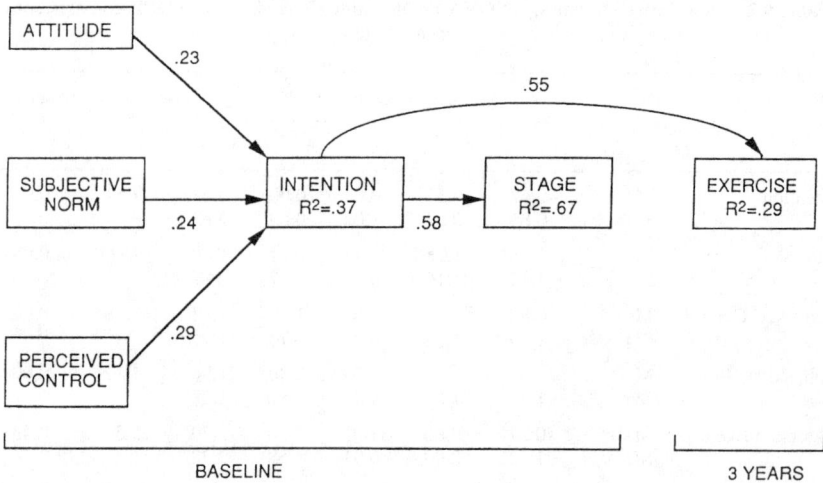

Figure 9.1 Path model showing relationships among baseline planned behavior constructs, baseline exercise stage, and current exercise behaviour. Paths that had nonsignificant ($p < 0.01$) standardized path coefficients were deleted.

stage, and current exercise behaviour (Figure 9.2). The results indicated support for TPB in understanding both exercise stage and behaviour over time but limited support for SCM as a predictive construct for exercise behaviour. Subjective norm, attitude, and perceived control all had effects on intention, and intention in turn mediated the effects of these constructs on both baseline and current exercise stage. These findings supported the second main hypothesis that intention would mediate the relationship between planned behaviour constructs and exercise stage. Neither baseline nor current exercise stage, however, completely mediated the effect of intention on current exercise behaviour as hypothesised. In fact, baseline exercise stage did not even have a direct effect on current exercise behaviour whereas baseline intention did. Thus the third main hypothesis was not supported.

DISCUSSION

The purpose of the present study was to examine an integrated model of the TPB, the SCM, and exercise behaviour in older persons over a three year period. Correlations, ANOVAS, and path analyses from the present study all indicated that TPB had a strong relationship with SCM and exercise behaviour but questioned the utility of including both intention and stage as predictors of exercise over time.

Findings from the present study showed that perceived behavioural control, attitude, and subjective norm were approximately equally important in predicting exercise intention at baseline. The direct effects of attitude and perceived behavioural control on intention have been well documented

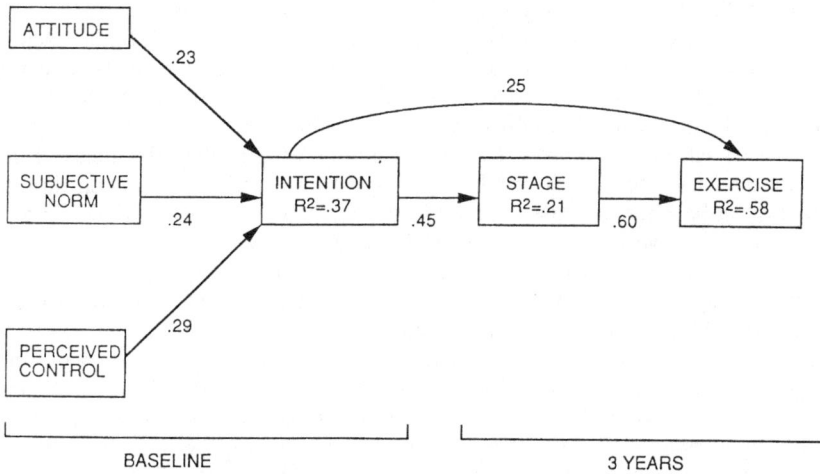

Figure 9.2 Path model showing relationships among baseline planned behaviour constructs, current exercise stage, and current exercise behaviour. Paths that had nonsignificant ($p < 0.01$) standardized path coefficients were deleted.

whereas the direct effect of subjective norm on intention is much less consistent (Godin, 1993; McAuley & Courneya, 1993). Perhaps subjective norm is more relevant for the formation of an intention in an older population because older persons may be less independent from the pressure of important others in their lives. The explained variance in intention of 37% is above the mean for exercise research but within the typical range reported in previous reviews (Godin, 1993; McAuley & Courneya, 1993). These results suggest that intention to exercise in older persons is influenced by a positive evaluation of exercise, perceptions of control over exercise, and perceived pressure from others. These results support a large body of literature showing the validity of the theory of planned behaviour in predicting exercise intention (Godin, 1993; McAuley & Courneya, 1993).

A second finding of the present study was that the TPB was shown to be a valid predictor of exercise stage three years later with the exception of subjective norm. These results are the first to show that the TPB can predict exercise stage over a significant time period. It seems remarkable that cognitive constructs measured at baseline can predict exercise stage three years later especially given the concerns raised over the time interval between cognitive and behavioural assessments (Ajzen, 1991). Some research has shown that the longer the time interval between assessments, the lower the correlations between cognitions and behaviour (e.g., Courneya & McAuley, 1993b; Davidson & Jaccard, 1979). A recent meta-analysis, however, has found that the intention-behavior relationship is not affected significantly by the elapsed time interval (Randall & Wolff, 1994). These present findings may attest to the relative stability of both cognitions and behaviour concerning exercise in an older population.

The path analyses supported the theoretical assertion that intention would mediate the effects of the other planned behaviour constructs on both baseline and current exercise stage. It seems impressive that the path analysis using current exercise stage showed that intention still mediated the effects of the baseline planned behaviour constructs even though exercise stage was assessed three years later (see Figure 9.2). These findings support the robustness of the mediational role that intention plays in predicting exercise stage even though intention at baseline was assessed with respect to a four week period whereas behaviour was measured for a typical week three years later.

The strength of the planned behaviour constructs in predicting exercise stage compares favourably to that of the 'why' constructs from the TTM. Results from the present study found planned behaviour constructs to explain 67% of the variance in baseline exercise stage and 21% of the variance in current exercise stage. Marcus et al. (1994) found the TTM constructs to explain 41% and 45% of the variance in baseline exercise stage in two separate analyses involving a main sample and a subsample. It seems clear that the planned behaviour constructs in the present study outperformed the TTM constructs from the Marcus et al. (1994) study in terms of explaining baseline exercise stage. It is likely that the addition of intention in the planned behaviour model is largely responsible for this improved predictive capacity. The Marcus et al. (1994) study did not provide any data concerning the predictive validity of the TTM constructs over time with respect to exercise stage and so a direct comparison is not possible. The figure of 21% in the present study seems acceptable given the three year time frame. Future research should attempt to predict exercise stage over various time periods to determine the stability of theoretical prediction over time.

The final objective of the present study was to combine the TPB and the SCM into a single theoretical model to predict current exercise behaviour. The only construct that did not have a significant zero order correlation with current exercise behaviour was subjective norm. The construct that correlated the strongest with current exercise behaviour was current exercise stage ($r = 0.72$) and the total path model using current exercise stage explained 58% of the variance in current exercise behaviour (see Figure 9.2). This finding compares favourably to the Marcus et al. (1994) cross-sectional data wherein exercise stage including the 'why' constructs from the TTM explained only 19% of the variance in behaviour. It is likely that the higher explained variance in the present study is due to the addition of the intention construct which had a direct effect on current exercise behaviour and also the validity of the self-report measure of exercise behaviour as argued earlier.

Nevertheless, baseline intention had a higher correlation with current exercise ($r = 0.49$) than did baseline exercise stage ($r = 0.35$) which was hypothesised to mediate the effect of intention on current exercise. Contrary to hypothesis, the path analyses did not support the mediational role of the exercise stage construct. In fact, the path model with baseline exercise stage showed that the construct had no direct effect on current exercise and the only significant path to current exercise was baseline intention.

Moreover, although the path model with current exercise stage showed a direct link between it and current exercise behaviour it did not fully mediate the effect of baseline intention measured three years earlier. These findings suggest that intention provides unique information concerning exercise behaviour that is not completely represented in the exercise stage construct. This finding is contrary to that reported by Marcus et al. (1994) who tested the 'why' constructs from the TTM which do not include attitude, subjective norm, and intention. The strength of the planned behaviour and stages of change constructs in predicting exercise behaviour compares favourably to that of the constructs of the TTM tested by Marcus et al. (1994). Results from the present study found that the TPB and the SCM together explained 29% of the variance in current exercise behaviour using baseline exercise stage. Marcus et al. (1994) found that the TTM explained 28% of the variance in physical activity in the longitudinal data set. Thus the model used in the present study explained the same variance in current exercise behaviour over a three year period as did the Marcus et al. (1994) model over a six month period. These data provide strong support for the long term predictive validity of theory of planned behaviour in the exercise domain although the necessity of including the stage construct in the model might be questioned.

One major issue arising from the present study is whether intention, stage, and behaviour need to be included in the same model or whether they are conceptually redundant with each other. Some researchers have suggested that the stage construct from the TTM is a combination of intention and behaviour with intention defining the first two stages of change and behavioural criteria defining the last three stages of change (Marcus et al., 1994). This definition of the stage construct seems insufficient for at least two reasons. First, the distinction between the first two stages is often defined and operationalised as 'seriously considering' or 'thinking about' a change as opposed to 'intending' to change (e.g., DiClemente et al., 1991; Marcus et al., 1994; Marcus & Owen, 1992; Marcus, Rakowski et al., 1992; Prochaska & DiClemente, 1983). Seriously considering and intending are two different psychological constructs. In fact, Weinstein (1988) includes them as two different stages in his Precaution Adoption Process Model. Second, Prochaska and Marcus (1994) noted that the preparation stage is the only stage that really combines intentional and behavioural criteria. The action and maintenance stages are distinguished by the length of time performing the behaviour at the appropriate level. More recent stage models, however, have made a much more explicit attempt to combine intention and behaviour into a stage construct (e.g., Booth et al., 1993; Godin et al., 1995; Nguyen et al., 1997). Theoretical and empirical research in the exercise domain is needed to determine the relative merits of including intention and behaviour as separate constructs in a model (such as in the TPB) versus combining them as part of a single stage construct (such as in the TTM and other stage models).

If future research continues to support the utility of the TPB for understanding 'why' exercise stage change has occurred, it might be fruitful to integrate the TPB constructs with the processes of change from the TTM to understand 'how' people change their exercise stage. Researchers might examine the relationships between the processes of change and the TPB constructs to determine 'how' people change their attitudes, subjective norms, perceptions of control, and intentions. A path model could be tested wherein the 'why' constructs from the TPB are hypothesised to be mediators between the 'how' constructs (i.e., processes of change) and stage of change. Such a model would likely provide important information for identifying interventions that are likely to help people change their exercise behaviour.

We have recently completed such a study and the results were consistent with our hypotheses (Courneya & Bobick, 1998). Specifically, hierarchical regression analyses showed that the TPB performed well in mediating the relationships between the processes and stages of change. Moreover, perceived behavioural control was predicted exclusively by behavioural processes of change whereas attitude was predicted by both cognitive and behavioural processes of change. It was concluded that the proposed integrated model produced important theoretical insights into how and why people successfully change their exercise behaviour.

If the results of these studies are replicated (i.e, the present study; Courneya, 1995a, Courneya & Bobick, 1998) there are important practical implications that follow. First, it seems clear that the social cognitive constructs contained within the TPB provide a more comprehensive explication of why people change exercise stages than the current social cognitive constructs contained within the TTM (i.e., pros, cons, self-efficacy, and temptation). As such, practitioners interested in exercise stage change should focus on interventions aimed at changing attitude, PBC, and subjective norm. Moreover, based on our other research (Courneya, 1995a; Courneya & Bobick, 1998), it appears that attitude is the key social cognitive construct that should be targeted for early to middle stage transitions (i.e., from precontemplation to action) whereas PBC is the key social cognitive construct that should be targeted for middle to later stage transitions (i.e., from contemplation to maintenance). Attitude may be influenced using both cognitive/experiential and behavioural/environmental processes of change whereas PBC will likely be altered primarily through the behavioural/environmental processes of change.

Despite the theoretical insights and improvements in design of the present study, there are a number of limitations that need to be taken into account when interpreting the findings and planning future research. One limitation is the measurement of subjective norm and intention. Subjective norm was measured by a single item and the time frame for the intention measure did not correspond with the behaviour. A second limitation is that the present study only examined exercise stage at two time points that were three years apart. A number of stage changes might have occurred during such a time interval. It would seem profitable to assess stage at multiple, shorter intervals (perhaps six months) to examine the predictive validity at different time points. A third limitation is that the present study was prospective and longitudinal but not experimental. The issue of causation is best inferred using experimental designs. Future studies might attempt interventions based on TPB and monitor exercise stage changes over time. Fourth, the path analysis approach taken in the present study, called 'theory trimming', does not test the proposed model explicitly nor does it compare it to other possible models. Other models may have provided a better fit to the data. Future research may wish to collect multiple measures of each construct and use the more powerful technique of structural equation analysis. Finally, the data collected were from a self-selected, motivated sample and relied exclusively on self report for assessment. Future research is needed to verify the results of this study using more diverse and reliable methods such as random sampling and behavioural observations.

REFERENCES

Ajzen, I. (1988). *Attitudes, Personality, and Behavior.* Chicago: Dorsey Press.

Ajzen, I. (1991). The theory of planned behavior. *Organizational Behavior and Human Decision Processes, 50,* 179–211.

Ajzen, I. & Driver, B. L. (1992). Application of the theory of planned behavior to leisure choice. *Journal of Leisure Research, 24,* 207–224.

Ajzen, I. & Fishbein, M. (1980). *Understanding Attitudes and Predicting Social Behavior.* Englewood Cliffs, NJ: Prentice-Hall.

Ajzen, I. & Madden, T. J. (1986). Prediction of goal-directed behavior. Attitudes, intentions, and perceived behavioral control. *Journal of Experimental Social Psychology, 22,* 453–474.

Bandura, A. (1986). *Social Foundations of Thought and Action.* Englewood Cliffs, NJ: Prentice-Hall.

Blair, S. N. (1984). How to assess exercise habits and physical fitness. In J. Matarazzo, S. Weiss, J. Herd & N. Miller (eds.), *Behavioral Health: A Handbook of Health Enhancement and Disease Prevention* (pp. 424–447). New York, NY. John Wiley & Sons.

Booth, M. L., Macaskill, P., Owen, N., Oldenburg, B., Marcus, B. H. & Bauman, A. (1993). Population prevalence and correlates of stages of change in physical activity. *Health Education Quarterly, 20,*431–440.

Buxton, K., Wyse, J., and Mercer, T. (1996). How applicable is the stages of change model to exercise behavior? A review. *Health Education Journal, 55,* 239–257.

Cardinal, B. J. (1995). The transtheoretical model of behavior change as applied to physical activity and exercise: A review. *Journal of Physical Education and Sport Sciences, 8(2),* 32–45

Courneya, K. S. (1994). Predicting repeated behavior from intention: The issue of scale correspondence. *Journal of Applied Social Psychology, 24,* 580–594.

Courneya, K. S. (1995a). Understanding readiness for regular physical activity in older individuals: An application of the theory of planned behavior. *Health Psychology, 14,* 80–87.

Courneya, K. S. (1995b). Perceived severity of the consequences of physical inactivity across the stages of change in older adults. *Journal of Sport and Exercise Psychology, 17,* 447–457.

Courneya, K. S. & Bobick, T. M. (in press). No evidence for a termination stage in exercise behavior change. Avante.

Courneya, K. S. & Bobick, T. M. (1998). Integrating the theory of planned behavior with the processes and stages of change: An application to physical exercise. *Manuscript submitted for publication.*

Courneya, K. S. & McAuley, E. (1995). Cognitive mediators of the social influence – exercise adherence relationship: A test of the theory of planned behavior. *Journal of Behavioral Medicine, 18,* 499–515.

Courneya, K. S. & McAuley, E. (1993a). Predicting physical activity from intention: Conceptual and methodological issues. *Journal of Sport and Exercise Psychology, 5,* 50–62.

Courneya, K. S. & McAuley, E. (1993b). Can short range intentions predict physical activity participation? *Perceptual and Motor Skills, 77,* 115–122.

Davidson, A. R. & Jaccard, J. J. (1979). Variables that moderate the attitude-behavior relationship: Results of a longitudinal survey. *Journal of Personality and Social Psychology, 37,* 1364–1376.

DiClemente, C. C., Prochaska, J. O., Fairhurst, S. K., Velicer, W. F., Velasquez, M. M. & Rossi, J. S. (1991). The process of smoking cessation: An analysis of precontemplation, contemplation, and preparation stages of change. *Journal of Consulting and Clinical Psychology, 59,* 295–304.

Dishman, R. K. (1990). Determinants of participation in physical activity. In C. Bouchard, R. J. Shephard, T. Stephens, J. R. Sutton and B. D. McPherson (eds.), *Exercise, Fitness, and Health. A Consensus of Current Knowledge* (pp. 75–101). Champaign, IL: Human Kinetics.

Dishman, R. K. (1991). Increasing and maintaining exercise and physical activity. *Behavior Therapy, 22* 345–378.

Dishman, R. K. & Sallis, J. F. (1993). Determinants and interventions for physical activity and exercise. In C. Bouchard, R. J. Shephard and T. Stephens (eds.), *Physical Activity, Fitness, and Health: Consensus Statement* (pp. 214–238). Champaign, IL: Human Kinetics.

Fishbein, M. & Ajzen, I. (1975). *Belief, Attitude, Intention, and Behavior: An Introduction to Theory and Research.* Reading, MA: Addison-Wesley.

Godin, G. (1993). The theories of reasoned action and planned behavior: Overview of findings, emerging research problems and usefulness for exercise promotion. *Journal of Applied Sport Psychology, 5,* 141–157.

Godin, G., Desharnais, R., Valois, P. & Bradet, R. (1995). Combining behavioral and motivational dimensions to identify and characterize the stages in the process of adherence to exercise. *Psychology and Health, 10,* 333–344.

Godin, G., Jobin, J. & Boullon, J. (1986). Assessment of leisure time exercise behavior by self-report: A concurrent validity study. *Canadian Journal of Public Health, 77,* 359–361.

Godin, G. & Shephard, R. J. (1985). A simple method to assess exercise behavior in the community. *Canadian Journal of Applied Sport Sciences, 10,* 141–146.

Jacobs, D. R., Ainsworth, B. E., Hartman, T. J. & Leon, A. S. (1993). A simultaneous evaluation of 10 commonly used physical activity questionnaires. *Medicine and Science in Sports and Exercise, 25* 81–91.

Janis, I. L. & Mann, L. (1977). *Decision-Making: A Psychological Analysis of Conflict, Choice and Commitment.* New York: Free Press.

Lee, C. (1993). Attitudes, knowledge, and stages of change: A survey of exercise patterns in older Australian women. *Health Psychology, 12,* 476–480.

Marcus, B. H., Eaten, C. A., Rossi, J. S. and Harlow, L. L. (1994) Self-efficacy, decision-making, and stages of change: An integrative model of physical exercise. *Journal of Applied Social Psychology, 24* 489–508.

Marcus, B. H., Emmons, K. M., Simkin-Silverman, L. R., Linnan, L. A., Taylor, E. R., Bock, B. C., Roberts, M. B., Rossi, J. S., & Abrams, D. B. (1998). Evaluation of motivationally tailored vs. standard self-help physical activity interventions at the workplace. *American Journal of Health Promotion, 12,* 246–253.

Marcus, B. H. and Owen, N. (1992) Motivational readiness, self efficacy and decision making for exercise. *Journal of Applied Social Psychology, 22,* 3–16.

Marcus, B. H., Rakowski, W. & Rossi, J. S. (1992). Assessing motivational readiness and decision making for exercise. *Health Psychology, 11,* 257–261.

Marcus, B. H., Selby, V. C., Niaura, R. S. & Rossi, J. S. (1992). Self-efficacy and the stages of exercise behavior change. *Research Quarterly for Exercise and Sport, 63,* 60–66.

Marcus, B. H. & Simkin, L. R. (1993). The stages of exercise behavior. *The Journal of Sports Medicine and Physical Fitness, 33*83–88.

McAuley, E. & Courneya, K. S. (1993). Adherence to exercise and physical activity as health-promoting behaviors: Attitudinal and self-efficacy influences. *Applied and Preventive Psychology,* 265–77.

Murphy, D. (1993). *Application of the Transtheoretical Model to Exercise Adherence.* Unpublished Master's thesis.

Nguyen, M. N., Potvin, L., & Otis, J. (1997). Regular exercise in 30- to 60-year-old men: Combining the stages-of-change model and the theory of planned behavior to identify determinants for targeting heart health interventions. *Journal of Community Health, 22,* 233–246.

Pedhauzer, E. J. (1982). *Multiple Regression in Behavioral Research.* New York: Holt, Rinehart, and Winston.

Prochaska, J. O. & DiClemente, C. C. (1983). Stages and processes of self change in smoking: Towards an integrative model of change. *Journal of Consulting and Clinical Psychology, 51*390–395.

Prochaska, J. O. & DiClemente, C. C. (1985). Common processes of self change in smoking, weight control, and psychological distress. In S. Shiffman and T. A. Willis (Eds.), *Coping and Substance Abuse* (pp. 345–363). New York: Academic Press.

Prochaska, J. O. & DiClemente, C. C. (1986). Toward a comprehensive model of change. In W. E. Miller and N. Heather (eds.), *Treating Addictive Behaviors* (pp. 3–27). London: Plenum Press.

Prochaska, J. O. & Marcus, B. H. (1994). The transtheoretical model: Applications to exercise. In R. K. Dishman (ed.), *Advances in Exercise Adherence* (pp. 161–180). Champaign, IL: Human Kinetics.

Prochaska, J. O. & Velicer, W. F. (1997). The transtheoretical model of health behavior change. *American Journal of Health Promotion, 12 (1),* 11–12.

Prochaska, J. O., Velicer, W. F., Rossi, J. S., Goldstein, M. G., Marcus, B. H., Rakowski, W., Fiore, C., Harlow, L., Redding, C. A., Rosenbloom, D., & Rossi, S. R. (1994) Stages of change and decisional balance for twelve problem behaviors. *Health Psychology, 13,* 39–46.

Randall, D. M. and Wolfe, J. A. (1994) The time interval in the intention-behavior relationship: Meta-analysis. *British Journal of Social Psychology, 33,* 405 –418.

Sallis, J. F. & Hovell, M. F. (1990). Determinants of exercise behavior. In K. B. Pandolph and J. O. Holloszy (eds.), *Exercise and Sport Sciences Rreviews, Vol. 18* (pp. 307–330). Baltimore, MD: Williams & Wilkins.

Sonstroem, R. J. (1988). Psychological models. In R. K. Dishman (ed.), *Exercise Adherence: Its Impact on Public Health* (pp. 125–153). Champaign, IL: Human Kinetics.

Tolson, H. (1980). An adjustment to statistical significance: W^2 *Research Quarterly for Exercise and Sport, 51,* 580–584.

Weinstein N. D. (1988). The precaution adoption process. *Health Psychology, 7,* 355–386.

CHAPTER TEN

A Critical Review of the Transtheoretical Model Applied to Smoking Cessation

Stephen SUTTON

Stage models of health behaviour are becoming increasingly popular in health psychology and health promotion (Weinstein, Rothman, & Sutton, 1998). Stage theories view behaviour change as a dynamic process involving movement through a sequence of discrete, qualitatively distinct stages. Different factors are assumed to be important at different stages. Hence, people in different stages are assumed to require different interventions to encourage or help them to move to the next stage in the sequence.

Current models of health behaviour that incorporate stage assumptions include: the transtheoretical model (TTM; Prochaska & DiClemente, 1986, 1992; Prochaska, DiClemente, & Norcross, 1992; Prochaska & Velicer, 1997) and variants of it (e.g., De Vries & Backbier, 1994; De Vries & Mudde, 1998, also this volume), the precaution adoption process model (Weinstein, 1988; Weinstein & Sandman, 1992), the health action process approach (Schwarzer, 1992; Schwarzer & Fuchs, 1996), and the health behaviour goal model (Gebhardt, 1997).

This chapter focuses on the TTM because it is the dominant model in the field. Nevertheless, many of the points made about the TTM also apply to other stage models of health behaviour. In the first part of the chapter, the TTM is briefly described and the definition and measurement of the central construct of stage of change are considered. The remainder of the chapter reviews the evidence for the TTM, focusing on longitudinal and experimental studies. The review is restricted to studies of smoking cessation which make up the majority of studies using these research designs. For a recent critique of the TTM applied to addictive behaviours in general, see Davidson (1998). Other, empirically based, critiques are referred to in the subsequent discussion.

THE TRANSTHEORETICAL MODEL

Although it is often referred to simply as the stages of change model, the TTM includes 15 different theoretical constructs drawn from different theories of behaviour change. These include the stages of change (which provide the basic organising principle), the 10 processes of change, the perceived pros and cons of changing, and self-efficacy and temptation. The TTM was an attempt to integrate these different constructs in a single comprehensive framework – hence the name transtheoretical.

In stage models, transitions between adjacent stages are the dependent variables, and the other theoretical constructs are variables that are assumed to influence these transitions – the independent variables. But Martin, Velicer, and Fava (1996) refer to the processes of change as independent variables and the pros, cons, self-efficacy, and temptation as dependent variables. It is not clear if they mean that the processes of change influence stage transitions by way of the pros, cons, self-efficacy, and temptation. Those who develop stage models should clearly specify the causal relationships between the constructs. A well-specified stage model would postulate a causal model for each forward stage transition. Indeed, this is a prerequisite for developing stage-based interventions. Simply having a method of classifying people into stages is not a sufficient basis for developing interventions; it is necessary to specify, or at least hypothesise, the factors that need to be changed in order to produce the desired stage transitions.

THE STAGES OF CHANGE

The number and names of the stages and their operational definitions have changed over the years. Farkas, Pierce, Gilpin, Zhu, Rosbrook, Berry, and Kaplan (1996) tabulated some of the different definitions used in the studies by Prochaska and colleagues between 1983 and 1991. They note that the different classifications have never been compared empirically. This lack of standardisation makes it difficult to compare results from different studies and to accumulate the research findings into a coherent body of knowledge.

The version of the TTM used most widely in recent years specifies five stages: precontemplation, contemplation, preparation, action, and maintenance (DiClemente, Prochaska, Fairhurst, Velicer, Velasquez, & Rossi, 1991). Table 10.1 gives the operational definitions. Using a 'staging algorithm', participants are classified into stages on the basis of their responses to a small number of questionnaire items. The first three categories contain the current smokers, the remaining two the ex-smokers; people who have never smoked are not represented in this scheme. Precontemplation, contemplation, and preparation are defined in terms of current intentions and past behaviour (whether or not the person has made a 24-hour quit attempt in the past year), whereas action and maintenance are defined purely in terms of behaviour; ex-smokers' intentions are not taken into account.

Prochaska et al., (1992) represented the stages of change as a spiral. People start at the bottom in precontemplation. They then move through the stages in order (contemplation, preparation, action, maintenance) but will typically relapse back into precontemplation. They may cycle and recycle through the stages several times before achieving successful long-term behaviour change. Prochaska and Velicer (1997) state that for smoking and exercise only about 15% of people regress all the way to the precontemplation stage; the vast

Table 10.1   Stage Definitions (from DiClemente et al., 1991)

Precontemplation
Currently smoking and 'not seriously considering quitting within the next 6 months'.

Contemplation
Currently smoking and 'seriously considering quitting within the next 6 months'; ' were not considering quitting within the next 30 days, had not made a quit attempt of 24 hr in the past year, or both.'

Preparation
Currently smoking, 'were seriously considering quitting in the next 6 months and were planning to quit within the next 30 days', and 'had made a 24-hr quit attempt in the past year.'

Action
Currently not smoking; quit in last 6 months.

Maintenance
Currently not smoking; quit > 6 months ago.

majority return to contemplation or preparation. Thus, the spiral model is not accurate in this respect.

Although the DiClemente et al., (1991) staging algorithm is presumably intended to divide current smokers into three homogeneous groups, close examination reveals that it creates in effect *six* different subgroups (Table 10.2; cf. Pierce, Farkas, Zhu, Berry, & Kaplan, 1996). The precontemplation stage includes two subgroups (labelled A and B in Table 10.2): those who have not made a quit attempt in the past year and those who have. The contemplation stage includes three subgroups. For instance, contemplation-C comprises those smokers who are planning to quit within the next 30 days but who are allocated to contemplation rather than to preparation because they have not made a quit attempt in the past year. Although the term 'intention' is used in Table 10.2 for simplicity, different versions of the staging questions used in different studies ask whether the smoker is 'intending to quit', 'seriously considering quitting', 'seriously thinking of quitting' or 'planning to quit' (e.g., compare DiClemente et al., (1991) with Prochaska & Goldstein (1991)). Such apparently small changes can have a large effect. For example, of 400 participants in a study of radon testing, 23.7% said they had 'planned' to test, but only 13.7% said they had 'decided' to test (Weinstein, Lyon, & Sandman, 1996).

Close inspection of the stage definitions reveal that they are logically flawed. First, a smoker cannot be in the preparation stage unless he or she has made a recent quit attempt. Thus, a smoker can never be 'prepared' for his or her first quit attempt (Sutton, 1996b). Second, smokers in contemplation subgroup-C cannot move directly to the next stage in the sequence (preparation). If they make an attempt to quit smoking, they move directly into the action stage. Similarly, if smokers in contemplation subgroup-A develop an intention to quit in the next 30 days and then make a quit attempt, they go directly to the action stage. Thus, *the stages of change are defined in such a way that some smokers cannot move directly to the next stage in the sequence.* (Compare with the following statement by Prochaska, DiClemente, Velicer, and Rossi (1992,

Table 10.2   The different subgroups of current smokers created by the DiClemente et al. (1991) staging algorithm

Stage of change	Intention to quit[a]	Quit attempt in past year
Precontemplation-A	No intention to quit in next 6 months	No
Precontemplation-B	No intention to quit in next 6 months	Yes
Contemplation-A	Intention to quit in next 6 months[b]	No
Contemplation-B	Intention to quit in next 6 months[b]	Yes
Contemplation-C	Intention to quit in next 30 days	No
Preparation	Intention to quit in next 30 days	Yes

[a] The term 'intention' is used for simplicity; the precise wording of the intention questions differs between studies – see text.
[b] But not in the next 30 days.

p. 825): 'Individuals who successfully leap over stages...may exist, but we have not yet found any'.) Third, consider a smoker in the preparation stage who made an unsuccessful quit attempt 11 months prior to assessment. If he or she retains the intention to quit in the next 30 days for a further month without making a new quit attempt, he/she will automatically regress to the contemplation stage (subgroup C). Similar logical problems beset the earlier algorithms devised by Prochaska, DiClemente, and colleagues.

Another problem with this and earlier staging algorithms is that the time periods are arbitrary. Changing the time periods would lead to different stage distributions. The use of arbitrary time periods casts doubt on the assumption that the stages are qualitatively distinct, that is, that they are true stages rather than *pseudostages* (Bandura, 1998, also this volume; Sutton, 1996a). Although it is unrealistic to claim that the full set of stages as defined by the DiClemente et al., (1991) algorithm are pseudostages on a single continuum, nevertheless subsets of the stages may behave like pseudostages. For instance, action and maintenance, which are distinguished purely and arbitrarily by whether or not the duration of abstinence exceeds six months, may behave like pseudostages. If the stages, or subsets of them, are pseudostages, there is no reason to expect different factors to influence different stage transitions.

Only one study to date has directly compared different staging algorithms for smokers. Using data from a large sample of smokers from the California Tobacco Survey, Farkas, Pierce, Gilpin, Zhu, Rosbrook, Berry, and Kaplan (1996) compared the DiClemente et al., (1991) algorithm with an earlier algorithm (described in a later section) which classified smokers into precontemplation, contemplation, and relapse stages. The two algorithms produced markedly different stage distributions. For example, the earlier algorithm classified almost half the sample in the most advanced stage (relapse) whereas the revised scheme placed only 16% in the most advanced stage (preparation). The two algorithms would lead to very different conclusions concerning the proportion of smokers for whom action-oriented programmes are appropriate. Farkas and colleagues also showed that the earlier stage measure provided better prediction of cessation and quit attempts assessed at

1–2 year follow-up than the revised algorithm and that both schemes allocated smokers with very different probabilities of quitting to the same stage (see also Pierce et al., 1996).

Other research groups have devised their own staging algorithms. For example, in the stage measure used by De Vries and Mudde (1998; also this volume), smokers in the precontemplation stage were defined as those who did not intend to quit smoking in the next six months, those in contemplation intended to quit smoking within six months but not within a month, and smokers in preparation intended to quit within one month (the definitions of action and maintenance were similar to those in Table 10.1). Although this scheme is logical and consistent, the time periods are arbitrary and the 'stages' may behave like pseudostages.

Although the great majority of applications of the TTM to smoking cessation have used staging algorithms, a number of other methods have been used to measure stages of change. These include the contemplation ladder (Biener & Abrams, 1991) and multi-dimensional questionnaires such as the University of Rhode Island Change Assessment (URICA; McConnaughy, Prochaska, & Velicer, 1983). Very few studies have used more than one method of stage measurement, so there is little evidence on how well they agree or the extent to which they yield consistent results when related to other variables. Multi-dimensional questionnaires have the problem that respondents can, and do, score highly on more than one 'stage'. This is inconsistent with the assumption that the stages are discrete (Sutton, 1996a).

REVIEW OF TTM STUDIES OF SMOKING CESSATION

In the remainder of this chapter, evidence for the validity of the TTM is reviewed. We focus on smoking cessation because most TTM studies have applied the model to this target behaviour, including those studies that have employed relatively strong research designs.

The vast majority of TTM studies have used a cross-sectional research design. Participants are classified into stages and compared on theoretically relevant variables. Finding significant differences between people in different stages is interpreted as supporting the theory. Unfortunately, these interpretations are frequently erroneous. In fact, certain common patterns of means are *inconsistent* with a stage model. In particular, linear increases or decreases across stages are not consistent with the stage model assumption that different causal factors are important at different stages and therefore provide evidence *against* the model rather than evidence for it (Sutton, in press; Weinstein, Rothman, & Sutton, 1998).

Other patterns of means, however, are consistent with stage model predictions. In particular, what we have called *discontinuity patterns* can, under certain assumptions, be regarded as diagnostic of a true stage model (Kraft, Sutton, & Reynolds, 1999; Sutton, in press; Weinstein, Rothman, & Sutton, 1998). Consider a model with three stages: I, II, and III. If a given theoretically relevant variable shows a significant increase between stage I and stage II but no difference between stages II and III, this would be an example of a discontinuity pattern. Predicting and finding different discontinuity patterns for different theoretically relevant variables can be interpreted as support for the notion of distinct stages. Even so, such evidence would constitute only very weak support because cross-sectional associations are open to different causal interpretations.

The review that follows is restricted to longitudinal and experimental designs which, in principle, should enable stronger inferences to be drawn. In particular, we focus on what Weinstein, Rothman, and Sutton (1998) refer to as Research Designs 2, 3 and 4, namely examination of stage sequences, longitudinal prediction of stage transitions, and experimental studies of matched and mismatched interventions. When using any of these designs to investigate stage model predictions, it has to be assumed that the measurement schedule provides a complete picture of the stage transitions that occur. If the measurement interval is too long or people move rapidly through stages, transitions will be missed (Weinstein, Rothman, & Sutton, 1998). It may be possible to 'fill in the gaps' by careful retrospective questioning at each follow-up, but no study to date has used this approach.

Examination of Stage Sequences

Longitudinal data can be used to examine sequences of transitions through the stages. However, few studies have measured stage membership on more than two occasions. An important exception is the study by Prochaska, Velicer, Guadagnoli, Rossi, and DiClemente (1991) which reported data on 544 smokers and ex-smokers (out of an initial sample of 960) who provided information about stage of change every six months over a two-year period (i.e., a total of five waves of measurement). Participants were classified on each occasion as being in the precontemplation (PC), contemplation (C), action (A), or maintenance (M) stages. The study was conducted before the preparation stage was introduced. The stages were defined as follows. Immotives or precontemplators 'currently smoked and were not considering quitting'. Contemplators 'were currently smoking but were considering quitting in the next year'. Relapsers ('individuals who initially quit on their own but then relapsed in the year prior to the study') were classified with the contemplators. (No justification is given for combining relapsers and contemplators; relapsers were in fact the largest group.) Recent quitters (those in the action stage) 'had quit smoking without formalized treatment in the past six months'. Finally, long-term quitters (maintainers) were individuals 'who initially quit on their own at least six months prior to the study'. The stage definitions are reported in more detail in another study that used the same dataset (DiClemente, Prochaska, & Gibertini, 1985); in this paper, it is made clear that neither immotives nor contemplators had attempted to quit in the past year. As Farkas, Pierce, Gilpin, Zhu, Rosbrook, Berry, and Kaplan (1996) point out, by contrast with the definition used by DiClemente et al., (1991) and in subsequent studies, in this definition behaviour was the primary classification variable which was used to assign smokers to the most advanced stage (relapse), with intention being used to divide the remaining smokers into precontemplators and contemplators.

Prochaska et al., (1991) did not report the sequences of movement through the stages in full, but it is possible to extract some key findings from their paper. In particular, 16% of participants showed a stable progression over the two years from one stage to the next in the sequence (e.g., precontemplation to contemplation) without suffering any reverses (e.g., PC-PC-PC-C-C). There were apparently no participants who showed a stable progression through three or more stages (e.g., PC-PC-C-C-A); two was the maximum. Twelve percent of participants moved backwards one or two stages (e.g., C-C-C-PC-PC). Thirty-six percent of participants showed a flat profile, that is they stayed in the same stage across the five waves of measurement (e.g., PC-PC-PC-PC-PC). The findings indicate that forward progressive movement through the stages is not the modal pattern of change among volunteer self-changers.

Findings such as these are not necessarily inconsistent with stage model predictions. Stage models can vary in terms of the sequences and transitions they allow (Sutton, 1997). At one extreme, a stage model may postulate an invariant and irreversible sequence: everyone moves through the same sequence and only forward transitions to the next stage are allowed. Bandura (1998; also this volume) criticises the TTM for violating these assumptions. However, while invariance and irreversibility may be appropriate for developmental stages, it seems unrealistic to insist on such strict assumptions for stages of health behaviour change.

Table 10.3 shows a matrix of transition probabilities for four stages of change. A transition probability is the conditional probability of moving from one specified stage to another in a given period of time. There are 16 transition probabilities in Table 10.3. The diagonal elements are the probabilities of

Table 10.3 Transition probabilities and models for four stages

		Time 2		
		PC	C	A	M
	PC	P_1	P_2	P_3	P_4
	C	P_5	P_6	P_7	P_8
Time 1					
	A	P_9	P_{10}	P_{11}	P_{12}
	M	P_{13}	P_{14}	P_{15}	P_{16}

Note: PC = Precontemplation; C = Contemplation;
A = Action; M = Maintenance. If the time interval is
6 months or less, P_4 and P_8 must be zero by definition.

Model I

P_5, P_9, P_{10}, P_{13}, P_{14}, P_{15} = 0 (No backwards movement)
P_3, P_4, P_8 = 0 (Only movement to next forward stage allowed; no skips)

Model II

P_3, P_4, P_8, P_9, P_{13}, P_{14} = 0 (Only movement to next stage or immediately preceding stage allowed; no skips in either direction)

staying in each of the four stages over the time period in question; those below the diagonal refer to transitions to earlier stages (backwards movement); those above the diagonal refer to forward transitions. The probabilities in each row sum to one. Note that, because of the definition of maintenance, if the time interval is six months or less then P_4 and P_8 must equal zero. Note also that it is assumed that all stage transitions are direct and do not involve passage through intermediate stages; for example, a person moving from PC at time 1 to A at time 2 is assumed not to pass through C or any other intervening stage.

Two models are specified below the transition matrix. Model I specifies no backwards movement and no skips (e.g., it is not possible to go directly from precontemplation to action in one time period). Thus all the below-diagonal probabilities are set to zero as well as the three probabilities in the upper right-hand corner. This model represents Bandura's ideal stage model. Model II is more realistic insofar as it also allows backwards movement to the immediately preceding stage (e.g., action to contemplation). Note, however, that this model is inconsistent with the spiral version of the stages of change (Prochaska et al., 1992). Like Model I, Model II assumes that the probabilities of moving between pairs of non-adjacent stages are all zero. Even though it is less restrictive than Model I, Model II can still be regarded as a stage model in that it specifies a discontinuity in the pattern of transition probabilities (another example of the discontinuity principle). Assuming there is some forwards movement over the specified time period, both models would predict what Prochaska (e.g., Prochaska & Velicer, 1997) calls a *stage effect*. For example, compared with precontemplation at time 1, contemplation at time 1 would be associated with a higher probability of being in action at time 2 ($P_7 > P_3$); or, put simply, early stages predict later stages. However, demonstrating a stage effect is not by itself strong evidence for a stage model; the full set of transition probabilities needs to be considered. Researchers who use stage models should test predictions about the pattern of transition probabilities under the assumption that no stage transitions have been missed.

If longitudinal data on stage membership are available on two (or more) occasions separated by an appropriate time interval, models for the transition probabilities can be estimated using latent transition analysis (LTA[1]; Collins & Wugalter, 1992). In multi-wave data, there will be a transition matrix for each adjacent pair of occasions.

Although several studies have reported transition probabilities (De Vries & Mudde, 1998, also this volume; Pallonen, Leskinen, Prochaska, Willey, Kääriäinen, & Salonen, 1994), in only two studies have these been formally analysed using latent transition analysis. Velicer, Martin, and Collins (1996; see also Martin et al., 1996) employed this technique to analyse the same dataset as Prochaska et al., (1991). They did not test either of the models in Table 10.3, but, of the models they did examine, one that allowed backwards movement to the immediately preceding stage and forwards movement to the next or the next-but-one stage provided the best fit. Movement to the next-but-one stage could indicate that some stage transitions were missed by the measurement schedule. Velicer et al. (1996) also used the same method to analyse stage transitions in an intervention study.

A number of studies have found that initial stage of change predicted cessation at follow-up (i.e., movement to the action or maintenance stage) over time periods ranging from one month to two years (e.g., De Vries & Mudde, 1998, also this volume; DiClemente et al., 1991; Farkas, Pierce, Zhu, Rosbrook, Gilpin, Berry, & Kaplan, 1996; Pallonen et al. 1994; Prochaska & Velicer, 1997). As noted above, on their own such stage effects do not provide strong evidence for a stage model. Nevertheless, these findings do suggest that stage measures may be of practical value in measuring progress towards smoking cessation.

However, they may not be the best measures for this purpose. In their sample of Californian smokers, Farkas, Pierce, Zhu, Rosbrook, Gilpin, Berry, and Kaplan (1996) showed that stage of change (assessed using the DiClemente et al., (1991) algorithm) was not a significant independent predictor of cessation at 1–2 year follow-up when used in a multivariable analysis with other factors (including baseline cigarette consumption and quitting history), and that these factors were better predictors than stage of change. In a later paper which used the same dataset, they proposed the 'quitting continuum' as an alternative to the stage measure (Pierce, Farkas, & Gilpin, 1998). They categorised current smokers at baseline into five 'levels' on the basis of combinations of factors known to predict smoking cessation (cigarette consumption, quitting history, intention to quit). Borrowing the terminology of the TTM, they labelled these levels precontemplation, contemplation, early preparation, intermediate preparation, and advanced preparation. Early preparation, for example, was defined by the combination of a high level of addiction (smoking ≥ 15 cigarettes/day), limited quitting history (a 1–6 day quit attempt in the past year), and an intention to quit in the next six months. Together with three levels of abstinence (action, early maintenance, advanced maintenance), this created an eight level quitting continuum which could be used to measure progress towards smoking cessation. The scheme was not entirely consistent. For example, contemplators at baseline were no more likely than precontemplators to be in cessation at 1–2 year follow-up.

In principle, many such quitting continua could be created with different numbers of levels, using either the same predictive factors categorised and combined in different ways or a different set of predictive factors. (In the earlier paper, they presented a different categorisation scheme). Alternative categorisations should be compared empirically. However, if progress towards quitting is conceptualised as a continuum, it is not clear why one should want to categorise smokers at all. An alternative approach would be to use a regression model to estimate an individual smoker's likelihood of quitting smoking or of making a forward transition.

While Pierce et al.'s quitting continuum is useful for measuring progress towards cessation, it is based on factors that *predict* but may not necessarily *influence* the likelihood of smoking cessation (see Fisher, 1996). One therefore needs to be cautious about drawing implications for intervention. For example, one criterion for being in the advanced preparation stage is having a strong quitting history. A strong quitting history may influence the likelihood of future smoking cessation, for instance by increasing the smoker's confidence. But it may simply be a *marker* for a high motivation to quit and/or a low level of addiction. If the latter interpretation is correct, interventions need to be directed at changing motivation and addiction (and the factors that influence them) rather than at strengthening the smoker's quitting history. What is required is a theory that explains the causal relationships between addiction level, quitting history, intention to quit, and subsequent smoking cessation (see Hughes, 1996, and Shiffman, 1996). The quitting continuum certainly does not imply, as Pierce et al., (1998) claim, that different interventions should be used at different levels on the continuum.

Longitudinal Prediction of Stage Transitions

As well as examining stage sequences, longitudinal data can be used to test whether different theoretically relevant variables predict stage transitions among people in different baseline stages. The assumption is that such predictors represent causal factors that influence stage movement. Stage models should specify, or hypothesise, the factors that influence transitions between each pair of adjacent stages. As we have noted, expositions of the TTM are not entirely clear and consistent in this regard. Analyses of longitudinal data should be stratified by stage and should compare people who move to the next stage in the sequence with those who remain in a given stage with respect to baseline characteristics. Prediction of movement to any more advanced stage and prediction of backward transitions may also be of interest.

Only four studies could be identified that used prospective analyses stratified by initial stage to examine predictors of stage transitions. The study by Perz, DiClemente, and Carbonari (1996) is not included here because the analyses were either not properly prospective or failed to stratify by stage.

Prochaska and colleagues (Prochaska, DiClemente, Velicer, Ginpil, & Norcross, 1985) reported the results of discriminant function analyses predicting movement between stages over a six-month interval in a large sample of smokers and ex-smokers. This appeared to be the same dataset used by Prochaska et al., (1991) except that in this paper relapsers were retained as a separate stage instead of being combined with contemplators. The predictor set comprised the 10 processes of change, the pros and cons, and self-efficacy and temptation. Most of the analyses predicted movement out of a given stage to three or four other stages, including earlier stages. This makes the findings somewhat difficult to interpret, especially as the means were not reported. However, the analysis for immotives (precontemplators) predicted movement to any more advanced stage compared with remaining in the immotive stage. It showed that immotives who changed stage tended to have relatively high scores on the self-reevaluation process and the cons of smoking but relatively low scores on the social liberation process and the pros of smoking.

DiClemente et al., (1985) reported an analysis of the same dataset, focusing on self-efficacy and temptation as predictors of movement out of the contemplation, recent quitting, and relapse stages (but not the immotive stage) over a 3–5 month follow-up period. Temptation score was not predictive of stage transitions. However, contemplators who became recent quitters had relatively high initial self-efficacy scores compared with those who remained in contemplation, regressed to the immotive stage, or moved to the relapse stage;

those who moved to the relapse stage (theoretically the next stage in the sequence in this version of the model) had similar self-efficacy scores to those who remained in contemplation. In addition, recent quitters who became long-term quitters had higher self-efficacy scores than those who remained recent quitters or moved to the relapse stage. Self-efficacy did not predict movement out of the relapse stage.

De Vries and Mudde (1998; also this volume) reported data on 918 smokers and ex-smokers in the Netherlands who were interviewed after a national mass-media based smoking cessation campaign and again 10 months later. Their stage measure was described in an earlier section. They found that higher pros of quitting predicted forward stage movement among both precontemplators and contemplators, although the latter effect was only marginally significant ($p < .10$). Lower cons of quitting predicted forward movement out of the precontemplation stage, but again this achieved only borderline significance. Pros did not predict forward stage movement among those in the preparation or action stages, and cons did not predict forward stage movement among those in the contemplation, preparation, or action stages. Higher self-efficacy strongly predicted forward stage movement among preparers but did not predict forward movement among those in the precontemplation, contemplation, or action stages. As well as using a different staging algorithm, the measures of pros, cons, and self-efficacy differed from those used by Prochaska et al., (1985) and DiClemente et al., (1985). Processes of change were not measured in this study.

The fourth study failed to find consistent predictors of stage movements in a sample of about 600 smokers who participated in the Working Well Trial (Herzog, Abrams, Emmons, Linnan & Shadel, 1999). These authors used the staging algorithm of DiClemente et al., (1991) and short forms of the standard scales for the pros and cons of smoking and the processes of change; the last was limited to two experiential processes (consciousness raising and self-reevaluation) and four behavioural processes (counterconditioning, reinforcement management, self-liberation, and stimulus control). In a series of logistic regression analyses, each of the 10 variables (pros, cons, each of the six processes of change, and two composite measures representing experiential and behavioural processes) was used to predict stage movements between baseline and follow-up for smokers in each of the three baseline stages (precontemplation, contemplation, preparation). Half the analyses predicted movement to the next stage in the sequence and half to any of the more advanced stages. Half of the analyses predicted movement from baseline to one-year follow-up; the other half predicted movement between baseline and two-year follow-up. Out of a total of 120 tests, only one was significant at the $p < .01$ level; contemplators moving into preparation, action, or maintenance at the two-year follow-up had significantly lower pros scores at baseline than did those remaining in contemplation. The authors note that had they (inappropriately) used $p < .05$ as the criterion for significance, this would have yielded seven significant results out of 120, a proportion consistent with chance. Furthermore, five out of the six additional results involved either the behavioural composite or the behavioural process self-liberation predicting movement out of the precontemplation or contemplation stages. As the authors point out, this is inconsistent with the TTM prediction that experiential processes are more important than behavioural processes at these early stages.

It is remarkable that so few prospective analyses of stage transitions have been reported in almost 20 years of research on the TTM. The four studies outlined above used different measures (e.g., three different staging algorithms were used) and no consistent findings emerged. Given the relatively long follow-up periods used in these studies, it is highly likely that stage transitions were missed. Future studies should use more frequent measurement of stage of change.

Experimental Studies

Stronger evidence that behaviour change follows a stage process would be to demonstrate consistently in experimental studies that stage-matched interventions are more effective than stage-mismatched interventions in moving people to the next stage in the sequence (Weinstein, Rothman, & Sutton, 1998). To date, there have been three studies that have compared matched and mismatched interventions using a stage perspective (Dijkstra, De Vries, Roijackers & van Breukelen, 1998; Quinlan & McCaul, 1999; Weinstein, Lyon, Sandman & Cuite, 1998). The first two studies were based on the TTM with smoking as the target behaviour and found little or no evidence for the stage model predictions. The third used a different stage model (the precaution adoption process model) applied to home radon testing; in this study, the stage model hypotheses were supported. Only the TTM studies are discussed here, but the reader is referred to the study by Weinstein, Lyon, Sandman, and Cuite (1998) as an excellent example of how to derive and test predictions from a stage model.

In the first TTM-based match-mismatch study, Dijkstra et al., (1998) compared the effectiveness of individually tailored letters designed either to increase the pros of quitting and reduce the cons of quitting (outcome information) or to enhance self-efficacy, or both. Smokers were categorised into four stages of change: preparers (planning to quit within the next month); contemplators (planning to quit within the next six months); precontemplators (planning to quit within the next year or in the next five years); and immotives (planning to quit sometime in the future but not in the next five years, to smoke indefinitely but cut down, or to smoke indefinitely without cutting down).

On the basis of two earlier cross-sectional studies (De Vries & Backbier, 1994; Dijkstra, De Vries, & Bakker, 1996), it was hypothesised that immotives would benefit most from outcome information only, preparers from self-efficacy enhancing information only, and the other two groups from both types of information. Thus, counterintuitively, precontemplators and contemplators were predicted to benefit from the same kind of information. A close examination of the cross-sectional studies reveals only partial empirical support for these hypotheses. In neither study was a distinction made between precontemplators and immotives. In the study by Dijkstra et al., (1996), there were no significant differences in self-efficacy between precontemplation and contemplation or between contemplation and preparation, but there was a significant increase between preparation and action and a further significant increase between action and maintenance – a discontinuity pattern which supports a qualitative distinction between pre-action and post-action stages. A plausible interpretation of the increase in self-efficacy from preparation to action (and of the further increase from action to maintenance) is that this is a *consequence* of the stage transition: those who succeed in quitting smoking, at least in the short term, experience an increased sense of self-efficacy as a consequence. An alternative interpretation is that self-efficacy *influences* the likelihood of moving from preparation to action (and from action to maintenance); in other words, smokers in the preparation stage who have, or come to have, higher levels of self-efficacy are more likely, as a consequence, to move to the action stage, leaving behind those with lower levels of self-efficacy. Unlike the first interpretation, this interpretation has direct implications for intervention. In particular, it supports the notion that smokers in the preparation stage need self-efficacy enhancing information but that such information would not be beneficial to those in the precontemplation or contemplation stages.

In this study the cons of quitting were similar across the precontemplation, contemplation, preparation, and action stages (although people in the maintenance stage had significantly lower scores than those in the first three stages). The pros of quitting, on the other hand, showed a significant increase between precontemplation and contemplation and between contemplation and preparation but a significant *decrease* from preparation to action. If we interpret these differences between stages as indicating that the pros of quitting have a causal influence on the likelihood of stage transition, these findings suggest that increasing the pros of quitting may be beneficial for smokers in both the precontemplation and the contemplation stages.

Overall, then, the findings from the Dijkstra et al., (1996) study can be interpreted as suggesting that smokers in the precontemplation and contemplation stages need information designed to increase the pros of quitting whereas those in the preparation stage need self-efficacy-enhancing information. There is no evidence that a combination of the two types of information would be especially beneficial to smokers in any of the three stages.

The other cross-sectional study by De Vries and Backbier (1994) was conducted on a sample of pregnant women and used a different stage definition. Current smokers were classified into precontemplators, contemplators, and relapsers (there was no preparation stage), and the first two 'stages' were created by dichotomising a 5-point intention to quit scale. The results showed a significant increase in self-efficacy between contemplation and action but apparently no difference between precontemplation and contemplation. A measure of attitude (beliefs about the consequences of smoking and quitting), by contrast, showed a significant increase between precontemplation and contemplation but apparently no significant difference between contemplation and action. If we treat attitude and self-efficacy as causal factors, these findings can be interpreted as suggesting that smokers in the precontemplation stage need information designed to change their attitude towards smoking/quitting while smokers in the contemplation stage need information designed to enhance their self-efficacy – indeed, the authors themselves came to this conclusion (p. 172). Again, there is no strong evidence that smokers in any of these stages would benefit from combined information (but also no evidence that combined information would be detrimental).

It is difficult to see how Dijkstra et al., (1998) arrived at their predictions on the basis of the findings from these two studies. In the event, the results of their match-mismatch study showed only weak evidence for a beneficial effect of stage-matched information. With respect to the likelihood of making a forward stage transition, assessed at 10 week follow-up, there were no significant differences between the three types of information among smokers in any of the four stages. However, preparers who received the self-efficacy-enhancing information only were significantly more likely to have quit smoking for seven days at follow-up than preparers in the outcome only condition. Combining immotives and precontemplators, the percentage of smokers who made a forward stage transition did not differ significantly between those who received stage-matched and stage-mismatched information. Among contemplators and preparers combined, the percentage who made a forward stage transition and the percentage who quit for seven days were higher among those who received the stage-matched information than among those who received the stage-mismatched information, but these comparisons were only marginally significant ($p < .10$).

Overall, the findings of this study indicated that personalised, individually-tailored letters were more effective than assessment only, at least in the short term. Whether the letters included information about outcome, self-efficacy, or both, made no difference.

Dijkstra et al., (1998) included a combined information condition in their study, because they predicted that it would be especially beneficial to precontemplators and contemplators. However, there are other reasons for including a combined intervention in a match-mismatch study. As Weinstein, Rothman, and Sutton (1998) point out, predictions can be derived from stage models about the relative effectiveness of combined matched and mismatched interventions compared with their separate components. For example, if intervention A influences the likelihood of moving from stage I to stage II and intervention B influences the likelihood of moving from stage II to stage III, the model would predict that a combined intervention (A+B) would be no better in moving people forward from stage II than the matched intervention (B) alone.

In the second TTM-based match-mismatch study, Quinlan and McCaul (1999) compared a stage-matched intervention, a stage-mismatched intervention, and an assessment-only condition in a sample of college-age smokers in the precontemplation stage (i.e., they were not planning to quit smoking in the next six months). The stage-matched intervention consisted of activities designed to encourage smokers to think more about quitting smoking. The stage-mismatched intervention consisted of action-oriented information and activities intended for smokers who are ready to quit smoking.

There was no significant difference at one month in the percentage who made a stage transition, and significantly more smokers in the stage-mismatched condition tried to quit smoking than in the stage-matched condition. The authors concluded that the findings failed to support the stage model prediction.

Quinlan and McCaul suggest that a mismatched intervention may have different effects depending on whether it is matched to a later stage in the sequence (as in their own study) or to an earlier stage. For example, although it may not be detrimental for smokers in the precontemplation stage to receive an intervention designed for those in the preparation stage, it may be counter-productive to give preparers an intervention designed for precontemplators. The Dijkstra et al., (1998) study provided very weak support for this hypothesis. Nevertheless, the hypothesis is worth testing in future studies.

Prochaska and DiClemente's research groups have not conducted any comparisons of stage-matched and stage-mismatched interventions. Instead, they have developed stage-matched interventions based on self-help manuals and individually-tailored computer-generated feedback reports (which they refer to as an 'expert system') and have tested these in several large randomised trials (Prochaska, DiClemente, Velicer, & Rossi, 1993; Velicer, Prochaska, Fava, Laforge, & Rossi, 1999). These are impressive studies but the analyses reported to date provide no information on the validity of the TTM.

For example, in the most recent study, Velicer et al., (1999) found that an interactive intervention based on the expert system combined with the stage-matched manuals outperformed a noninteractive intervention using the manuals alone. Stage of change was not used as an outcome measure in this paper; nor were the results analysed by baseline stage of change. If it could be shown that the interactive intervention achieved its greater efficacy through changes in the relevant theoretical variables (pros and cons of quitting, self-efficacy and temptation, and the processes of change), resulting in a greater number of forward stage transitions, this would provide support for the TTM. But no such process analysis has been reported to date.

Finally, it should be noted that the notion of individually tailored interventions is not specific to the TTM in particular or to stage models in general. Such interventions can be based on continuum models such as the theory of reasoned action (Fishbein & Ajzen, 1975) or on models that emphasise factors other than social cognitions such as nicotine dependence.

CONCLUSIONS

The notion that behaviour change involves movement through a sequence of qualitative stages is an important idea which deserves further consideration. It is unfortunate that the model that has dominated the field is surrounded by a 'thicket of problems', to use Bandura's (1998) phrase. Although Bandura's insistence that stage models of behaviour change must incorporate the assumptions of invariance and irreversibility is unrealistic, there remain a number of serious problems with the TTM itself and with much of the research based on it:

1. Much more attention needs to be paid to basic measurement issues. The lack of standardisation of measures, particularly of the central construct of stages of change, makes it difficult, if not impossible, to accumulate the findings into a coherent body of knowledge. Investigators who devise new staging

algorithms should at least compare them empirically with existing algorithms. The staging algorithms for smoking devised by the originators of the TTM are logically flawed and based on arbitrary time periods.

2. A stage measure that showed strong predictive validity (early stages predicting movement to later stages) would be useful for measuring progress towards smoking cessation. However, continuous measures may provide more sensitive measures of progress. Furthermore, stage effects are not on their own strong evidence for a stage model. Stage models make predictions about particular patterns of transition probabilities which can be tested if the full set of probabilities are estimated over relatively short time periods under the assumption that no stage transitions have been missed.

3. The TTM is not adequately specified. It is important to specify clearly the causal relationships among the different constructs. We need a causal model for each stage transition. This is a prerequisite for developing stage-matched interventions.

4. The vast majority of studies on the TTM have used a cross-sectional design. This situation is certainly not unique to research on the TTM and is probably inevitable given that cross-sectional studies are relatively easy and inexpensive to conduct. The main problem with cross-sectional associations involving dynamic variables such as cognitions is that they are open to different causal interpretations. The problems are compounded in research on the TTM because researchers often assume, erroneously, that finding differences between people in different stages supports the model. In fact, the best we can do in cross-sectional research on stage models is to predict and look for particular discontinuity patterns.

5. There is considerable confusion in the literature concerning the nature of stage models and how they should be tested. Researchers who use the TTM or other stage models should make model-specific predictions and test them using the designs and analyses outlined in this chapter and elsewhere (Sutton, in press; Weinstein, Rothman, & Sutton, 1998).

6. Existing evidence from prospective and experimental studies applying the TTM and its variants to smoking cessation is insufficient and equivocal. It certainly does not justify the exaggerated claims sometimes made for the model (e.g., Prochaska, 1994).

NOTES

1. LTA extends previous approaches to analysing discrete latent variables (latent class theory and Markov techniques) to models that include both static and dynamic latent variables such as stage membership. In the simplest case where there is only a single indicator of stage membership, no latent class (discrete grouping variable such as experimental versus control condition), and only two time points, LTA provides estimates of two types of parameters: the proportion of the population in each stage at each occasion of measurement; and the probabilities of being in each of the stages at Time 2 conditional on stage membership at Time 1 (i.e., the transition probabilities). LTA can be used to ascertain how well a particular theoretical model fits the data. Goodness-of-fit statistics can be used to compare competing models. LTA requires specialist software; a Windows version of the programme can be downloaded from http://methcenter. psu.edu.

REFERENCES

Bandura, A. (1998). Health promotion from the perspective of social cognitive theory. *Psychology and Health*, 13, 623–649.

Biener, L., & Abrams, D. B. (1991). The contemplation ladder: Validation of a measure of readiness to consider smoking cessation. *Health Psychology*, 10, 360–365.

Collins, L. M., & Wugalter, S. E. (1992). Latent class models for stage-sequential dynamic latent variables. *Multivariate Behavioral Research*, 27, 131–157.

Davidson, R. (1998). The transtheoretical model: A critical overview. In W. R. Miller, & N. Heather (Eds.), *Treating Addictive Behaviors* (2nd ed., pp. 25–38). New York: Plenum.

De Vries, H., & Backbier, E. (1994). Self-efficacy as an important determinant of quitting among pregnant women who smoke: The Ø-pattern. *Preventive Medicine*, 23, 166–174.

De Vries, H., & Mudde, A. N. (1998). Predicting stage transitions for smoking cessation applying the attitude-social influence-efficacy model. *Psychology and Health*, 13, 369–385.

DiClemente, C. C., Prochaska, J. O., Fairhurst, S. K., Velicer, W. F., Velasquez, M. M., & Rossi, J. S. (1991). The process of smoking cessation: An analysis of precontemplation, contemplation, and preparation stages of change. *Journal of Consulting and Clinical Psychology*, 59, 295–304.

DiClemente, C. C., Prochaska, J. O., & Gibertini, M. (1985). Self-efficacy and the stages of self-change of smoking. *Cognitive Therapy and Research*, 9, 181–200.

Dijkstra, A., De Vries, H., & Bakker, M. (1996). Pros and cons of quitting, self-efficacy, and the stages of change in smoking cessation. *Journal of Consulting and Clinical Psychology*, 64, 758–763.

Dijkstra, A., De Vries, H., Roijackers, J., & van Breukelen, G. (1998). Tailored interventions to communicate stage-matched information to smokers in different motivational stages. *Journal of Consulting and Clinical Psychology*, 66, 549–557.

Farkas, A. J., Pierce, J. P., Gilpin, E. A., Zhu, S-H., Rosbrook, B., Berry, C., & Kaplan, R. M. (1996). Is stage-of-change a useful measure of the likelihood of smoking cessation? *Annals of Behavioral Medicine*, 18, 79–86.

Farkas, A. J., Pierce, J. P., Zhu, S-H., Rosbrook, B., Gilpin, E. A., Berry, C., & Kaplan, R. M. (1996). Addiction versus stages of change models in predicting smoking cessation. *Addiction*, 91, 1271–1280.

Fishbein, M., & Ajzen, I. (1975). *Belief, Attitude, Intention, and Behavior: An Introduction to Theory and Research*. Reading, MA: Addison-Wesley.

Fisher, E. B. (1996). Prediction, causation, description, and natural history of smoking cessation. *Addiction*, 91, 1285–1287.

Gebhardt, W. A. (1997). *Health Behaviour Goal Model*. Leiden: University of Leiden.

Herzog, T. A., Abrams, D. B., Emmons, K. M., Linnan, L., & Shadel, W. G. (1999). Do processes of change predict smoking stage movements? A prospective analysis of the transtheoretical model. *Health Psychology*, 18, 369–375.

Hughes, J. R. (1996). My dad can predict better than your dad: So what? *Addiction*, 91, 1284–1285.

Kraft, P., Sutton, S. R., & Reynolds, H. M. (1999). The transtheoretical model of behaviour change: Are the stages qualitatively different? *Psychology and Health*, 14, 443–450.

Martin, R. A., Velicer, W. E., & Fava, J. L. (1996). Latent transition analysis to the stages of change for smoking cessation. *Addictive Behaviors*, 21, 67–80.

McConnaughy, E. N., Prochaska, J. O., & Velicer, W. F. (1983). Stages of change in psychotherapy: Measurement and sample profiles. *Psychotherapy: Theory, Research and Practice*, 20, 368–375.

Pallonen, U. E., Leskinen, L., Prochaska, J. O., Willey, C. J., Kääriäinen, R., & Salonen, J. T. (1994). A 2-year self-help smoking cessation manual intervention among middle-aged Finnish men: An application of the transtheoretical model. *Preventive Medicine*, 23, 507–514.

Perz, C. A., DiClemente, C. C., & Carbonari, J. P. (1996). Doing the right thing at the right time? The interaction of stages and processes of change in successful smoking cessation. *Health Psychology*, 15, 462–468.

Pierce, J. P., Farkas, A. J., & Gilpin, E. A. (1998). Beyond stages of change: The quitting continuum measures progress towards successful smoking cessation. *Addiction*, 93, 277–286.

Pierce, J. P., Farkas, A., Zhu, S-H., Berry, C., & Kaplan, R. M. (1996). Should the stage of change model be challenged? *Addiction*, 91, 1290–1292.

Prochaska, J. O. (1994). Staging: A revolution. *Annals of Behavioral Medicine*, 16, 19.

Prochaska, J. O., & DiClemente, C. C. (1986). Toward a comprehensive model of change. In W. R. Miller & N. Heather (Eds.), *Treating addictive behaviors: processes of change* (pp. 3–27). New York: Plenum.

Prochaska, J. O., & DiClemente, C. C. (1992). Stages of change in the modification of problem behaviors. *Progress in Behavior Modification*, 28, 184–218.

Prochaska, J. O., DiClemente, C. C., & Norcross, J. C. (1992). In search of how people change: Applications to addictive behaviors. *American Psychologist*, 47, 1102–1114.

Prochaska, J. O., DiClemente, C. C., Velicer, W. F., Ginpil, S., & Norcross, J. C. (1985). Predicting change in smoking status for self-changers. *Addictive Behaviors*, 10, 395–406.

Prochaska, J. O., DiClemente, C. C., Velicer, W. F., & Rossi, J. S. (1992). Criticisms and concerns of the transtheoretical model in light of recent research. *British Journal of Addiction*, 87, 825–828.

Prochaska, J. O., DiClemente, C. C., Velicer, W. F., & Rossi, J. S. (1993). Standardized, individualized, interactive, and personalized self-help programs for smoking cessation. *Health Psychology*, 12, 399–405.

Prochaska, J. O., & Goldstein, M. G. (1991). Process of smoking cessation: Implications for clinicians. *Clinics in Chest Medicine*, 12, 727–735.

Prochaska, J. O., & Velicer, W. F. (1997). The transtheoretical model of health behavior change. *American Journal of Health Promotion*, 12, 38–48.

Prochaska, J. O., Velicer, W. F., Guadagnoli, E., Rossi, J. S., & DiClemente, C. C. (1991). Patterns of change: Dynamic typology applied to smoking cessation. *Multivariate Behavioral Research*, 26, 83–107.

Quinlan, K. B., & McCaul, K. D. (1999). *Matched and mismatched interventions with smokers: Testing a stage theory*. Manuscript submitted for publication.

Schwarzer, R. (1992). Self-efficacy in the adoption and maintenance of health behaviours: Theoretical approaches and a new model. In R. Schwarzer (Ed.), *Self-efficacy: Thought control of action* (pp. 217–243). Washington, DC: Hemisphere Publishing Corporation.

Schwarzer, R., & Fuchs, R. (1996). Self-efficacy and health behaviours. In M. Conner & P. Norman (Eds.), *Predicting Health Behaviour* (pp. 163–196). Buckingham: Open University Press.

Shiffman, S. (1996). 'Addiction *versus* stages of change models' vs. 'Addiction *and* stages of change models'. *Addiction*, 91, 1289–1290.

Sutton, S. R. (1996a). Can 'stages of change' provide guidance in the treatment of addictions? A critical examination of Prochaska and DiClemente's model. In G. Edwards & C. Dare (eds.), *Psychotherapy, Psychological Treatments and the Addictions* (pp. 189–205). Cambridge, England: Cambridge University Press.

Sutton, S. R. (1996b). Further support for the stages of change model? *Addiction*, 91, 1281–1292.

Sutton, S. R. (1997). Transtheoretical model of behaviour change. In A. Baum, C. McManus, S. Newman, J. Weinman, & R. West (eds.), *Cambridge Handbook of Psychology, Health and Medicine* (pp. 180–183). Cambridge, England: Cambridge University Press.

Sutton, S. R. (in press). Interpreting cross-sectional data on stages of change. *Psychology and Health.*

Velicer, W. F., Martin, R. A., & Collins, L. M. (1996). Latent transition analysis for longitudinal data. *Addiction*, 91, S197–S209.

Velicer, W. F., Prochaska, J. O., Fava, J. L., Laforge, R. G., & Rossi, J. S. (1999). Interactive versus noninteractive interventions and dose-response relationships for stage-matched smoking cessation programs in a managed care setting. *Health Psychology*, 18, 21–28.

Weinstein, N. D. (1988). The precaution adoption process. *Health Psychology*, 7, 355–386.

Weinstein, N. D., Lyon, J. E., & Sandman, P. M. (1996). *Pilot study of radon testing interventions.* Unpublished manuscript, Department of Human Ecology, Rutgers University.

Weinstein, N. D., Lyon, J. E., Sandman, P. M., & Cuite, C. L. (1998). Experimental evidence for stages of health behavior change: The precaution adoption process model applied to home radon testing. *Health Psychology*, 17, 445–453.

Weinstein, N. D., Rothman, A. J., & Sutton, S. R. (1998). Stage theories of health behavior: Conceptual and methodological issues. *Health Psychology*, 17, 290–299.

Weinstein, N. D., & Sandman, P. M. (1992). A model of the precaution adoption process: Evidence from home radon testing. *Health Psychology*, 11, 170–180.

Section 5 –
Self-Regulation and Health Goals

CHAPTER ELEVEN

The Emergence and Implementation of Health Goals

Peter M. GOLLWITZER and Gabriele OETTINGEN

Health goals focus on the promotion of health and the prevention of illness. Accordingly, they specify desired health outcomes, such as a healthy blood pressure and weight, and are concerned with the respective health enhancing and disease preventing behaviours. The most prominent health-enhancing and disease preventing behaviours (see Taylor, 1991) are exercising, dieting, accident prevention as well as preventive self-examination (e.g., of breasts or testicals). Health goals may not only specify health enhancing and disease preventing behaviours, they may also be targeted at discouraging health compromising behaviours, such as alcohol and drug abuse, smoking, 'Type A' behaviour, risky diets as well as dangerous sports. For people who suffer from an acute or chronic illness or are plagued by a disability (Johnston, 1996), health goals may also focus on the management of these hardships. These behaviours may range from the efficient use of health services, improving patient-practitioner interactions, coping with pain, complying with medical regimens, effective rehabilitation exercises, and specific management of disabilities.

The current literature on the self-regulatory determinants of health behaviours primarily focuses on motivational variables. The health belief model (Hochbaum, 1958; Rosenstock, 1966, 1974) lists general health values, specific beliefs about vulnerability to a particular disorder, and beliefs about the consequences of this disorder. For example, a person may consider changing her diet to include low cholesterol foods, if she values health, feels personally threatened by the possibility of heart disease and believes that the threat of heart disease is severe. Whether or not a health threat leads to the actual implementation of the respective health behaviours, however, further depends on whether a person believes that these behaviours will reduce the experienced threat. This in turn is determined by both the belief that the specific measure can be effective and the belief that the benefits of the health behaviour exceed its costs.

The theory of reasoned action (Fishbein, 1980) also specifies the motivational determinants of values and expectancies. Attitudes towards health behaviours are based on beliefs about the likely outcomes of these behaviours (outcome expectations) and the evaluations of these outcomes (outcome values). In addition, subjective norms are said to play a role. They derive from what other people think one should do (expectation) and the motivation to comply with these normative references (value). In a recent extension of this theory by Ajzen, called the theory of planned behaviour, a further motivational determinant is added: perceived behavioural control over the respective behaviour (Ajzen, 1985). Bandura (1977, 1986), in his social-cognitive theory of behaviour, has referred to this latter variable as self-efficacy beliefs. An important aspect of the Ajzen and Fishbein models is the proposal that the listed determinants affect behaviour by the mediation of a behavioural intention. The behavioural intention construct captures the individual's commitment or goal to perform the specified behaviour. The strength of this goal (or behavioural intention) is said to be dependent on the strengths of the motivational variables listed, and the translation of the intention into behaviour is the more effective, the stronger the intention.

At first glance it appears that Ajzen and Fishbein have transcended the assumption that behaviour is solely dependent on motivational variables (expectations and values) by introducing the concept of behavioural intention (or goal). However, a closer look reveals that the effective translation of intention into behaviour is a function of the strength of the behavioural intention, which is still solely determined by motivational variables. This implies that the individual cannot perform over and above the strength of her intention, which means that volitional strategies play no role over and above the individual's motivation. This conceptualisation is unfortunate, when predicting health behaviours. Usually such behaviours are not highly motivated to begin with (e.g., reducing alcohol consumption or switching from a high fat to a low fat diet), as the respective beliefs are seldom strongly held and the respective values or perceived incentives are mostly low. Moreover, during the attempt to implement health goals the individual is confronted with compromising distractions and temptations (e.g., professional obligations for a person with the goal to exercise regularly or social drinking for a person who has set the goal to abstain from alcohol) and often gets in conflict with bad health habits (e.g., a high calorie diet).

In summary, a self-regulatory view of the control of health behaviours needs to spell out the strategies that go beyond the strength of a person's intention (or goal commitment) and thus motivation. These strategies may relate to how the goal is framed or to volitional skills necessary for effectively translating a given intention into goal-directed behaviour.

MODERN GOAL THEORIES AND THE CONTROL OF GOAL ATTAINMENT

Modern goal theories assume that whether or not people meet their goals depends on both how goal content is framed and how people regulate goal-directed activities (Gollwitzer & Moskowitz, 1996). *Content theories* of goal pursuit focus on the thematic properties of the set goal and how these affect the regulation of goal pursuit and actual goal attainment. Such theories attempt to explain differences in goal-directed behaviours in terms of what is specified as the goal by the individual, because the content characteristics of the goal are expected to affect a person's goal pursuit. Goal content has been considered both in terms of the different needs on which it is based (e.g., autonomy versus materialistic needs, Deci & Ryan, 1991; Kasser & Ryan, 1993) as well as in terms of implicit theories (e.g., entity theories versus incremental theories of ability or morality, Dweck, 1991, 1996). Numerous other aspects of goal content have been suggested, such as specific/abstract (Emmons, 1992; Locke & Latham, 1990), proximal/distal (Bandura & Schunk, 1981), and positive versus negative outcome focus (Higgins, Roney, Crowe, & Hymes, 1994).

Self-regulation theories of goal striving, however, focus on the question of how people overcome certain implementation problems. Setting a goal is just a first step towards goal attainment which is followed by a host of implementation problems that need to be solved successfully. These problems are manifold as they pertain to initiating goal-directed actions and bringing them to a successful ending. Various theoretical approaches have delineated useful self-regulatory strategies, and addressed questions of why and how these strategies are effective. Typical self-regulatory problems of goal pursuit are, for example, warding off distractions (see implemental mindsets, Gollwitzer, 1990; various action control strategies, Kuhl, 1984; Kuhl & Beckmann, 1994), flexibly stepping up efforts in the face of difficulties (see effort mobilisation, Wright & Brehm, 1989), compensating for failures and shortcomings (see self-regulation of motivation, Bandura, 1991; discrepancy reduction, Carver & Scheier, 1981; symbolic self-completion, Wicklund & Gollwitzer, 1982), and negotiating conflicts between goals (see intelligent pursuit of life tasks, Cantor & Fleeson, 1994; conflict resolution in the face of contradictory personal strivings, Emmons & King, 1988).

All these theoretical approaches to the analysis of goal pursuit can, in our view, be profitably applied to the pursuit of health goals. People should benefit more from setting themselves health goals based on autonomy needs (e.g., losing weight for the purpose of self-actualisation; Kasser & Ryan, 1993) as compared to materialistic needs (e.g., losing weight to be attractive to high status people). Goals based on incremental theories of health (i.e., health can be maintained and enhanced by effort and learning; Dweck, 1996) should be more profitable than goals based on entity theories (i.e., health is conceived of as a fixed capacity which people have a certain amount of). In addition, health goals that are framed specifically (e.g., exercising 20 minutes a day; Locke & Latham, 1990), proximally (e.g., exercising during the upcoming weekend; Bandura & Schunk, 1981), and with a positive outcome focus (e.g., deciding to exercise; Higgins et al., 1994) should lead to better health performances than goals that are framed abstractly (e.g., exercising a lot), distally (e.g., exercising during the upcoming summer), and with a negative outcome focus (e.g., deciding not to be lazy). Similarly, self-regulation theories of goal pursuit inform us how people who have set themselves health goals can maximise the translation of these goals into behaviour. In the next section of this chapter we will present a particular self-regulation theory of goal-pursuit, the model of action phases (Heckhausen, 1991, Chap. 6; Gollwitzer, 1990, 1993), and explore whether and how the self-regulatory strategies discovered within this theoretical framework (mindsets and implementation intentions) are relevant to the regulation of people's health goals.

The Model of Action Phases

The model is based on the conceptual distinction between the motivational issue of goal setting and the volitional (wilful) issue of goal striving (Lewin, Dembo, Festinger, & Sears, 1944). It is assumed that the principles guiding goal selection and those guiding goal achievement are qualitatively different (Kuhl, 1984). The model provides a temporal perspective that starts with the awakening of people's wishes prior to goal setting and extends to the evaluative thoughts people have once goal striving has led to some kind of outcome. The sequence of events within this comprehensive time frame is spelled out in terms of four successive, concrete tasks that need to be accomplished in order to promote wish fulfilment. The first of these tasks consists of deliberating wishes and setting preferences in the predecisional phase. People cannot act on all of their wishes at once – some wishes may contradict each other, others are too difficult to implement – and life is simply too short to follow all of one's wishes. As a consequence, people have to decide which of the many wishes they prefer to pursue and preferences are established by employing the evaluative criteria of feasibility and desirability. A wish's feasibility (e.g., to keep an athletic body) is determined by reflecting on the chances that it can be realised (e.g., 'Do I possess the necessary skills and talent, time and equipment, access to relevant opportunities?'). Desirability relates to the expected value of wish fulfilment (i.e., the likelihood of the positive and negative consequences of having achieved the desired wish, such as an anticipated positive or negative self-evaluation, evaluation by others, progress towards some important life goal, excitement of acting on the wish, and external costs or rewards). The perceived feasibility and desirability of a wish are not fixed and depend on whether the wish is scrutinised in the context of other complimentary (e.g., getting to know people) or contradictory (e.g., spending more time on one's work) wishes.

The model suggests, however, that progress towards fulfilling a wish will not occur simply through judging a wish high in feasibility and desirability. Rather, progress demands a decision to act on a given wish. The model speaks of a transition from wishes and desires to binding goals, the latter being accompanied by a feeling of determination or obligation to fulfil the implied wish. Forming a goal commitment, however, is just a prerequisite for making progress towards wish fulfilment. Once a decision has been made, the next task is to promote the initiation of goal-directed actions. This may be quite simple when the necessary goal-directed actions are well practiced or routine. However, difficulties may arise when people are still undecided about where and how to act (e.g., when a person has set herself the goal to exercise). In such cases the execution of goal-directed actions has to be prepared. The model of action phases speaks of this period prior to the initiation of goal-directed action as the preactional phase. To advance further on the way from wishes to action, individuals should reflect and decide on when, where, and how to act, thus creating plans for action. With the initiation of goal-directed behaviours individuals enter the actional phase that comprises the task of bringing goal-directed behaviours to a successful conclusion. To serve this purpose effectively, the individual should flexibly respond to situational opportunities and demands, and when hindrances are encountered, she should readily increase her efforts. The final action phase, called postactional, is characterised by the task of evaluating goal achievement by comparing what has been achieved to what was desired; in this stage the individual assesses whether the desired outcomes have been attained or whether it is necessary to continue striving.

In summary, the model of action phases attempts to delineate distinct tasks within the course of wish fulfilment. In temporal order these tasks are as follows: setting preferences between or among wishes, making plans for goal-directed actions, bringing initiated actions to a successful ending, and evaluating action outcomes. The model's primary objective is to identify potential problems people may encounter when attempting to translate wishes and desires into reality. By doing so, the model has stimulated further concepts that more directly touch self-regulatory processes helping people to overcome these problems. These are the concepts of mindsets and implementation intentions.

The Concept of Mindsets

This concept was suggested by the Würzburg school of thought (Külpe, 1904; Watt, 1905). It was used to explain the experimental observation that instructing participants to solve a specific task creates a related cognitive set that furthers the solution of the task at hand. Apparently, when a person becomes involved with a given task, relevant cognitive procedures are activated and hence become more easily accessible. When this idea is applied to the model of action phases, it follows that different mindsets (i.e., general cognitive orientations with distinct features) should emerge when people become involved with the different tasks associated with the various action phases, and these mindsets should be endowed with cognitive features that facilitate the respective task at hand.

In various studies (for a summary, see Gollwitzer, 1990) it has been demonstrated that participants who had been asked to deliberate a personal wish developed a different cognitive orientation (i.e., a deliberative mindset) than participants who had been induced to plan the implementation of a personal goal (i.e., an implemental mindset). Comparing the features of the deliberative with the implemental mindsets, it became apparent that the different cognitive orientations were functional for solving the respective tasks, that is, setting preferences between wishes and initiating goal-directed actions. From a self-regulation point of view these findings imply that people can acquire these beneficial mindsets by getting involved with intensive deliberation or intensive planning.

The Concept of Implementation Intentions

In the preactional phase people face the task of initiating goal-directed actions. As long as the implementation of a chosen goal does not follow habitualised routes, an individual has to make further decisions. This time the choice is not among wishes, but among competing ways of realising a chosen wish (i.e., a goal). Such a decision takes the format of 'I intend to do x, when situation y is encountered' and its result can be referred to as an *implementation intention* (Gollwitzer, 1993). In an implementation intention, an anticipated future situational cue (opportunity) is linked to a certain goal-directed behaviour. Holding implementation intentions commits the individual to performing certain goal-directed behaviours when the critical situation is actually encountered.

Implementation intentions should not be confused with goal intentions. *Goal intentions* are a result of a decision among competing wishes and desires. Such decisions take the format of 'I intend to achieve x', whereby the x specifies a desired end-state, such as the execution of a concrete behaviour or the attainment of a desired outcome. Accordingly, the consequence of having formed a goal intention is a feeling of commitment to achieve this end-state. Hierarchically, goal intentions are superior to implementation intentions; the latter are formed in the service of the former.

From a self-regulatory point of view, the formation of implementation intentions promotes the initiation of goal-directed action by specifying anticipated situational cues and linking them to specific to-be-performed goal-directed behaviours. Gollwitzer (1993; 1999) assumes that implementation intentions delegate the control of this behaviour to the critical situational cues. As a consequence, these situational cues are more easily detected, more readily attended to, and more efficiently recalled. In the presence of these cues, the specified behaviour becomes elicited automatically. Action initiation is immediate, demands little cognitive capacity, and is started even when the critical situation has not been consciously processed. Furnishing goal intentions with implementation intentions, therefore, transforms the self-regulation of goal pursuit from conscious and effortful regulation into direct control through environmental cues.

PROBLEMS OF GOAL IMPLEMENTATION

Problems of goal implementation can be classified into two categories. The first set of problems involves getting started (remember the task of the preactional phase in the action phase model). For a number of reasons (to be spelled out below), people miss good opportunities to act and thus delay goal achievement. The second set of problems involves ensuring that, once started, goal pursuits are successfully completed. People often give up in the face of difficulties, fail to ward off distractions, and have trouble resuming goal pursuit once disruptions have occurred. How can implementation intentions and implemental mindsets alleviate such problems?

Getting Started: Facilitative Effects of Implementation Intentions

Goals that are furnished with implementation intentions should show a comparatively higher completion rate. As Lewin and his collaboraters observed (Lewin, 1926; Mahler, 1933; Ovsiankina, 1928), once a goal-directed action has been started, chances for its eventual completion are substantially raised.

Accordingly, we ran two studies exploring whether or not implementation intentions raise the completion rate of longer-term projects (Gollwitzer & Brandstätter, Studies 1 and 2; 1997). In the first study, we asked college students prior to Christmas break to each name two projects they intended to achieve during their vacation, one difficult to implement and the other easy to implement. For both types of projects participants indicated such goals as writing a seminar paper, settling an ongoing family conflict, or engaging in sports activities. When we asked participants whether they had formed intentions on where and when to get started (i.e., implementation intentions), about two thirds – again for both types of goals – responded positively.

After Christmas vacation we contacted the participants and checked on project completion. For projects that were difficult to implement, two out of three of the participants who had formed implementation intentions had carried it out. Participants without implementation intentions, however, mostly failed to complete their projects (only one quarter were successful). For the projects that were easy to implement, completion rate was very high (four out of five), regardless of whether or not participants had formed implementation intentions. Participants had also been asked to indicate how they perceived certain qualities of the named projects (e.g., importance of project completion, likelihood of potential obstacles, perceived closeness to project completion). On the basis of this data it could be confidently ruled out that the assessment of implementation intentions was a surrogate for goal quality variables which might have produced the observed pattern of completion rates.

The findings of the above study were corroborated in an analogous experiment in which the experimenters set participants a goal that was difficult to implement (Gollwitzer & Brandstätter, 1997, Study 2). In this experiment all participants were asked, again prior to Christmas break, to write a report on how they spent Christmas Eve. This report was to be written no later than 48 hours after the event and then sent to the experimenters who were supposedly conducting a demographic study on how people spend their holidays in modern times.

Half of the participants were randomly chosen and then instructed to form implementation intentions. They were given a questionnaire that asked them to specify when and where they intended to write the report during the critical 48 hours. The other half of the participants were not requested to pick a specific time and place for implementing this project. When participants' reports arrived in the mail after Christmas, they were analysed in terms of the dates when they were written. It turned out that three-quarters of the implementation intention participants wrote the report in the requested time period, whereas only one-third of the control participants managed to do so. It would be tempting to explain this finding in terms of obedience to the authority of the experimenter – the experimenters, being aware of this problem, however, granted participants absolute anonymity.

Given that most health promoting and disease preventing projects are subjectively perceived as difficult or unpleasant to implement (e.g., starting to regularly exercise for a fifty year old person; changing one's unhealthy diet, to which one has adhered to for one entire life; engaging in difficult rehabilitation activities after a stroke; walking for patients with arthritis, etc.), implementation intentions should have a substantial impact on translating health goals into action. Indeed, women who had set themselves the goal of performing breast self-examination (BSE) during the next month (Orbell, Hodgkins, & Sheeran, 1997) greatly benefited from forming implementation intentions. Participants were university students or administrative staff who were first asked to indicate how strongly they intended to perform BSE during the next month. To create relevant implementation intentions, participants were asked to write down where they would perform BSE in the next month and at what time of the day. Of the participants who had reported strong intentions to perform BSE during the next month, 100% did so when they had been induced to form additional implementation intentions. If no additional implementation intentions were formed, however, the strong goal intention alone only produced 53% of goal completion.

How do implementation intentions facilitate action initiation? Initiation of goal-directed action can fail for a number of reasons: when people are highly absorbed in an ongoing activity, wrapped up in demanding ruminations, gripped by an intense emotional experience, or simply tired, they may not seize an available opportunity to act on their goals, simply because the opportunity fails to attract attention (e.g., a restaurant that offers low cholesterol food for the person with the health goal of reducing her cholesterol level). The reason for this is that attention is focused on other things that have nothing to do with the question of how to achieve the intended goal. But even when people search for appropriate opportunities in a given situational context, they may not detect it simply because it is not obvious at first sight (e.g., when in a club offering social activities people fail to recognise the available sports opportunities). In addition, the initiation of goal-directed action often becomes a problem, because people fail to respond to opportunities which present themselves only for a short moment (e.g., when a migrane patient fails to take his medication at the onset of symptoms). In such cases, immediate initiation of appropriate goal-directed behaviour is required.

Gollwitzer (1993) theorised that implementation intentions which specify anticipated situational cues and link them to concrete goal-directed behaviours are ideally suited to alleviate these problems. By forming implementation intentions the mental representation of the anticipated situational cue becomes highly activated and thus easily accessible. This has attentional, perceptual, and behavioural consequences that should alleviate the problems listed above.

First, regarding the attentional consequences, it was observed in a dichotic-listening task (Bargh, 1982; Johnston & Dark, 1986) that critical words describing the anticipated situational cues were highly disruptive to focused attention. Participants' performance of shadowing (i.e., efficient repeating of the words presented to the attended channel) was severely hampered when critical words were presented to the non-attended channel. Apparently, even when efforts are made to direct attention to the shadowing task, the critical words still managed to attract attention as indicated by the weakened shadowing performance. In dichotic listening research the critical situational cues are presented to participants in terms of verbal descriptions only. In real life, when a person enters a situational context that entails such critical cues not just as words, their potential to attract attention and thus to disrupt focused attention should be even stronger. This implies that opportunities to act as specified in implementation intentions will not easily escape people's attention even when people focus on other things (e.g., worries, strong emotions, the conscious pursuit of competing goals) besides the respective goal pursuit.

Second, to assess the perceptual processes of implementation intentions, an experiment by Steller (1992) employed the embedded figures test (Gottschaldt, 1926; Witkin, 1950). This test consists of complex geometrical figures (b-figures) that contain a smaller partial figure (a-figure). The a-figure is hidden within the b-figures according to Gestalt principles and is thus difficult to detect. Still, following from the idea that implementation intentions lead to heightened accessibility, and thus better detection of a-figures, it was observed that participants showed enhanced detection when they had formed implementation intentions that used the a-figure as the critical situational cue.

Third, the postulated behavioural readiness as a result of forming implementation intentions was demonstrated in a series of three experiments. In the first experiment (Gollwitzer & Brandstätter, 1997, Study 3) participants were induced to form implementation intentions that specified good opportunities to present counterarguments to a series of racist remarks made by a confederate. When participants were finally allowed to counterargue, implementation intention participants initiated their counterarguments more immediately when these good opportunities arose than mere goal intention participants. In a second experiment (Brandstätter, 1992, Study 2) which involved a button pressing task embedded as the secondary task in a dual task paradigm, participants were induced to form the goal intention to press a button as fast as possible whenever numbers appeared on the screen but not when letters were shown. Participants in the implementation intention condition were asked to form the further intention to press the button particularly fast when the number 3 was presented. Implementation intention participants showed a substantial increase in speed (and the number 3 led to faster reactions than the other numbers) as compared to a control group and this effect was independent of whether the simultaneously demanded primary task was easy or difficult to perform. Apparently, the immediacy of responding as induced by implementation intentions is effortless in the sense that it does not put much cognitive load on limited processing resources, and thus persists even when the cognitive demands of the primary task in a pair of tasks are high. In a third experiment (Malzacher, 1992) it was observed that the goal-directed behavior specified in an implementation intention is triggered without any conscious intent once the critical situational context is encountered. Participants in a study employing a retaliation paradigm modelled on Zillman and Cantor (1976), formed the goal intention to respond to an insult by the experimenter in the form of a complaint spoken directly to the transgressor. Some participants also formed implementation intentions of the following form: 'As soon as I see the experimenter again, I will tell her what an unfriendly person she is'. In a subsequent, supposedly independent cognitive experiment, participants were asked to read a series of successively presented adjectives as quickly as possible from a screen. The adjectives were either positive or negative words, suitable for describing people. Shortly before (about 100 msec) each adjective, either a neutral face or the face of the unfriendly experimenter were subliminally presented (presentation time was less than 10 msec). Negative adjectives presented directly after the face of the unfriendly experimenter tended to be read faster than those presented directly after the neutral face, and positive adjectives were read much more slowly after the unfriendly experimenter's face than after the neutral face. This data pattern was only observed for implementation intention participants and failed to show up for mere goal intention participants. Apparently, the situational cues specified in an implementation intention directly elicit cognitive processes without conscious intent, in this case the activation of relevant knowledge and the inhibition of irrelevant knowledge, which facilitates the initiation of the intended action. The mere formation of a goal intention is not sufficient to produce this effect.

In summary, it appears that implementation intentions lead to the heightened activation of the mental representation of the specified situational cues. As a consequence, these cues are more easily detected and more readily attended to. In addition, the reported findings on the behavioural readiness induced by implementation intentions suggests that the commitment which people attach to the behaviour-situation contingency that is proclaimed in their implementation intention creates strong links which normally can only be attained through frequent and consistent situation-response pairings. As this latter procedure leads to the automatic, direct environmental control of behaviour (Bargh, 1992, 1994), one could argue that implementation intentions also achieve this effect. In other words, implementation intentions may be conscious mental acts that set up contingencies which will then lead to the automatic, environmental control of behaviour.

From the perspective of health psychology, these effects of implementation intentions are important, as the crucial objective of any intervention in health behaviour is to first initiate behavioural control by first helping the client set positive health goals and then transforming this conscious behavioural control to automatic and thus habitual behavioural control. This habitualisation of goal-directed behaviour may be particularly difficult in the case of health behaviours, because such behaviours may be unpleasant and thus do not suggest themselves for frequent and consistent execution. But habitual action initiation can also be achieved by the simple mental act of forming implementation intentions. In the study on performing BSE (Orbell et al., 1997), this became evident. Whereas old habits were the best predictors of performing BSE in the next month for participants who had not formed implementation intentions, the predictive power of old habits was nil when participants had formed implementation intentions. Apparently, implementation intentions had created 'new habits.' This interpretation is supported by the finding that all of the implementation intention participants performed BSE exactly in that situation and at the time they had specified.

Are the effects of implementation intentions independent of the respective goal intentions? As the Orbell et al. observations and other findings reported above (for details, see Gollwitzer, 1993) demonstrate, implementation intentions formed in the service of goal intentions have a substantial effect on effective goal pursuit over and above the mere goal intentions. If one follows Ajzen's and Fishbein's theorising, the strength of the goal intention represents a person's motivation to reach the goal. Consequently, the effects of mere motivation on action can be enhanced by implementation intentions.

However, the question remains whether implementation intentions are still effective when the goal intentions on which they are based are weak or have been either completed or abandoned. From a functional point of view, this should not be the case. As soon as no relevant goal exists, implementation intentions should not evince their typical effects. An experiment by Seehausen, Bayer, and Gollwitzer (1994) supports this view. When participants were told that the goal intention would no longer have to be implemented, the typical effects of implementation intentions (in this case the postulated heightened accessibility of the situational cues was measured by a recall test) did not vanish immediately, but were completely gone after 48 hours. In addition, it was observed that varying the strength of participants' commitments to their implementation intentions had an effect. When participants were told that they were the kind of people who would benefit from rigidly adhering to their plans versus the kind of person who would benefit from staying flexible, the former participants showed strong implementation intention effects whereas the latter failed to do so.

In summary, feeling strongly about achieving the goal intention appears to be a prerequisite for the effects of implementation intentions. On the basis of such strong goal commitments, it is the forming and holding of highly mandated links between situational cues and goal-directed behaviours that produce implementation intention effects. For the successful implementation of health goals this implies that people need to set and hold strong health goals and furnish them with implementation intentions to which they feel highly committed.

Is behavioural control through implementation intentions truly habitual? The neuropsychological literature reports that patients with a frontal lobe injury have problems with the conscious control of their actions (e.g., Shallice, 1982), whereas the control of habitual actions is not impeded. Lengfelder (1994) explored the assumption that implementation intentions automatise action initiation by employing the dual task paradigm described above (Brandstätter, 1992, Study 2) with a sample of frontal lobe patients. As expected, implementation intentions managed to speed up action initiation with these patients. Most interestingly, this effect was even stronger when patients showed a weak performance on the Tower of Hanoi problem, a classic measure of a person's aptitude for conscious action control. These findings support the argument that implementation intentions induce direct, automatic action control. Implementation intentions are an effective self-regulatory tool even, and in particular for frontal lobe patients, and should, therefore, be included in rehabilitation programmes. Moreover, relying on implementation intentions as a self-regulatory tool seems to be crucial when a break-down of the conscious control of action is anticipated; for example, when people have to face strong emotional experiences, intensive ruminations, intricate problem solving, or strong pain, all of which are likely concomitant circumstances of acute and chronic illnesses.

Can implementation intentions break bad habits? The automatic action control associated with implementation intentions has an interesting implication for the control of unwanted habitual responses. When certain behaviours, goals, and cognitive concepts are repeatedly and consistently instigated in the same situational context, they fall under the direct control of the respective situational cues (Bargh & Gollwitzer, 1994). If people want to inhibit such cues, goals, or cognitive concepts, they may turn to implementation intentions as a self-regulatory tool. In this case, implementation intentions will have to link the critical situational cues to antagonistic behaviours, goals, and concepts. This should create competition between the unwanted habitual response and the aspired to antagonistic response. The competition should be won by the intended antagonistic response, when the link created by the implementation intention is stronger than the link established through repeated and consistent pairing of the critical situational cues with the habitual response. Gollwitzer and collaborators (Gollwizer & Schaol, 1998) are currently exploring the inhibiting factors of implementation intentions on the suppression of the so-called automatic activation of stereotypes (i.e., the gender stereotype and the elderly stereotype). This line of thought seems particularly relevant for the suppression of bad health habits. For example, a person, who has formed the health goal of adhering to a low calorie diet, must not only focus on the initiation of goal-directed behaviours (i.e., eating low calories foods) but also on inhibiting relevant bad habits, such as indulging in chocolate and other high calorie foods when they are presented. For this purpose the person may form implementation intentions such as, 'as soon as I see chocolate, I will ignore it!'.

Getting Started: Facilitative Effects of Implemental Mindsets

The effects of implementation intentions we have discussed so far are very specific. They only relate to the particular situations and behaviours specified. However, forming implementation intentions should also have more general effects. As pointed out above, intensive involvement with planning the implementation of one's goals creates a so-called implemental mindset. The features of this special cognitive orientation also help people to act by alleviating a crucial problem of getting started. Often people fail to implement a goal even though the situational context would allow it because they experience doubts about the feasibility or the desirability of the goal. Numerous mindset experiments suggest that implemental mindsets suppress such doubts. As a consequence, people in an implemental mindset should more readily seize any goal-relevant opportunities.

Positive illusions. Gollwitzer and Kinney (1989) primed a group of university student participants into an implemental mindset by asking them to plan the implementation of a personal decision they had already made (e.g., to move from home or have a medical check-up). More specifically, participants had to divide this project into five steps, and to list when, where, and how they intended to initiate goal-directed actions for each of these steps (i.e., form implementation intentions). A second group of participants were primed into a deliberative mindset. These participants were asked to contemplate the pros and cons of an unresolved personal problem (e.g., should I move from home, should I have a medical check-up?). Subsequent to the mindset manipulations, both groups of participants were moved on to a supposedly second experiment, where participants had to work on an Alloy and Abramson type (1979) contingency learning task. A third group of participants (control group) immediately started to work on this task, which involved attempts to gain control over frequent but uncontrollable target light onset by either pressing or not pressing a button. Implemental mindset participants' illusion of control tended to be greater than that of control participants and was much greater than that of deliberative mindset participants.

Taylor and Gollwitzer (1995) extended this research by encompassing other indications of positive illusions, such as optimistic self concept (e.g., athletic ability, social self-confidence, self-respect) as well as perceived invulnerability to more or less controllable risks (e.g., addiction to prescription drugs and having a drinking problem versus losing a partner to an early death and developing diabetes, as rated by a similar college student sample). When using the same type of mindset manipulation, implemental mindset participants described their own personal qualities and skills more positively than those of the average college student, and they did this to a larger degree than both deliberative mindset and control participants. The same pattern of data emerged for perceived invulnerability to both more or less controllable risks. Finally, implemental mindset participants reported themselves to be in a better mood than both deliberative mindset and control participants. The differences in mood did not account, however, for the differences in self-perception and perceived invulnerability to risks. These findings suggest that individuals in an implemental mindset are quite certain of the feasibility of their goals. They believe themselves to be very capable, rather invulnerable to both more and less controllable risks and in control of uncontrollable action outcomes (see the study by Gollwitzer & Kinney). This abundant optimism associated with the implemental mindset should supress doubts about being able to reach a set goal and so favour the effective initiation of goal-directed actions. As has been shown many times, optimism about the feasibility of goals – even if it is illusionary – leads to more successful goal achievement than pessimism (for reviews, see Bandura, 1991; 1997; Carver & Scheier, 1989; Oettingen, 1997; Taylor & Brown, 1988; Seligman, 1991).

It has been argued that unrealistic optimism about controllable health risks is counterproductive for setting health goals (Schwarzer, 1994; Weinstein, 1980, 1982). This makes sense, as a person who does not accept a risk will not protect herself by forming respective health goals. When people already have set health goals, however, being optimistic about avoiding health risks should feed into people's efforts to implement their goals like any other optimism does (e.g., illusion of control, high outcome expectation, strong self-efficacy expectation).

It appears, then, that involving oneself with the planning of set goals and thus working up an implemental mindset with its consequent optimism is a powerful self-regulatory tool. It remains an open question, however, whether people who are facing a severe health threat are also capable of working up optimism via implemental mindsets. In a recent study, we put severely depressed patients (mean BDI > 28) who were either out-patients or hospitalised into an implemental mindset by having them plan (in the way described above) the performing of a daily chore. When implemental participants were subsequently asked to gain control over frequent uncontrollable outcomes in a contingency learning task, they reported a striking illusion of control that substantially exceeded that observed in control participants and participants who had been cued into a deliberative mindset. It would seem, therefore, that implemental mindsets do create optimism effects even in people who are chronically pessimistic. This recommends implemental mindsets as a self-regulatory tool for people who have reason to have a pessimistic outlook on themselves and the world.

Unequivocal behavioral orientation. Continuously deliberating the desirability of the chosen goal anew should hamper the efficient initiation of goal-directed actions as doubts about the goal's desirability might be raised. Therefore, it is interesting to ask whether the implemental mindset directs a person's thoughts away from the deliberative issue of estimating the expected value of the goal towards the implementational issues of when, where, and how to act on the goal. Gollwitzer, Heckhausen, and Steller (1990) report two studies suggesting that implemental mindsets favour the processing of information relevant to executing a person's goals and hamper the processing of expected-value-related information. Planning apparently orients people towards issues of implementation as processing of implementation-related information becomes easier, whereas the opposite is true for expected-value-related information.

If participants who have started to plan the execution of a goal (e.g., to terminate an unhappy relationship) are forced to think about its expected value by being asked why they would pursue the chosen goal (Taylor & Gollwitzer, 1995; Study 3), they do not think equally about the pros and cons, but rather strongly favour pros over cons. In addition, they think more about implementation-related issues than about the expected value of the set goal. Apparently, planning discourages people from returning to the deliberation of a chosen goal by focussing them on both, the pros of their choice and the implied implementational issues. These findings should also apply to health goals: for example, a person, who has started to plan the implementation of the goal to stop smoking should develop an unequivocal behavioural orientation that makes redeciding more difficult.

Completion of Goal Pursuit: Positive Effects of Implemental Mindsets and Implementation Intentions

Volitional problems are not only associated with getting started. When the first steps towards goal achievement are successfully implemented, further obstacles may be encountered. First, people may have to step up their efforts when unexpected increases in task difficulties threaten successful task performance. Second, people may have to ward off distractions, because most situations allow for more than one goal pursuit; that is, people need to prevent the primary goal pursuit from being derailed. Third, if people fail at these problems, a further volitional problem arises: the interrupted goal pursuit needs to be resumed. Can planning alleviate these volitional problems?

Effort mobilisation. Energization theory (Wright, 1996) holds that as perceived task difficulty increases, so does a person's effort – at least up to a certain point. This cutoff point describes a person's potential motivation and is reached rather early with unattractive tasks, but much later with attractive tasks. As implemental mindsets make people feel very positive about the expected value of their goals, it follows that people in an implemental mindset should reach the cutoff point comparatively later and therefore show high persistence in the face of difficulties. But effort mobilisation may also be achieved via implementation intentions. If a person anticipates the critical difficulty and links it to a behavioural response that implies heightened effort, the initiation of this behaviour should be facilitated once the difficulty is encountered. In other words, an implementation intention that links an anticipated difficulty with the behavioural response associated with high effort should lead to effort mobilisation in the presence of this difficulty. For example, a person with the goal to abstain from drinking alcohol may form implementation intentions to politely but firmly reject a drink when it is offered by the host of a dinner party.

Warding off distractions. Kuhl (for reviews see Kuhl & Beckmann, 1985, 1994) has applied his theory of action control to the issue of warding off distractions. The theory distinguishes a number of different mental strategies (e.g., attention control and emotion control) which are assumed to effectively shield a person's ongoing goal pursuit from distractions stemming from potential alternative pursuits. Action-oriented people are found to use these strategies more effectively than state-oriented people, as the latter tend to become wrapped up in ruminations about past failures and desired successes or in the deliberation of a decision.

Can planning also strengthen a person's shielding off an ongoing goal pursuit? Gollwitzer and Bayer (1999) report experiments where participants were placed into an implemental or deliberative mindset and then asked to work on certain cognitive tasks. In the first study, a so-called central-incidental memory task was employed, in later studies displays with modified Mller-Lyer-figures were presented. Implemental mindset participants showed a comparatively worse recognition performance for peripherally presented incidental information, and the implemental mindset produced more illusions associated with a narrow field of attention. The results of these studies suggest that planning creates a certain closed-mindedness which is based on a narrow field of attention. This effect of planning transported via the implemental mindset should facilitate warding off all kinds of distractions (even unanticipated distractions), because the goal currently pursued commonly takes centre stage, whereas distractions originate from the periphery.

But planning can also focus on particular anticipated distractions. Implementation intentions that specify a feared distraction as the situational cue to which a protective response is linked should provide an effective strategy for escaping these distractions. This has been shown some time ago by

Patterson and Mischel (1976) who equipped children with specific plans to escape the temptations of 'Mr. Clown Box' while they were trying to complete the boring task of putting as many pegs into a pegboard as possible. Mr. Clown Box asked the children to disrupt their task and press his nose, and displayed various distractive stimuli (e.g., attractive toys in an illuminated window). When the children had formed temptation-inhibiting plans ('When Mr. Clown Box says to look at him and play with him, then I just won't look at him, and will say, "I am not going to look at Mr. Clown Box!"'), they were very successful in warding off the distractions of Mr. Clown Box and showed an enhanced pegboard performance as compared to control children who were not equipped with such a plan. Interestingly, so-called task facilitative plans ('When Mr. Clown Box says to look at him and play with him, I'll just look at my pegboard, and say, "I am going to look at my work!"') did not show any effects.

Schaal (1993; Gollwitzer & Schaal, 1998) recently replicated these findings with adults who were asked to solve as many arithmetic problems presented on a computer screen as possible. These problems were simple but demanded much attention. On top of this screen a TV-terminal was mounted showing very attractive award winning commercials in random intervals. Participants were requested to form disruption-inhibiting implementation intentions ('As soon as a commercial comes on, I will ignore it!') or task-facilitating implementation intentions ('As soon as a commercial comes on, I will concentrate on my work!'). The control participants solely set the goal not to let themselves be distracted from working on the arithmetic problems (i.e., they formed a goal intention). As in the Patterson and Mischel study, the way in which the response part of the implementation intention was phrased mattered. Distraction-inhibiting implementation intentions were superior to both task-facilitating implementation intentions and goal intentions. Future research may clarify why distraction-inhibiting implementation intentions are more effective than task-facilitating implementation intentions.

It appears, therefore, that distraction-inhibiting implementation intentions could be powerful self-regulatory tools for people who have set themselves health goals, in particular when the successful pursuit of these goals is threatened by frequent distractions. Think of the person who has formed the health goal of eating low-calorie food. Any table that holds tastier high calorie foods provides a host of distractions. Forming distraction-inhibiting implementation intentions should provide a chance to stick to the goal of eating low-calorie food.

Resumption of disrupted goal-pursuit. Many goal pursuits are long-lasting and therefore often get interrupted. To resume the disrupted goal pursuit is particularly difficult when many incomplete goal pursuits rival each other. Such conflict may produce inactivity with all of the goal pursuits at hand. The question addressed in a recent study was whether placing people in an implemental mindset reduces such conflict.

Pösel (1994) asked participants to start two delayed goal pursuits by writing a letter for each of these projects. However, when participants had addressed each of the two letters, they were disrupted and put in an implemental, deliberative, or no mindset by a different experimenter. When participants returned to the first experimenter, they were allowed to complete the incomplete letters which were still sitting on the desk. Pösel observed that there was no difference between participants with respect to the latency with which participants grabbed one of the letters. However, the implemental mindset participants started to write faster as compared to the deliberative mindset and the control group. Apparently, the implemental mindset helps participants to shield the resumption of an interrupted task from competing unfinished business. This finding parallels the observations reported in the subsection (above) on warding off distractions, which suggests that implemental mindset participants are characterised by a narrowed field of attention.

For people who have set themselves health goals, conflicts between unfinished business may be prevalent and hinder resumption. For instance, the goal of exercising regularly may conflict with other unfinished business (e.g., professional tasks). Being in an implemental mindset should reduce such conflicts and thus focus the individual's mind so that both projects can be pursued effectively (in turn or successively) without feeling disturbed by the other project.

Conclusions and Prospects for Future Research on Goal Implementation

Given that a person feels highly committed to a goal, does planning how to achieve this goal help goal attainment? Our analysis strongly suggests that people can derive additional volitional benefits from planning. First, initiating goal-directed behaviours is facilitated, because planning creates a perceptual readiness which guides people's attention towards relevant opportunities and goal-related means. In addition, it sets up a special behavioural readiness to respond effectively once these opportunities and means are encountered. Illusory optimism and the unequivocal behavioural orientation associated with planning also suppress disfunctional doubts about the goal's feasibility and desirability. Second, bringing an initiated goal pursuit to successful completion is facilitated, because planning helps to mobilise effort in the face of difficulties and to ward off distractions. Moreover, if disruptions to goal-directed actions occur, planning furthers effective resumption.

The experiments presented have demonstrated that many of the beneficial effects of planning are based on the cognitive features of the implemental mindset. The task that leads to the implemental mindset is planning the execution of goal-directed behaviours. The form of planning we have used to induce implemental mindsets has been committing oneself to plans that specify when, where, and how the most important behavioural steps of goal attainment are to be executed; all of this has been requested with projects which demand intensive planning. Future research may want to address the question of whether other forms of planning are equally suited to produce implemental mindsets. In addition, health psychologists may want to explore how people who have set themselves health goals are best taught to produce implemental mindsets so that they can be used as an effective self-regulatory tool in everyday life.

The experiments discussed have also demonstrated that many of the beneficial effects of planning are based on the various cognitive processes originating from implementation intentions. The strength of these effects should be dependent on the strength of the links that are created between anticipated situational cues and goal-directed behaviours. The Seehausen et al. (1994) experiment reported above hints at commitment or strong willing as a crucial variable of strengthening these links ('I really want to stick to my implementation intention as specified!'). Apparently, the strength of the link specified in an implementation intention is dependent on the strength of willing a person manages to mobilise when she connects situational cues with goal-directed behaviours. This is why strong implementation intention effects can only be observed on the basis of strong goal intentions: one cannot expect strong acts of willing on the basis of weak goal intentions.

Future research may want to address whether the strong implementation intention effects observed in the present research are dependent on concretely specifying the situational cues and the respective behaviours. Perhaps more abstract definitions would suffice. For the health psychologist it will be important to not only focus on strengthening the commitment to set health goals but also to teach people to furnish their health goals with strong implementation intentions.

THE EMERGENCE OF GOALS

In the action phase model goals are conceived of as transformed wishes in the sense that they are transformed into a binding commitment. The action phase model also specifies the criteria that predict which of the many wishes and desires a person holds are most likely to be turned into goals. It is assumed that feasible and attractive wishes have the best chance, but the model does not explain how wishes are turned into binding commitments and thus cannot specify beneficial self-regulatory procedures that help people to move from wishes to goals.

One might argue that wishes by themselves are guiding people's behaviours as long as they are describing attractive, desirable end-states. A closer look at this proposition, however, reveals that wishes (e.g., 'I wish I had a slim body', 'I wish I would be a non-smoker', 'I wish I had better health') are not just ineffective in guiding outcome-related behaviours, they even hinder the attainment of the desired outcomes. In the next section, we will report a series of studies that attest to the harmful quality of indulging in positive fantasies about one's personal future, that is, in one's wishes and desires.

The Harmful Effects of Indulging in Positive Fantasies

Researchers commonly analyse people's thinking about the future in terms of expectations, that is, judgements about the likelihood of future events. Whether these expectations are conceptualised as control beliefs, self-efficacy beliefs, outcome expectations, or expectations of future life in general (Bandura, 1997; Scheier & Carver, 1992; Seligman, 1991; Taylor & Brown, 1988), they are held to reflect a person's past experiences and therefore are considered to be powerful predictors of a person's future. Thoughts about the future, however, do not necessarily have to be beliefs about how likely or unlikely a certain desired event will occur, or that a certain behaviour will be performed. People can also spontaneously imagine their desired successes, experience them in their minds' eye, and construct and reconstruct their mental images of future events to their liking; in their daydreams they fancy masterful performances and blissful experiences. Fantasies more easily escape the grip of reality than expectations, because fantasies are not constrained by the cognitive mechanisms that make people acknowledge factual information (Klinger, 1971, 1990; Singer, 1966). Accordingly, individuals may indulge in spontaneous positive fantasies about the future, even though a critical analysis of past performances or assessing the statistical likelihoods would lead to low expectations of success.

But how does fantasising about one's personal future affect a person's readiness to act on her desires? Positive fantasies of success constitute an anticipation of already having reached the success and thus an anticipatory consumption of the various associated positive consequences or experiences. In a positive fantasy a person may vividly experience the desired future event and may colour it more brightly and joyfully than reality would ever permit. Therefore the need to act may be diminished and the thorny path towards enacting the fantasy overlooked. Consequently, no action plans on how to achieve the fantasies may be formed and no precautions for unforeseen hindrances taken. This should reduce the chances of success as a lack of action plans has been linked to decreased performance (see above). In summary, because positive fantasies imply anticipatory consumption of success, no need to act towards implementing the success is experienced and no concern with how to act originates. All of this should hinder successful performances. In comparison, negative fantasies should prevent anticipatory consumption and thus should not be associated with the mental consequences described above and the respective negative performances. An overweight person, for example, who indulges in positive fantasies of losing weight and obtaining a slim body should be less prepared for the necessary actions and attaining the desired outcomes than an overweight person who allows for thoughts about the burden of her overweight body and the hardships of dieting.

Various correlational studies were conducted to test these hypotheses. Different life domains were chosen that affect people's living a productive and healthy life (i.e., romantic and professional success, recovery from chronic and acute illness, and weight loss; Oettingen, 1996, 1997). In all of these studies the positive nature of participants' fantasies about the future were assessed long before (up to four years) the respective successes were measured (e.g., getting a job).

Participants' expectations about achieving the desired success were also assessed, to set the predicted negative relation between fantasies and success against the classic finding that thinking about the future in terms of expectations relates positively to success (for a summary, see Bandura, 1997). Because expectations (in contrast to fantasies) are beliefs about the likelihood of future events which reflect a person's performance history, high expectations of success signal that a given desired event is likely to be attained and thus stimulate people's efforts to realise the desired success.

Weight loss. Oettingen and Wadden (1991) assessed expectations of weight loss as well as weight and food related fantasies in 25 obese women who had enrolled in a weight reduction programme. A semi-projective procedure was used to assess the positivity of patients' fantasies. Each patient was asked to imagine herself vividly as the main character in four weight and temptation-related scenarios. Two stories were designed to elicit fantasies about the participants' weight loss, whereas the other two stories described encounters with tempting foods. Each story had an open ending which participants were asked to complete in writing by describing the stream of thoughts that occurred to them. Immediately after describing the mental images, participants rated the positivity of their fantasies as well as their imagined body shape. Weight loss was measured three times, at 4 months, 1 year, and 2 years later. Both, fantasies and expectations, predicted weight loss, albeit in opposite directions. After 1 year, patients with positive fantasies lost about 11 kilogram less than those with negative fantasies, and patients with positive expectations lost about 12 kilogram more than those with negative expectations. After 2 years, the respective differences were 12 and 15 kilograms. The observed results stayed unchanged when participants' weight loss aspirations (in kilograms) and the expected value of reaching the aspired weight loss were covaried. The results demonstrate that indulging in positive fantasies of getting a slim body and resisting food temptations hinders the actual attainment of weight loss.

A closer look at the individual fantasies participants reported revealed that participants with positive fantasies daydreamed that weight loss had occurred without much effort. For example, one participant who rated her fantasies as very positive imagined herself in a bathing suit being critically appraised by her friends: 'I'll be shining!'. Participants with negative fantasies, however, created food and weight-related problems in their minds' eye and simulated solutions, thus preparing themselves for upcoming hindrances and unforeseen obstacles.

Recovery from chronic and acute illness. In a conceptual replication of the weight loss study, out-patient children suffering from chronic asthma and gastrointestinal disease as well as cancer (leukemia and lymphoma) were contacted, and fantasies, expectations, and disease activities were measured (see Oettingen, 1996, 1997). Positive fantasies concerning patients' future lives were assessed by 12 scenarios which pertained to the domain of health, interpersonal relations, and school achievement. A typical scenario read: 'Imagine you have been invited to sleep over at a friend's house, but since you have been sick for the past couple of days, your mother calls the doctor to see if you are well enough to go. She hangs up the phone and ....'. After the children had completed the scenarios in writing, they rated the positivity of their images. Expectations were operationalised by using the Children's Attributional Style Questionnaire, which assesses to what extent hypothetical positive events are perceived as stable, global, and internal when compared to negative events (Seligman, Peterson, Kaslow, et al., 1984). An optimistic explanatory style conveys a person's sense that she will eventually be able to deal with the situation at hand and thus indicates positive expectations.

When disease activity for chronic illnesses (i.e., peak flow measures for asthmatic children and prescription scores for children with gastrointestinal disease) were assessed several months later, and corrected for the respective measures at the time of the assessment of fantasies and expectations, the pattern of results was the same as in the weight loss study. The more positive the children's fantasies were, the worse their disease activity; the reverse relationship was again observed for expectations. With respect to the children with leukemia and lymphoma, we asked the physician in charge to rate probability of survival at two points in time: when fantasies and expectations were obtained and four years later. Positive fantasies in response to health scenarios hampered recovery rate, whereas expectations showed a close to zero correlation.

Professional success. In a third study students who were completing their university education and prepared to enter the job market were asked to report about their spontaneous positive and negative fantasies related to the upcoming transition into work life (see Oettingen, 1996, 1997). They then had to indicate how often they recently had experienced such positive and negative fantasies, respectively. From these reports we constructed an index that captured the relative frequency of positive over negative fantasies. As in the other studies, participants were also asked to report their expectations of finding a job. Two years later, participants were contacted again and asked how many jobs they had been offered and what their present salary was. Positive fantasies hampered professional success as measured by both variables, whereas high expectations facilitated it. This pattern of data held even after the incentive value of getting a job was statistically controlled for.

Summary. These results suggest that indulging in positive fantasies about the future is not only maladaptive for health promoting and disease preventing behaviours such as losing weight, but also for the recovery from chronic and acute illnesses. This implies that self-help books (e.g., Kirk, 1994; Simonton, Matthews-Simonton, & Creighton, 1978) that advise the health conscious person to think positively about her health (or a slim body, athletic fitness, successful dieting and exercising), hoping to induce health promoting responses and to reduce health compromising responses are therefore likely to fail. Dwelling on positive fantasies inhibits rather then promotes self-regulation.

Apparently, the self-help literature has failed to make the distinction between thinking about the future in terms of spontaneous fantasies versus expectations. It correctly took notice of repeated empirical demonstrations of the beneficial effects of high expectations of success. As these are based on a person's performance history, they are certainly powerful predictors of behaviour, but cannot be changed at will and thus do not qualify as an ubiquitous self-regulatory tool. To increase expectations of success one needs to change one's performance history; simply fantasising about great performances will not suffice. On the other hand, fantasising is not restricted by reality, and can therefore be used excessively. No wonder, then, that self-help books focus on the fantasy-type of positive thinking: it is readily accessible and thus seduces one to think of it as a potential self-regulatory tool. The problem is that the effects on behaviour and success are just opposite to what is known of positive thinking in terms of expectations. Thus, the health psychologist must encourage the transformation of positive fantasies about the future into binding health goals. In the next section, we will explore mental procedures that instigate this transformation process.

The Transformation of Positive Fantasies into Goals

Why were positive fantasies about the future more harmful to success than negative fantasies? Participants with positive fantasies failed to perceive the occurrence of hardships in their minds' eye and did not feel a need to act towards realising their fantasies. This speculation is supported by the data collected in the context of professional success. Participants with positive fantasies reported to have sent out fewer job applications than participants with negative fantasies; at the same time, they reported having refrained from making commitments that potentially would conflict with starting the desired job and having already prepared themselves for changes in their private relationships that would result from accepting the hoped for job offer. Apparently, participants generating positive fantasies took their successes for granted. They presumptuously perceived themselves as already having obtained the desired job offer, and thus failed to tackle the adverse reality that needs to be changed if success is actually to be attained.

These observations suggest an answer to the question of how positive fantasies about the future might be stripped of their consumptive qualities and turned into binding goals. If positive fantasies are mentally contrasted with reflections about the negative reality that stands in the way of fantasy fulfilment, a person should feel a need to act. Positive fantasies are now experienced as something to be achieved in real life and thus should no longer allow indulgence and premature consumption. Moreover, whereas reflections on the negative reality point to the necessity to act and provide clues on how to actually implement fantasies in real life, positive fantasies give action the necessary direction. In other words, mentally contrasting the positive fantasies with reflections on the negative reality should turn the fantasies into behavioural goals. For example, an overweight person who contrasts her positive fantasies with reflections about the respective negative reality (e.g., her impulsive eating behaviours, her liking of high-calorie foods, social drinking, and her distaste for physical exercise), should no longer be able to indulge in her fantasies of a slim body, because they appear as something to be obtained in real life.

One further crucial precondition is required. When people start to experience a positive fantasy as something to be realised and the negative reality as something to be changed, they must also acknowledge the probability that this can be achieved. Accordingly, their expectations of success should ultimately determine whether mental contrasting leads a person to adopt binding goals.

Only if subjective probabilities (i.e., expectations of success) are high and the person sees a reasonable chance to reach her desired fantasies in real life, should she commit herself to the respective behavioural goals. If the subjective probabilities are low, the person faces the unattractive option of having to dismiss her fantasies. As mentally contrasting has turned these fantasies into something to be achieved, they can no longer be consumed and enjoyed presumptuously; and if the prospects of actually achieving them are bleak, it does not make sense to attempt their realisation.

On the contrary, a person who enjoys her positive fantasies without contrasting them with reflections on negative reality does not experience a need to act and therefore will not consider subjective probabilities of success when acting. Such a person should not show intensive goal striving when expectations are high, and should not show disengagement when expectations are low. As compared to the individual who mentally contrasts fantasy and reality, there should be no difference in her engagement regardless of whether subjective probabilities of success are high or low. Similarly, a person who only dwells on the negative reality should also fail to set herself goals, because without positive fantasies action lacks necessary direction and reality is not experienced as something to be changed. Subjective probabilities of success should again not be considered, and engagement in any of the respective behaviors should not reflect the strength of expectations.

This line of thought implies that people who are requested to mentally contrast their positive fantasies with reflections on the negative reality should act according to their expectations. In case of positive expectations, strong goals should emerge and intensive goal pursuit should be observed when the situational context allows for it. In case of negative expectations, people should decide to stay passive and therefore no goal pursuit should be observed even when people face good opportunities to act. Pure dreamers and pure worriers, in contrast, should neither set themselves goals when expectations are high nor intentionally refrain from goal-pursuit when expectations are low. When relevant opportunities arise, they are merely pulled by their positive fantasies or pushed by their worries about the negative reality. Therefore a middle level of engagement with respect to relevant actions (i.e., to change reality in the direction of fantasy fulfilment) should be observed irrespective of the level of subjective probabilities of success.

These ideas were tested in a series of experiments. In each of the studies a fantasy-reality contrast condition was established and compared to both a positive fantasy only group and a group who only reflected on negative aspects of reality. The fantasy only group was established by inducing participants to excessively fantasise about a desired positive future. The reality only group was created by requesting participants to intensely ruminate about aspects of the present negative reality that stands in the way of fantasy fulfilment. In the fantasy-reality contrast condition participants were encouraged to face the contradiction between the desired future and the experienced present reality. In all studies participants' readiness to realise their positive fantasies about the future was assessed; this was done immediately after the experimental manipulations and again some time later (up to two weeks) to provide participants with ample opportunities to get started.

Interpersonal relationships. In the first experiment (Oettingen, Pak & Schretter, 1999), female students were asked to name the interpersonal matter that was presently most important to them (e.g., participants mentioned matters such as settling a conflict with my partner, getting to know somebody) and to judge the likelihood that it would result in a happy ending. Then they were asked to list positive aspects of the happy ending (e.g., feelings of being cared for, being needed) and negative aspects of the present reality that stand in the way (e.g., being impulsive, being shy). In the fantasy-reality contrast group participants had to select two aspects of both, the happy ending and the negative reality. To achieve a fantasy-reality contrast, participants were asked to alternate between generating spontaneous thoughts and images for positive aspects of wish fulfilment and negative aspects of reality, beginning with a positive aspect. Thus two positive and two negative aspects had to be reflected on intermittently. In the fantasy only group participants had to pick four positive aspects of wish fulfilment and indulge in respective fantasies; while in the reality only group, participants had to pick four negative aspects of reality and ruminate about them. Immediately afterwards participants were asked by use of a mood questionnaire how energised and active they felt, and two weeks later they were asked if and when they had acted to realise their fantasies.

Participants felt most energised and initiated actions earliest in the fantasy-reality contrast group, when they held high expectations of success; in the case of low expectations participants felt least energised and initiated actions most sluggishly. On both of these dependent variables the other two groups, the fantasy only and the reality only group, scored in between regardless of whether participants held low or high expectations. The results of various additional statistical analyses confidently ruled out the possibility that this pattern of data might be a consequence of a change in the level of expectations or expected values caused by the different mental manipulations.

For the health psychologist who wants to help people to turn their wishes to get rid of bad health habits (e.g., smoking too much) into effective health goals, these findings have important implications. First, it does not suffice to intensify people's fantasies about a positive future of having overcome this problem. Second, it does not help to make people dwell on their present shortcomings in dealing with the problem. Instead, people need to be encouraged to mentally contrast their positive fantasies with reflections on the respective negative reality. However, this needs to be preceded with strengthening people's expectations of success. Many approaches to boosting people's expectations could be used (e.g., pointing out past successes, having people vicariously experience successes of similar others, praise by a professional, or simply providing detailed information on how to effectively deal with the problem; see Bandura, 1986). The present study is concerned with fantasies originating from ongoing concerns. But perhaps new fantasies can also be turned into goals by the mental procedure of contrasting positive fantasies with reflections on the negative reality. This would have important implications for instigating health goals because it would allow infatuations (e.g., with fashionable trends such as eating Japanese foods, taking fitness vacations, or using the bike instead of the car) to be translated into a binding goal of regular dieting or exercising. The following study considers this issue.

Combining work and family life. In a second study participants were female doctoral students who were approaching a critical age for being able to have children (Oettingen, in press). They were asked to produce positive fantasies about their professional and private lives several years from now, let these mental images pass in front of their minds' eye, and then describe them in writing. Most of the participants daydreamed about having both a professional career and a child. To measure expectations of success, participants were requested to rate their confidence that their fantasies would come true. Thereafter the fantasy-reality contrast, the positive fantasy, and the negative reality groups were established. All participants read lively reports from working mothers who described the daily hassles of combining work and family life. In the fantasy-reality contrast group participants were encouraged to read these statements carefully and to create associations to these negative reports. In this way participants who had just fantasised positively were forced to contrast these fantasies with the respective negative reality. In the fantasy only group participants were encouraged to trivialise the mothers' complaints; participants were told that the mothers came up with these statements as an excuse, that is, they were trying to conceal personal problems. Participants were asked to find out what each mother was trying to conceal; in this way participants were encouraged not to take the reported negative reality seriously. In the reality only group participants were induced to ruminate about the negative reality by being asked to relate the mothers' reports about the experienced hardships to participants' own problems, that is, to the question of why they had failed to start a family.

Two weeks later participants were asked how committed they were to the goal to combine work and family life, how much effort they would be willing to exert towards achieving this goal, and whether they had started to think about the implementation of this goal. The same pattern of results emerged as were observed in the previous experiment. Participants in the fantasy-reality contrast group who had high expectations of success again showed the strongest indications that they now had adopted a firm goal of combining work and family life (i.e., they reported the strongest feelings of commitment, the highest willingness to exert effort, and the highest frequency of relevant mental simulations), whereas participants with low expectations in the same group showed the least indications. Participants in both the positive fantasy only and the negative reality only group scored in between whether they held high or low expectations of success.

Summary. In both experiments participants with high expectations in the fantasy-reality contrast group showed immediate and long-term responses that are commonly found with people who have already set themselves goals (i.e., participants felt energised, they felt committed to attaining the desired outcomes, they planned the implementation of these outcomes, and initiated relevant actions without delay). Apparently, the mental contrasting of positive fantasies about the future with reflections on the negative reality makes people with high expectations turn their fantasies into goals. This mental contrasting thus qualifies as a self-regulatory tool for the transformation of a person's wishes and desires into goals.

Conclusions and Prospects for Future Research on Goal Emergence

It is important to remember that the self-regulatory tool of mental contrasting yields the opposite results for people who have high versus low expectations. It is only for people with high expectations that mental contrasting leads to goal emergence, for people with low expectations, a pronounced passivity is the result. For health goals to arise it seems important, therefore, to first strengthen people's expectations of success. For instance, if stress coping is at issue, people should be first taught (or should teach themselves) about the basic techniques of stress management in order to acquire a strong sense of competence (i.e., high expectations) with respect to coping with stress.

A further implication pertains to people who only ruminate about the negative aspects of reality and thus might be caught up in a depressed state of mind. Using the self-regulatory tool of mental contrasting with these people involves explicitly fostering the intrusion of positive fantasies. If these efforts to intersperse positive fantasies into their negative ruminations are successful, the mental contrasting procedure should lead to the emergence of goals and consequently alleviate the depressive state of mind: Goals are known to provide meaning (Emmons, 1986; Frankl, 1959), and efforts to attain the goal are associated with optimistic expectations (Taylor & Gollwitzer, 1995).

The reported findings make another point that is not directly related to goal emergence, but is relevant to increasing people's knowledge and procedural competence about how to effectively perform health promoting and disease preventing behaviours (e.g., programmes on stress coping, healthy nutrition). The reported experimental findings suggest that people do not consult their expectations of success when they are wrapped up in positive fantasies or lost in ruminations on the negative reality. Therefore even if programmes designed to increase people's competence are successful, they may not affect people's actual health behaviours. For example, an increase in competence (e.g., how to adhere to a low cholesterol diet) should yield respective behaviours only when people have contrasted their positive fantasies (e.g., about a long productive and healthy life) with reflections on the negative reality (e.g., the present poor health condition and bad health habits).

From an applied perspective it will be important to explore how the contrasting procedure can be induced most effectively. Contrasting positive fantasies about the future with reflections on the negative reality forces people to either set the goal to implement the fantasy or to forget the fantasy, and, therefore, contrasting should be experienced as aversive. As a consequence, it seems necessary to explicitly encourage people to contrast and discourage them from dreaming or ruminating. In positive fantasisers one has to disrupt the fantasies by pointing to the negative reality and by discouraging the fantasisers' rationalisations (e.g., downward comparisons, dehumanisation of people who provide negative feedback) that down play this negative reality. For ruminators, on the other hand, it is important to instil lively positive fantasies and to intersperse them into their repetitive ruminations.

Health psychologists might also want to know how often the contrasting procedure has to be applied to induce stable goals. In the present experiments one application was enough to produce long lasting effects and thus stable goals. Repeated applications were not necessary, but this may not always be the case. Also, some people might be less suited to benefit from the mental contrasting procedure. It is possible that visualisers (e.g., Horowitz, 1978) find it more difficult to apply the described contrasting procedure than verbalisers, because it is easier for visualisers to protect their fantasies from the critical objections stemming from reality. Finally, future research on the emergence of goals should also address the issue of setting avoidance goals. In the experiments presented above the contrasting procedure was employed to induce approach goals only (e.g., resolving an interpersonal conflict). How would the contrasting procedure have to be restructered to foster the emergence of avoidance goals (e.g., to stay away from high calorie foods or alcohol)? In other words, is the contrasting procedure also applicable to goals that specify the avoidance of health compromising behaviours? Oettingen (1997, 1999) suggests contrasting negative fantasies about the future (e.g., developing an overweight body, looking ugly and feeling horrible) with reflections on the positive reality (e.g., the present relatively slim and healthy body, looking nice and feeling well). Again, the crucial prerequisite for goals to emerge has to be kept in mind. One has to ensure that people have high expectations of success, which should relate this time to the likelihood of avoiding the unwanted future state. Accordingly, one has to teach people efficient ways of avoiding high calorie foods and alcohol before contrasting their negative fantasies about the future with reflections on the positive reality. Results from research on fear appeals are in line with this emphasis on high expectations. Scaring people by pointing to the negative consequences of their health compromising behaviors stimulates change only if reassuring instructions on how to avoid the danger are also added to the threatening message (Leventhal, 1970; Rogers, 1983).

GENERAL CONCLUSION

Modern goal theories make the claim that a person's behaviour is not solely determined by motivational variables (expectations, values). The self-regulatory strategies people employ are said to make an additional contribution in the sense that a strong motivation can be enhanced by volition. This has been exemplified in the present chapter by analysing how effectively implemental mindsets and implementation intentions help people overcome classic problems of goal pursuit, such as initiating goal-directed actions and bringing them to a successful conclusion. Implemental mindsets and implementation intentions trigger various cognitive processes (e.g., perceptual and attentional processes) which in turn facilitate successful goal pursuit. As a consequence, it is suggested that people who have set themselves health goals may in a self-regulatory effort, actively create implemental mindsets and form implementation intentions which in turn trigger passive cognitive processes that foster goal achievement. In this way, the wilful act of forming implementation intentions puts the individual's goal pursuit on automatic pilot.

Modern goal theories are mute to the question of how goals emerge. There has been recent theorising on this issue, however, that focuses on the manner in which people think about the future. Assuming that a person's wishes and desires are the substance from which goals grow, one might expect that intensifying wishes and desires by positive fantasising is the prominent route to goal emergence. The research discussed above clearly contradicts this view by demonstrating that positive fantasising about desired outcomes (e.g., weight loss) has adverse effects. People's positive fantasising about their wishes and desires can, however, promote goal emergence, if it is contrasted with reflections on negative aspects of the present reality. This mental contrasting procedure qualifies as a powerful self-regulatory tool for people who would benefit from setting themselves stable health goals.

ACKNOWLEDGEMENTS

The studies described in this paper and its preparation were supported in part by research grants and awards from the German Science Foundation, the Humboldt Foundation, and the Max Planck Society. We thank Charles Abraham, John Bargh, and two anonymous reviewers, for their helpful comments on an earlier draft of this chapter.

REFERENCES

Ajzen, I. (1985). From intensions to actions: A theory of planned action. In J. Kuhl & J. Beckman (eds.), *Action Control: From Cognition to Behavior* (pp. 11–39). New York: Springer.

Alloy, L. B. & Abramson, L. Y. (1979). Judgment of contingency in depressed and nondepressed students: Sadder but wiser? *Journal of Experimental Psychology: General, 108,* 441–485.

Bandura, A. (1977). Self-efficacy: Toward a unifying theory of behavioral change. *Psychological Review, 84,* 191–215.

Bandura, A. (1986). *Social Foundations of Thought and Action: A Social Cognitive Theory.* Englewood Cliffs, NJ: Prentice Hall.

Bandura, A. (1991). Self-regulation of motivation through anticipatory and self-reactive mechanisms. In R. A. Dienstbier (ed.), *Nebraska Symposium on Motivation: Vol. 38. Perspectives on Motivation* (pp. 69–163). Lincoln, NE: University of Nebraska Press.

Bandura, A. (1997). *Self-Efficacy: The Exercise of Control.* New York: Freeman.

Bandura, A. & Schunk, D. H. (1981). Cultivating competence, self-efficacy and intrinsic interest through proximal self-motivation. *Journal of Personality and Social Psychology, 41,* 586–598.

Bargh, J. A. (1982). Attention and automaticity in the processing of self-relevant information. *Journal of Personality and Social Psychology, 43,* 425–436.

Bargh, J. A. (1992). Being unaware of the stimulus versus unaware of its interpretation: Does subliminality per se matter to social psychology? In R. Bornstein & T. Pittman (Eds.), *Perception Without Awareness* (pp. 236–255). New York: Guilford Press.

Bargh, J. A. (1994). The four horseman of automaticity: Awareness, intention, efficiency, and control of social cognition. In R. S. Wyer. Jr. & T. K. Srull (eds.), *Handbook of Social Cognition (2nd ed.)*. Hillsdale, NJ: Erlbaum.

Bargh, J. A. & Gollwitzer, P. M. (1994). Environmental control of goal-directed action: Automatic and strategic contingencies between situations and behavior. In W. Spaulding (ed.), *Nebraska Symposium on Motivation: Vol. 41. Integrative Views of Motivation, Cognition, and Emotion* (pp. 71–124). Lincoln, NE: University of Nebraska Press.

Brandstätter, V. (1992). *Der Einflu? von Vorsätzen auf die Handlungsinitiierung. Ein Beitrag zur willenspsychologischen Frage der Realisierung von Absichten*. Franfurt: Peter Lang.

Cantor, N. & Fleeson, W. (1994). Social intelligence and intelligent goal pursuit: A cognitive slice of motivation. In W. Spaulding (ed.), *Nebraska Symposium on Motivation: Vol. 41. Integrative views of motivation, cognition, and emotion* (pp. 125–180). Lincoln, NE: University of Nebraska Press.

Carver, C. S. & Scheier, M. F. (1981). *Attention and Self-Regulation: A Control-Theory Approach to Human Behaviors*. New York: Springer.

Carver, C. S. & Scheier, M. F. (1989). Expectancies and coping: From test anxiety to pessimism. In R. Schwarzer, H. M. Van der Ploeg & C. D. Spielberger (eds.), *Advances in Test Anxiety Research* (Vol. 6, pp. 3–11). Amsterdam: Swets & Zeitlinger.

Deci, E. L. & Ryan, R. M. (1991). A motivational approach to self: Integration in personality. In R. Dienstbier (ed.), *Nebraska Symposium on Motivation: Vol. 38. Perspectives on Motivation* (pp. 237–288). Lincoln, NE: University of Nebraska Press.

Dweck, C. S. (1991). Self-theories and goals: Their role in motivation, personality, and development. In R. Dienstbier (ed.), *Nebraska Symposium on Motivation: Vol. 38. Perspectives on Motivation* (pp. 199–255). Lincoln, NE: University of Nebraska Press.

Dweck, C. S. (1996). Implicit theories as organizers of goals and behavior. In P. M. Gollwitzer & J. A. Bargh (eds.), *The Psychology of Action: Linking Cognition and Motivation to Behavior* (pp. 69–90). New York: Guilford.

Emmons, R. A. (1986). Personal strivings: An approach to personality and subjective well-being. *Journal of Personality and Social Psychology, 51*, 1058–1068.

Emmons, R. A. (1992). Abstract versus concrete goals: Personal striving level, physical illness, and psychological well-being. *Journal of Personality and Social Psychology, 62*, 292–300.

Emmons, R. A., & King, L. A. (1988). Conflict among personal strivings: Immediate and long-term implications for psychological and physical well-being. *Journal of Personality and Social Psychology, 54*, 1040–1048.

Fishbein, M. (1980). A theory of reasoned action: Some applications and implications. In M. M. Page (ed.), *1972 Nebraska Symposium on Motivation*. Lincoln: University of Nebraska Press.

Frankl, V. E. (1959/1984). *Man's Search for Meaning*. New York, NY: Washington Square Press.

Gollwitzer, P. M. (1990). Action phases and mind-sets. In E. T. Higgins & R. M. Sorrentino (Eds.), *Handbook of Motivation and Cognition: Foundations of Social Behavior*. (Vol. 2, pp. 53–92). New York: Guilford.

Gollwitzer, P. M. (1991). *Abwägen und Planen*. Göttingen: Hogrefe.

Gollwitzer, P. M. (1993). Goal achievement: The role of intentions. In W. Stroebe & M. Hewstone (eds.), *European Review of Social Psychology* (Vol. 4, pp. 141–185). Chichester, UK: Wiley.

Gollwitzer, P. M. (1999). Implementation intentions: Strong effects of simple plans. *American Psychologist, 54*, 493–503.

Gollwitzer, P. M. & Bayer, U. (1999). Deliberative versus implemental minnows in the control of action. In S. Chailxen & Y. Trope (eds.), *Dual process theories in social psychology* (pp. 403–422). New York: Guilford.

Gollwitzer, P. M. & Schaal, B. (1998). Metacognition in action: The importance of implementation intentions. *Personality and Social Psychology Review, 2*, 124–136.

Gollwitzer, P. M. & Brandstätter, V. (1997). Impementation intentions and effective goal pursuit. *Journal of Personality and Social Psychology, 73*, 186–199.

Gollwitzer, P. M., Heckhausen, H. & Steller, B. (1990). Deliberative vs. implemental mind-sets: Cognitive tuning toward congruous thoughts and information. *Journal of Personality and Social Psychology, 59*, 1119–1127.

Gollwitzer, P. M. & Kinney, R. F. (1989). Effects of deliberative and implemental mind-sets on the illusion of control. *Journal of Personality and Social Psychology, 56*, 531–542.

Gollwitzer, P. M. & Moskowitz, G. B. (1996). Goal effects on action and cognition. In E. T. Higgins & A. W. Kruglanski (eds.), *Social Psychology: A Handbook of Basic Principles* (pp. 361–399). New York: Guilford Press.

Gottschaldt, K. (1926). Über den Einfluß der Erfahrung auf die Wahrnehmung von Figuren. I. Über den Einflu? gehäufter Einprägung von Figuren auf ihre Sichtbarkeit in umfassenden Konfigurationen. *Psychologische Forschung, 8*, 261–317.

Heckhausen, H. (1991). *Motivation and Action*. Heidelberg: Springer.

Higgins, E. T., Roney, C. J. R., Crowe, E., & Hymes, C. (1994). Ideal versus ought predilections for approach and avoidance: Distinct self-regulatory systems. *Journal of Personality and Social Psychology, 66*, 276–286.

Hochbaum, G. (1958). *Public participation in medical screening programs (DHEW Publication No. 572, Public Health Service)*. Washington, DC: U.S. Government Printing Office.

Horowitz, M. J. (1978). *Image Formation and Cognition*. New York: Appleton-Century-Crofts.

Johnston, M. (1996, May). Models of disability. *The Psychologist*, 205–210.

Johnston, W. A. & Dark, V. J. (1986). Selective attention. *Annual Review of Psychology, 37*, 43–75.

Kasser, T. & Ryan, R. M. (1993) A dark side of the American dream: Correlates of financial success as a central life aspiration. *Journal of Personality and Social Psychology, 65*, 410–422.

Kirk, C. C. (1994). *Taming the Diet Dragon*. St. Paul, Mn: Llewellyn.

Klinger, E. (1971). *Structure and Functions of Fantasy*. New York: Wiley.

Klinger, E. (1990). *Daydreaming: Using Waking Fantasy and Imagery for Self-Knowledge and Creativity*. Los Angeles: Tarcher.

Külpe, O. (1904). Versuche über Abstraktion. In F. Schuhmann (ed.*)*, *Bericht über den 1. Kongreß für Experimentelle Psychologie* (pp. 56–71). Leipzig: Barth.

Kuhl, J. (1984). Volitional aspects of achievement motivation and learned helplessness: Toward a comprehensive theory of action control. In B. A. Maher & W. B. Maher (eds.) *Progress in Experimental Personality Research* (pp 99–171). New York: Academic Press.

Kuhl, J. & Beckmann, J. (eds.). (1985). *Action Control: From Cognition to Behavior*. Berlin: Springer.

Kuhl, J. & Beckmann, J. (eds.). (1994). *Volition and Personality: Action versus State Orientation*. Seattle: Hogrefe Huber.

Lengfelder, A. (1994). *Die Bedeutung des Frontalhirns beim Abwägen und Planen*. Unpublished doctoral dissertation, Ludwig-Maximilians-Universität, München.

Leventhal, H. (1970). Findings and theory in the study of fear communications. In L. Berkowitz (ed.), *Advances in Experimental Social Psychology* (Vol. 5, pp. 119–186). New York: Academic Press.

Lewin, K. (1926). Vorsatz, Wille und Bedürfnis. *Psychologische Forschung, 7*, 330–385.

Lewin, K., Dembo, T., Festinger, L. A. & Sears, P. S. (1944). Level of aspiration. In J. M. Hunt (ed.), *Personality and the Behavior Disorders* (Vol. 1, pp. 333–378). New York: Ronald.

Locke, E. A. & Latham, G. P. (1990). *A Theory of Goal Setting and Task Performance.* Englewood Cliffs, NJ: Prentice Hall.

Mahler, W. (1933). Ersatzhandlungen verschiedenen Realitätsgrades. *Psychologische Forschung, 18*, 27–89.

Malzacher, J. T. (1992). *Erleichtern Vorsätze die Handlungsinitiierung? Zur Aktivierung der Vornahmehandlung.* Unpublished doctoral dissertation, Ludwig-Maximilian-Universität, München.

Oettingen, G. (1996). Positive fantasy and motivation. In P. M. Gollwitzer & J. A. Bargh (eds.), *The Psychology of Action: Linking Cognition and Motivation to Behavior* (pp. 236–259). New York: Guilford.

Oettingen, G. (1997). *Psychologie des Zukunftsdenkens: Erwartungen und Phantasien.* Göttingen: Hogrefe.

Oettingen, G. (1999). Free fantasies about the future and the emergence of developmental goals. In J. Brandstädter & R. M. Lerner (Eds.), *Action and self-development Theory and research through the life span* (pp. 315–342). Thousand Oaks: Sage.

Oettingen, G., Pak, H., & Schnetter, K. (1999). Turning free fantasies about the future into binding goals. Manuscript submitted for publication.

Oettingen, G. & Wadden, T. A. (1991). Expectation, fantasy, and weight loss: Is the impact of positive thinking always positive? *Cognitive Therapy and Research, 15*, 167–175.

Oettingen, G. (in press). Expectancy effects on behavior depend on self-regulatory thought. *Social Cognition.*

Orbell, S., Hodgkins, S. & Sheeran, P. (1997). Implemantation intentions and the theory of planned behavior. *Personality and Social Psychology Bulletin, 23*, 945–954.

Ovsiankina, M. (1928). Die Wiederaufnahme unterbrochener Handlungen. *Psychologische Forschung, 11*, 302–379.

Patterson, C. J. & Mischel, W. (1976). Effects of temptation-inhibiting and task-facilitating plans of self-control. *Journal of Personality and Social Psychology, 33*, 209–217.

Pösel, I. (1994). *Wiederaufnahme unterbrochener Handlungen: Effekte der Bewußtseinslagen des Abwägens und Planens.* Unpublished master's thesis, Universität Regensburg.

Rogers, R. W. (1983). Cognitive and psychological processes in fear appeals and attitude change: A revised theory of protection motivation. In J. Cacioppo & R. Petty (eds.), *Social Psychophysiology: A Sourcebook* (pp. 135–176). New York: Guilford.

Rosenstock, I. M. (1966). Why people use health services. *Milbank Memorial Fund Quarterly, 44*, 94ff.

Rosenstock, I. M. (1974). The health belief model and preventive health behavior. *Health Education Monographs, 2*, 354–386.

Schaal, B. (1993). *Impulskontrolle: Wie Vorsätze beherrschtes Handeln erleichtern.* Unpublished master's thesis, Ludwig-Maximilian-Universität, München.

Scheier, M. F. & Carver, C. S. (1992). Effects of optimism on psychological and physical well-being: Theoretical overview and empirical update. *Cognitive Therapy and Research, 16*, 201–228.

Schwarzer, R. (1994). Optimism, vulnerability, and self-beliefs in health-related cognitions: A systematic overview. *Psychology and Health, 9*, 161–180.

Seehausen, R., Bayer, U. & Gollwitzer, P. M. (1994, September*). Experimentelle Arbeiten zur vorsätzlichen Handlungsregulation.* Paper presented at the biannual meeting of the German Psychological Association, Hamburg.

Seligman, M. E. P. (1991). *Learned Optimism.* New York: Knopf.

Seligman, M. E. P., Peterson, C., Kaslow, N. J., Tanenbaum, R. L., Alloy, L. B., & Abramson, L. Y. (1984). Attributional style and depressive symptoms among children. *Journal of Abnormal Psychology, 93*, 235–238.

Shallice, T. (1982). Specific impairments of planning. *Philosophical Transactions of the Royal Society of London (Biological Science), B 298*, 199–209.

Simonton, O. C., Matthews-Simonton, S. & Creighton, J. (1978). *Getting Well Again.* Los Angeles, CA: Tarcher.

Singer, J. L. (1966). *Daydreaming.* New York: Random House.

Steller, B. (1992). *Vorsätze und die Wahrnehmung günstiger Gelegenheiten.* München: Tuduv.

Taylor, S. E. (1991). *Health Psychology (2nd ed.).* New York: McGraw-Hill.

Taylor, S. E. & Brown, J. D. (1988). Illusion and well-being: A social psychological perspective on mental health. *Psychological Bulletin, 103*, 193–210.

Taylor, S. E. & Gollwitzer, P. M. (1995). Effects of mindset on positive illusions. *Journal of Personality and Social Psychology, 69*, 213–226.

Watt, H. J. (1905). Experimentelle Beiträge zu einer Theorie des Denkens. *Archiv für die gesamte Psychologie, 4*, 289–436.

Weinstein, N. D. (1980). Unrealistic optimism about future life events. *Journal of Personality and Social Psychology, 39*, 806–820.

Weinstein, N. D. (1982). Unrealistic optimism about susceptibility to health problems. *Journal of Behavioral Medicine, 5*, 441–460.

Wicklund, R. A. & Gollwitzer, P. M. (1982). *Symbolic Self-Completion.* Hillsdale, NJ: Erlbaum.

Witkin, H. A. (1950). Individual differences in ease of perception of embedded figures. *Journal of Personality, 19*, 1–15.

Wright, R. A. (1996). Brehm's theory of motivation as a model of effort and cardiovascular response. In P. M. Gollwitzer & J. A. Bargh (eds.), *The Psychology of Action: Linking Cognition and Motivation to Behavior.* New York: Guilford.

Wright, R. A. & Brehm, J. W. (1989). Energization and goal attractiveness. In L. A. Pervin (Ed.), *Goal Concepts in Personality and Social Psychology* (pp. 169–210). Hillsdale, NJ: Erlbaum.

Zillman, D. & Cantor, J. R. (1976). Effect of timing of information about mitigating circumstances on emotial responses to provocation and retaliatory behavior. *Journal of Experimental Social Psychology, 12*, 38–55.

CHAPTER TWELVE

Goal Setting and Goal Pursuit in the Regulation of Body Weight

Richard P. BAGOZZI and Elizabeth A. EDWARDS

An important distinction in the study of purposive behaviour is frequently made between goal setting and goal striving (e.g., Heckhausen & Gollwitzer, 1987). The former addresses the motivational bases for forming a goal, whereas the latter concerns the volitional processes in goal pursuit.

Perhaps the most comprehensive framework for explaining purposive behaviour can be found in the model of action phases which specifies four stages, plus transitions between stages (e.g., Gollwitzer, 1990, 1996; see also Heckhausen, 1991, pp. 175–188). The first, or 'predecisional' stage, is initiated by wishes and desires and consists of the contemplation of possible goals and the setting of preferences amongst them. The culmination of the predecisional stage is the formation of a goal intention, the decision or choice to pursue a goal (where the goal is to attain an outcome or perform a behaviour). The goal intention serves as a transition to the 'preactional' phase, wherein decision makers 'reflect and decide on *when*, *where*, *how*, and *how long* to act' (Gollwitzer, 1996, p. 290, emphasis in original). The preactional phase 'ends' with action initiation, which in turn serves as a transition to phase three: the 'actional' phase. Action initiation refers to implementation intentions, which are intentions to perform particular behaviours in the service of the goal intention. The aim of the actional phase is to attain the goal by implementing and controlling instrumental acts. Finally, stage four, the 'post actional' phase, is an appraisal of goal attainment or failure in the light of one's wishes and desires and concludes with a decision to continue with goal pursuit or disengage from it.

Until quite recently, researchers in the subarea of psychology that deals with attitudes have not considered goal setting and goal striving (c.f., Bagozzi, 1992). Instead, the well-known theory of reasoned action (Ajzen & Fishbein, 1980) and the theory of planned behaviour (Ajzen, 1985) scrutinise only a small part of the larger phenomenon of purposive behaviour. Namely, these theories focus primarily upon antecedents of goal intentions (where the goal is to perform an action), and then only on a subset of key antecedents. The theories of reasoned action and planned behaviour consider neither implementation intentions and its antecedents nor the processes related to goal attainment or failure (Ajzen & Fishbein, 1980, pp. 29–30, 111; Fishbein & Stasson, 1990, p. 177).

Understandably, the theories of reasoned action and planned behaviour have been infrequently applied to the achievement of outcome goals, and when they have, typically very small amounts of explained variance result. A case in point is the self-regulation of body weight, which is the subject of the present study. Netemeyer, Burton, and Johnston (1991) found, for example, that the theories of reasoned action and planned behaviour accounted for 4.2 and 7.9 per cent of the variance in weight loss, respectively. Likewise, Schifter and Ajzen (1985) found that 19.4 per cent of the variance in weight loss was explained in their test of the theory of planned behaviour. Of particular interest for our concerns are the findings in both Netemeyer et al., (1991) and Schifter and Ajzen (1985) that intentions failed to significantly predict weight loss. This suggests that either weight loss is nonvolitional or perhaps processes intervening between intentions and weight loss function to fulfil one's volitions, thus making intentions a more distal cause of weight loss which would be difficult to detect when regressing weight loss directly on intentions.

More defensible, theoretically, is the application of the theories of reasoned action and planned behaviour to specific actions leading to body weight maintenance, such as exercising and dieting (e.g., Conner & Sparks, 1996). Here the theories have fared much better. Consider first exercising, where the majority of research has been conducted to date. Godin (1993) reviewed 12 studies in which the theory of reasoned action was used to predict exercise behaviours and found that the average relationship between intention and behaviour was .54, implying that on average about 29 per cent of the variance in exercising was accounted for. Godin (1993) found mixed support for the theory of planned behaviour. Although perceived behavioural control significantly predicted intentions in all 8 studies examined (where between 4 and 20 per cent additional variance (average = 8 per cent) was explained beyond that accounted for by attitudes), only one study of six found a significant effect for perceived behavioural control on exercising (for an additional contribution to explained variance of 3 per cent). More recently, Bagozzi and Kimmel (1995) reported that 41 and 46 per cent of the variance in intentions and 4 and 12 per cent of the variance in exercising were attributable to the theories of reasoned action and planned behaviour, respectively. Likewise in their test of the theory of planned behaviour, Conner and Norman (1996) found that 44 and 53 per cent of the variance was explained in intentions and behaviour, respectively.

The theories of reasoned action and planned behaviour have been applied much less frequently to dieting behaviours. Bagozzi and Kimmel (1995) found that 59 and 64 per cent of the variance in intentions and 25 and 28 per cent of the variance in dieting were explained by the theories of reasoned action and planned behaviour, respectively. However, perceived behavioural control did not significantly predict either dieting intentions or actual dieting under the theory of planned behaviour. In contrast, Conner and Norman (1996) found that perceived behavioural control significantly predicted both intentions and behaviours for a range of specific dieting behaviours. The explained variance in intentions and dieting behaviours ranged from 40–57 per cent and 26–39 per cent, respectively.

In sum, although the theories of reasoned action and planned behaviour are not designed to explain the achievement of outcome goals, they do apply to the prediction of both goal intentions (where the goal is to perform an action) and specific acts in the service of goal pursuit. The purpose of the present chapter is to develop and test a broader model of goal setting and goal pursuit with respect to the regulation of body weight. The specific approach taken herein builds on Gollwitzer's (1990, 1996) model of action phases and on the similar theory of self-regulation found in Bagozzi (1992).

The chapter is organised in two parts. Part one presents an operationalisation and test of many aspects of the model of action phases, by use of structural equation models in a field study. Focus is upon a molar representation of goal setting and goal striving in the advancement of goal achievement. Part two takes a more fine-grained stance and explores the bases of goal setting. The hierarchical cognitive schemas of people are investigated with respect to their reasons for desiring to lose or maintain their body weights. Multiple regression is used to test the dependence of attitudes, subjective norms, goal efficacy, and desires on subgoals and linkages amongst subgoals in people's cognitive schemas in part two.

PART I: A MODEL OF GOAL ACHIEVEMENT

Figure 12.1 presents a schematic of the theory of self-regulation to be applied to the maintenance of body weight. Let us describe the stages.

The role of attitudes and subjective norms as instigators of intentions has been criticised recently by Bagozzi (1992), who argued that these variables provide reasons for forming intentions but do not supply sufficient motivational content for producing intentions. The motivational impetus for intentions was hypothesised to reside in desires. Gollwitzer's (1990, p. 289) summary of the predecisional phase captures well the role of desires in goal setting: 'preferences are set between wishes by deliberating their desirability and feasibility'. However, he did not develop what desires are, per se, and how they function as determinants of goal intentions, nor did he consider nondeliberative desires.

There are at least two main types of desires: volitive and appetitive (Bagozzi, 1992, pp. 185–186; see also Davis, 1984; Nagel, 1970, p. 29, makes a similar distinction but uses the terms, motivated and unmotivated, respectively). A volitive desire can be construed as one based on deliberations and arrived at as a personal decision. Wants and wishes are common synonyms of volitive desires. In Figure 12.1, attitudes toward anticipated success and failure in goal attainment, attitudes toward the process of goal pursuit, and subjective norms reflect certain kinds of deliberations that can stimulate volitive desires (Bagozzi & Warshaw, 1990). The deliberations are implicit in the consideration of beliefs and evaluations about the consequences of goal achievement, failure, and pursuit (for attitudes toward success, failure, and process, respectively) and normative beliefs of, and motivation to comply with, specific individuals (for subjective norms). We can think of attitudes and subjective norms as summarising or integrating the cognitive and evaluative content of the consequences of goal outcomes and the process of goal pursuit. To the extent that these outcomes and the process are valued, a volitive desire for a goal will be energised.

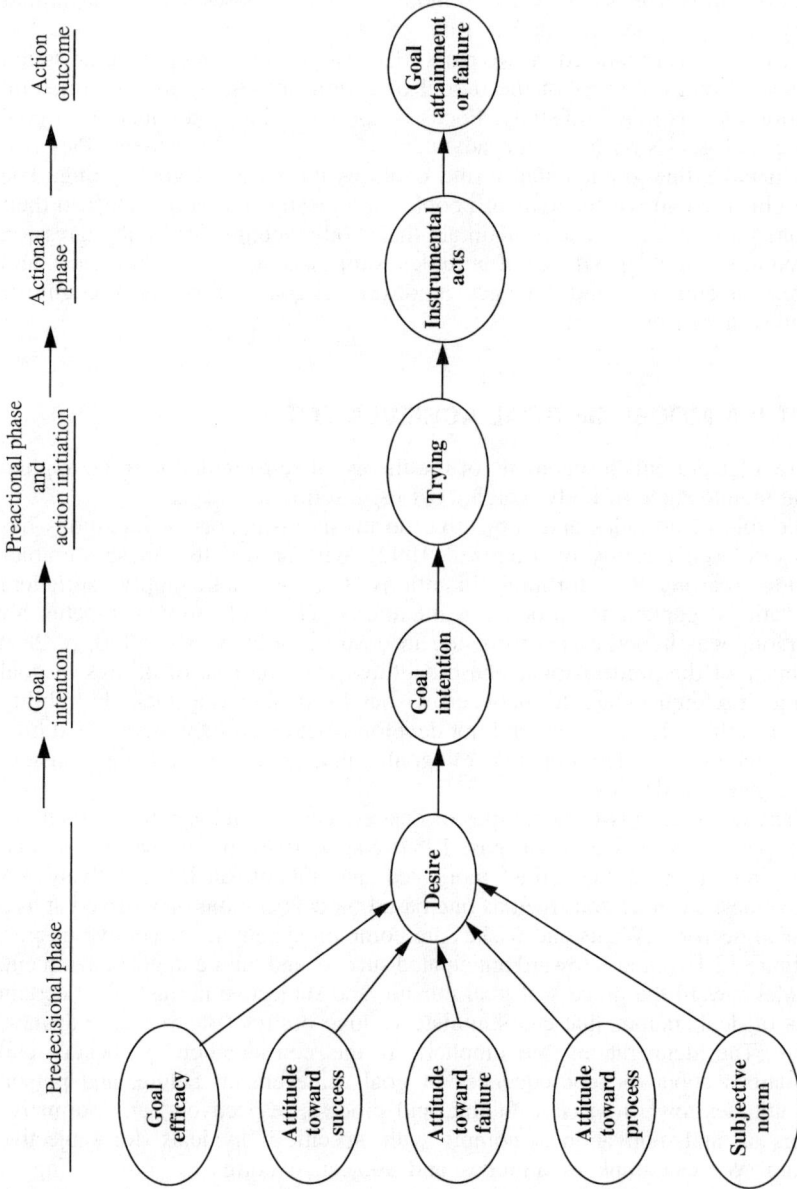

Figure 12.1 A Framework for self-regulation of body weight

Not all desires for a goal, however, are based on deliberations. The desire to pursue a goal can arise, as well, through appetitive desires, whereby needs or drives directly serve to inform one that he or she has a desire for an object or outcome or to perform an action. Unlike volitive desires which are motivated, an appetitive desire is unmotivated, yet serves to motivate the individual having it. Common synonyms for appetitive desires are craving, hungering, longing, and yearning. Being unmotivated, appetitive desires do not have antecedents, per se, but rather serve as originators of volitional behaviours in their own right. Nevertheless, antecedents may function to help one become aware of one's appetitive desires and in this sense can be thought to 'free up' the desire.

Another antecedent of desires not shown in Figure 12.1 and not considered empirically herein is emotion. When one achieves a goal, experiences a pleasant event, or anticipates achieving a goal or experiencing a pleasant event, and conversely when one fails to achieve a goal, experiences an unpleasant event, or anticipates failing to achieve a goal or experiencing an unpleasant event, appraisals of these happenings or possibilities will lead to specific emotions, depending on the nature of the phenomena, and specific coping responses will follow (Bagozzi, 1992, pp. 186–189, 191–194). The coping responses will frequently begin with desires to initiate goal pursuit or not, or to regulate goal pursuit or abandon it once it has begun, depending on the circumstances. Bagozzi, Baumgartner, and Pieters (1998) report a study finding that appraisals of the consequences of achieving or not achieving body weight goals led to positive and negative anticipatory emotions, which in turn influenced volitions in the service of goal pursuit. The volitions next affected goal-directed behaviours, and these determined the degree of subsequent goal attainment. Positive and negative goal-outcome emotions then fed-back to reinforce the meaning of goal attainment for respondents.

When anticipatory emotions arise from conscious appraisals, they can influence volitive desires. When appraisals happen automatically and are nonconscious, the resulting emotions either function as surrogate appetitive desires or else free-up self-conscious appetitive desires. It is possible that attitudes and subjective norms can also form as a function of nondeliberative processes and free up appetitive desires. For example, attitudes and subjective norms might develop through classical conditioning or instrumental learning and operate as secondary or learned drives.

The final antecedent of desires shown in Figure 12.1 is goal efficacy. Goal efficacy refers to the perceived likelihood of goal achievement, given that one decides to try to achieve a goal. It is similar to self-efficacy (e.g., Bandura, 1991) and perceived behavioural control (e.g., Ajzen, 1991) except that, instead of performance of a behaviour, it refers to goal achievement. In addition, goal efficacy rests on more complex cognitive processes than does either self-efficacy or perceived behavioural control. The latter address only a person's self-appraisal of the ability to perform an act. Goal efficacy entails an estimate of not only one's ability to perform instrumental acts but also the likelihood that these acts will lead to goal attainment. Goal efficacy estimates require the decision maker to take into account personal and situational factors and relate these to the likelihood that goal attainment will occur. In this sense, goal efficacy encompasses both self-efficacy and response efficacy. We expect goal efficacy to positively influence desires. Low goal efficacy should not stimulate volitive desires or at best will be associated with unrealistic desires with little hope of fulfilment. High goal efficacy should influence volitive desires that have reasonable chances of accomplishment.

A desire of sufficient intensity, in the case of a decision to pursue a single goal or not, or a desire for a goal of greater intensity than desires for other goals, in the case of a choice amongst goals, will motivate a goal intention. A goal intention is a self-commitment to realise a desired end state and might be expressed linguistically in the form, 'I intend to pursue x!' (Gollwitzer, 1993, p. 150). Formation of a goal intention terminates deliberative processes in the predecisional phase, at least temporarily, and inaugurates goal pursuit.

The inauguration of goal pursuit takes the form of trying, i.e., mental and physical activities leading up to and regulating the instrumental acts directly producing goal attainment. For purposes of discussion, we can describe three processes which comprise trying: decisions with respect to means, planning and control of goal-directed behaviours, and maintenance of commitment (Bagozzi, 1992).

After a person forms an intention to pursue a goal, he or she is faced with the problem of how to reach that goal. We can think of the choice of the means to pursue the goal as the integration of three appraisal processes. One of these is the degree of self-confidence one has for performing each of the alternative instrumental acts in one's means-choice set and is similar to self-efficacy (Bandura, 1991). The second is the appraisal of the likelihood that the initiation of each means will lead to goal achievement and is termed instrumental beliefs. The third is the pleasantness-unpleasantness of each means. Bagozzi, Baumgartner, and Yi (1992) hypothesised and found that the choice of means to implement coupon usage goals in a sample of consumers depended on a three-way interaction between self-efficacies, instrumental beliefs, and affect towards means.

Another aspect of trying concerns the implementation of means. Given a goal intention and choice of means, further commitment is needed in the form of explicit implementation intentions. Occasionally, a goal intention leads immediately to an implementation intention and actual implementation behaviours. This occurs, for example, in seemingly impulsive purchases made in the supermarket, in scripted actions such as ordering a meal in a restaurant, or in habitual behaviours such as seeing the automobile fuel gauge on empty and then proceeding straightaway to a petrol station.

More frequently, a significant gap in time exists between formation of goal intentions and the opportunity for goal attainment. An important mechanism for initiating trying is the formation of an implementation intention wherein a person dedicates him or herself to goal pursuit in accordance with future contingencies. The implementation intention can be expressed linguistically as, 'I intend to initiate behaviour x whenever the situational conditions y are met!' (Gollwitzer, 1993, p. 152). Specific plans may be made for activating an implementation intention. Monitoring activities may be performed to ensure that the intention is executed according to plan; monitoring is also done after initiation of goal-directed behaviours to assess progress. Guidance and control procedures are needed as well so as to execute changes in plans, modifications in goal-directed behaviours, or new actions to realise a goal.

The final class of processes involved in trying include those mental activities needed to maintain, or disengage from, commitment to goal and/or implementation intentions. Situational and interpersonal factors serve to distract or tempt people in ways potentially thwarting the initiation of instrumental acts and goal achievement. Likewise given a disruption in goal pursuit, one may need to recommit oneself and reactivate intentions and goal-directed behaviours to maintain progress toward goal attainment. This aspect of trying is both dispositional (e.g., action versus state orientation, Kuhl, 1992) and overtly purposive (i.e., entailing decision making and volitions).

In sum, trying is an omnibus term for a set of volitional, motivational, and conative processes needed to transform a goal intention into action. As shown in Figure 12.1, trying influences instrumental acts, which are goal-directed behaviours. Exercising and dieting are the principle instrumental acts investigated herein for the goal of losing or maintaining one's body weight.

METHOD

Subjects and Procedure

One hundred and seventeen undergraduate students responded to two questionnaires administered a month apart. On the first wave, answers were obtained to questions about goal efficacy, attitudes toward success, attitudes toward failure, attitudes toward the process of goal pursuit, subjective norms, desires, goal intentions, and other measures not pertinent to the study at hand. Before providing these responses, respondents indicated whether their personal goal for the forthcoming month was to 'lose weight', 'maintain my current weight', or 'gain weight', or whether 'I have no goal one way or the other with respect to my weight'. This was done both to direct respondents to subsequent questions worded in accordance with their personal goal and to avoid confounding those who had no goal or whose goal was to gain weight (and therefore would entail different volitions and goal-directed behaviours) with those who wished to lose or maintain their body weights.

Respondents to wave 1 were unaware that they would be solicited later for their reactions and therefore the chances for across time self-presentational and consistency biases should have been minimised. At wave 2 a month later, respondents provided information on the nature and extent of trying, goal-directed behaviours performed, and goal achievement. The 117 respondents represented a response rate across waves of 77 per cent.

Measures

Goal efficacy was measured with the item, 'Assuming I *try* to *lose* [*maintain* my current*] weight during the next four weeks, it is …'. A seven-point semantic differential scale was used, anchored with 'unlikely' and 'likely'. Beneath each response alternative was 'extremely', 'quite', 'slightly', 'neither', 'slightly', 'quite', and 'extremely', respectively.

Attitudes toward success were measured with two seven-point semantic differential items: 'unpleasant-pleasant' ·and 'bad-good'. The items were introduced with the statement, 'My *trying and succeeding* to *lose* [*maintain* my current] weight during the next four weeks would make me feel...'. The same seven response alternatives were used as employed for the goal efficacy items.

Attitudes toward failure and *attitudes toward the process* of body weight maintenance were also each indicated by responses to seven-point 'unpleasant-pleasant' and 'bad-good' semantic differential items. The former was introduced by, 'My *trying but failing* to *lose* [*maintain* my current] weight during the next four weeks would make me feel...', while the latter was elicited with, 'Considering the things I would have to do to *lose* [*maintain* my current] weight during the next four weeks (for example, exercising, dieting, etc.), my attitude toward doing these things can be described as making me feel...'. Again the same seven response alternatives were used as employed for the goal efficacy items.

Subjective norms were measured with a seven-point 'disapprove-approve' item in response to the statement, 'Most people who are important to me would ['disapprove-approve'] of my losing weight'. The measure was introduced with, 'Please indicate the degree to which most people who are important to you would approve or disapprove of your losing weight sometime during the next four weeks (circle number closest to their level of approval):'.

Desires were measured with two items introduced by the statement, 'Please express your overall felt, *subjective urge* to *lose* [*maintain* your current] weight during the next four weeks on the following two items:'. The first measure was a seven-point 'false-true' item and was worded, 'I *want* to lose [maintain my current] weight during the next four weeks'. The same seven response alternatives were used as employed for the goal efficacy items. The second measure of desires asked respondents to indicate their degree of desire in response to, 'My *desire* to lose [maintain my current] weight during the next four weeks can be best expressed as...'. Six response alternatives were provided: 'no desire at all', 'very weak desire', 'weak desire', 'moderate desire', 'strong desire', and 'very strong desire'.

Goal intentions were measured with two seven-point semantic differential items. The first was worded as follows: 'Please express how likely it is that you *intend* to lose [maintain your current] weight during the next four weeks: 'I *intend* to lose weight during the next four weeks'. Responses were recorded with 'unlikely-likely' formats. The second item stated, 'Please indicate your extent of disagreement or agreement with the following statement: 'I *plan* to lose weight during the next four weeks'. A 'disagree-agree' format was used. The seven response alternatives in each case were the same as used for goal efficacy.

Trying was indicated by three items: two measuring mental trying, and one reflecting 'physical energy'. All three were expressed on five-point scales: 'not at all', 'very little', 'moderate amount', 'very hard', and 'extremely hard', and were introduced with the query, 'How hard did you try to lose [maintain your] weight during the past four weeks in the sense of ...'. Then the following three senses of trying were presented along with the response alternatives: 'maintaining your *will power* and *self discipline* to lose [maintain your] weight', 'devoting *time for planning* with respect to however you went about trying to lose [maintain your] weight', and 'expending a lot of *physical energy*'.

Instrumental acts were measured with regard to sets of goal-directed behaviours corresponding to dieting and exercising. People were asked, 'How *frequently* did you do each of these [goal-directed behaviours] during the past four weeks?'. The following five-point response alternatives were used to record responses: 'never or very infrequently', 'infrequently', 'neither infrequently nor frequently', 'frequently', and 'very frequently'. For dieting, the following five items were employed: 'avoiding snacks between meals and in the evenings', 'cutting down on fatty or starchy foods (e.g., sweets, bread, potatoes)', 'decreasing food intake by eating lighter meals, not having seconds, or not overeating', 'taking diet pills, liquid diet formula, or medications to control weight', and 'fasting (i.e., purposefully skipping one or more meals a day)'. For exercising, the following two items were utilised: 'doing exercises (e.g., jogging, callisthenics, weight lifting, aerobics)' and 'participating in sports (e.g., swimming, tennis, basketball, etc.)'.

Goal attainment was measured with two items. The first used a seven-point semantic differential scale with response alternatives, 'I lost a lot of weight', 'I lost a moderate amount of weight', 'I lost a small amount of weight', 'I maintained my weight', 'I gained a little bit of weight', 'I gained a moderate amount of weight', and 'I gained a lot of weight'. The second measure was a self-report of the amount of weight in pounds lost or gained over the previous four weeks. A more stringent test of the theory could have been performed if actual changes in weight had been measured objectively.

Analytical Procedures

Structural equation models were used to operationalise the model shown in Figure 12.1 and test hypotheses. The LISREL8 program was employed to estimate parameters and compute goodness-of-fit measures (e.g., Jöreskog & Sörbom, 1989).

Figure 12.2 presents the latent variables actually tested in the theory of self-regulation. Two measures each were used as separate indicators in the structural equation model for attitudes towards success, failure, and the process; desires, intentions, mental trying, and goal attainment. One measure each was used for subjective norms, physical trying, and dieting and exercising.

Following common practice, three goodness-of-fit measures were employed to appraise the correspondence between the model in Figure 12.2 and the data. One of these is the chi-square test which can be used to assess the discrepancy between a hypothesised model and data. A nonsignificant chi-square goodness-of-fit test ($p \geq .05$) suggests that a model is a reasonable representation of the data. Because the chi-square test is sensitive to sample size and can lead to rejection of a model differing in a trivial way from data for large samples, and conversely can result in the acceptance of a model with important differences from the data for small sample sizes, it is prudent also to examine other measures of fit. In addition, the chi-square test does not provide an indication of the degree of fit, such as is available with indices normed from 0 to 1.

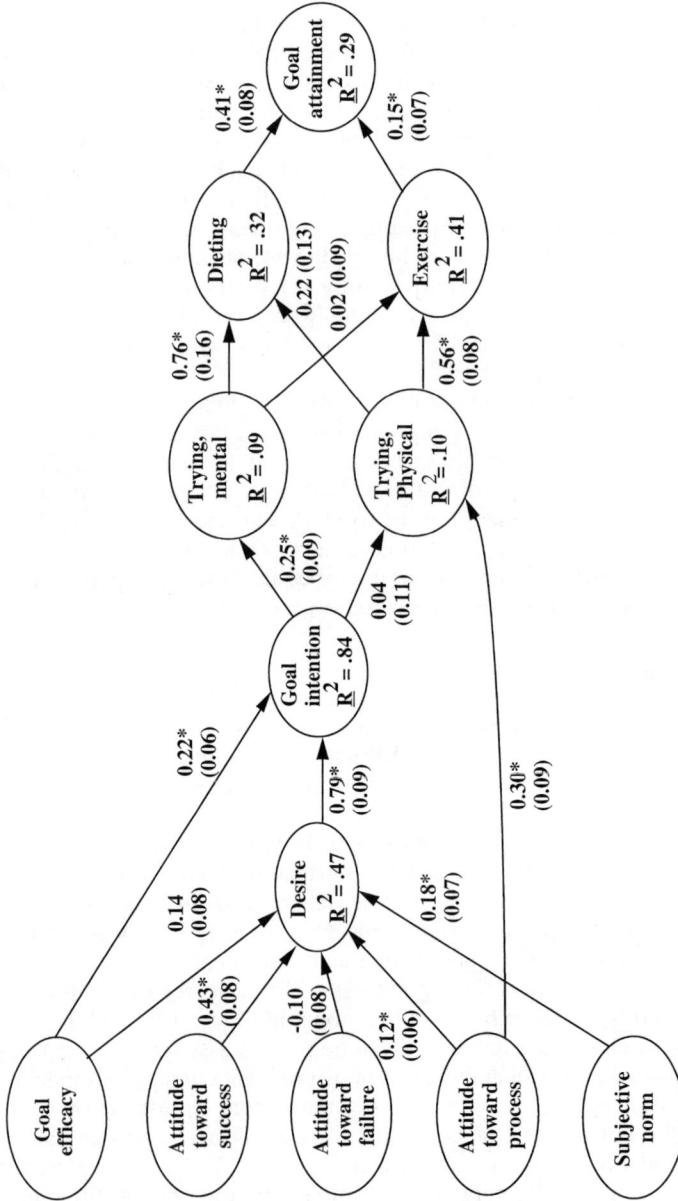

*Significant at p < .05 level or better.   Standard errors in parentheses .

Figure 12.2   Findings for test of theory of self-regulation

As a consequence, we chose as a second goodness-of-fit measure the comparative fit index (CFI). The CFI is an incremental fit index that compares a hypothesised model to the model that assumes all variables are uncorrelated (i.e., to a model where only error variances are estimated). The CFI is normed in the population and thus has values bounded by zero and 1. It also provides an unbiased estimate of its corresponding population value and is independent of sample size. Values for the CFI greater than or equal to .90 are generally considered satisfactory from a practical standpoint (Bentler, 1990).

The third goodness-of-fit measure employed is the root mean squared error of approximation (RMSEA). The RMSEA assesses model discrepancy per degree of freedom. Values of the RMSEA less than or equal to .08 represent a reasonable fit (Browne & Cudeck, 1993).

RESULTS

Reliability

Internal consistency reliabilities of measures were computed by use of the formula, $\rho = (\Sigma\lambda_i)^2/[(\Sigma\lambda_i)^2 + \Sigma\theta_i]$, where λ_i is the ith factor loading on a latent variable of interest, θ_i is the error variance corresponding to λ_i, and the standardised solution is assumed. This method for computing reliability is similar to Cronbach alpha, except, rather than assuming that each item has equal weight as in alpha, the items are weighted by their respective factor loadings.

For the variables with multiple measures, the following reliabilities resulted: attitudes toward success ($\rho = .94$), attitudes toward failure ($\rho = .93$), attitudes toward process ($\rho = .87$), desire ($\rho = .86$), goal intentions ($\rho = .85$), mental trying ($\rho = .73$), and goal attainment ($\rho = .80$).

Structural Equation Model

The findings for the model in Figure 12.2 show that χ^2 (132, $N = 117$) = 205.92, $p \cong .00$. The RMSEA = 0.07 and CFI = 0.94. On balance, therefore, the model fits satisfactorily.

Attitude toward success ($\gamma = 0.43$, s.e. = 0.08), attitude toward the process ($\gamma = 0.12$, s.e. = 0.06), and subjective norm ($\gamma = 0.18$, s.e. = 0.07) all influence desire significantly, as hypothesised (see Figure 12.2). The more positive the attitudes toward goal attainment and the process of goal pursuit and the stronger the felt normative pressure from significant others, the stronger the desire to pursue the goal. Nearly half of the variance in desire is accounted for by these antecedents ($R^2 = 0.47$).

Attitude toward failure does not significantly influence desire, although the coefficient is in the predicted direction ($\gamma = -0.10$, s.e. = 0.08). Inspection of the correlations between the measures of attitude toward failure and desire reveal that they are negatively and significantly correlated, as expected (average $r = -0.267$, $p < .05$; thus the more negative the attitude toward failure, the less the desire to pursue the goal). Apparently, multicollinearity accounts for the imprecision in parameter estimate ($\gamma = -0.10$, s.e. $= 0.08$), as the correlations between measures of attitude toward failure and subjective norm (average $r = -0.306$) exceed the correlations between measures of attitude toward failure and desire.

Goal efficacy did not significantly influence desire, contrary to expectations, although the coefficient ($\gamma = 0.14$, s.e. $= 0.08$) is in the predicted direction and is significant at the $p < 0.10$ level. Rather than being channelled through desire, per se, goal efficacy does have a significant direct effect on goal intention ($\gamma = 0.22$, s.e. $= 0.06$). The more likely that one believes that he or she would achieve the goal, if one tried to do so, the stronger the goal intention.

In addition to goal efficacy, goal intention is a function of desire, as hypothesised ($\beta = 0.79$, s.e. $= 0.09$). The greater the desire for a goal, the stronger the goal intention. The antecedents to goal intention explain a considerable amount of variation in the construct ($R^2 = 0.84$).

Goal intention significantly affects mental trying, according to theory ($\beta = 0.25$, s.e. $= 0.09$). The stronger the goal intention, the greater the will power and self-discipline and the more time devoted to planning goal pursuit. However, goal intention does not influence physical trying, although the coefficient is in the predicted direction ($\beta = 0.04$, s.e. $= 0.11$). Physical trying is nevertheless significantly influenced by attitude toward the process of goal pursuit ($\beta = 0.30$, s.e. $= 0.09$). The more favourable one's attitude toward the things needed to accomplish a goal, the more physical energy expended in trying to pursue the goal. The levels of explained variance are, however, modest for mental trying ($R^2 = 0.09$) and physical trying ($R^2 = 0.10$).

With respect to goal-directed behaviours, it can be seen in Figure 12.2 that actual dieting is a function of mental trying ($\beta = 0.76$, s.e. $= 0.16$) but not physical trying ($\beta = 0.22$, s.e. $= 0.13$). By contrast, actual exercising is a function of physical trying ($\beta = 0.56$, s.e. $= 0.08$) but not mental trying ($\beta = 0.02$, s.e. $= 0.09$). Hence, the greater the will power and self-discipline and the more time devoted to planning goal pursuit, the more frequently the various dieting behaviours were undertaken. Likewise, the greater the physical energy expended in preparation to lose or maintain one's body weight, the more frequently one engaged in various exercise behaviours. The explained variances in dieting and exercising were moderately high: $R^2 = 0.32$ and $R^2 = 0.41$, respectively.

Finally, goal attainment can be seen in Figure 12.2 to be influenced by the performance of dieting and exercise behaviours. Dieting ($\beta = 0.41$, s.e. $= 0.08$) and exercising ($\beta = 0.15$, s.e. $= 0.07$) both contributed to goal attainment and together explained a moderate amount of variance ($R^2 = 0.29$).

DISCUSSION

The current research presents one of the first field studies of purposive behaviour that investigates goal setting, goal striving, and goal attainment in a health context. This study operationalised variables from two similar frameworks; namely, the theory of self-regulation (Bagozzi, 1992) and the model of action phases (Gollwitzer, 1990, 1996; Heckhausen & Gollwitzer, 1987).

Previous research tended to examine only subprocesses found in purposive behaviour. For example, the theories of reasoned action (Ajzen & Fishbein, 1980) and planned behaviour (Ajzen, 1985) deal primarily with goal intentions (where the goal is to perform an action) and a limited set of their antecedents and only obliquely address the achievement of outcome goals; the theory of trying (Bagozzi & Warshaw, 1990) addresses goal striving as an aggregate construct and introduces additional antecedents but does not consider the subprocesses under trying which activate instrumental acts.

The model presented in Figure 12.1 and tested in Figure 12.2 shows the central role played by goal intention as a transition between the predecisional phase, which is primarily motivational, and the preactional phase, which is volitional. The principle motivational variable in the predecisional stage is desire. Indeed, desire is the main instigator of goal intention. One must have a desire for a goal before an intention to achieve it will form. Tests of direct paths from the exogenous variables to intentions confirm this in that no direct paths were significant, except for the path from goal efficacy to goal intention ($\chi_d^2(4) = 10.91, p < .05$). Thus consistent with findings in an experimental study performed by Gollwitzer, Heckhausen, and Ratajczak (1990), the formation of goal intentions is a function of the desirability and feasibility of the goal.

It has been argued that attitudes and subjective norms are neither necessary nor sufficient for a goal intention to form (Bagozzi, 1992). A goal intention can arise in the absence of attitudes and subjective norms, such as when an appetitive desire bursts forth or anticipatory emotions press one to cope by setting a goal. Likewise, attitudes and subjective norms are not sufficient for the formation of a goal intention because, while they provide reasons for having a goal, they may not supply the requisite self-awareness of a motive to pursue it.

Attitudes and subjective norms will influence goal intention only when a decision maker concludes that the goal is desirable and this arises as a result of weighing the desirability entailed by favourable attitudes and normative pressure against any other countervailing reasons not to pursue a goal that may come to mind (e.g., moral criteria or the presence of competing desires). In a sense, a decision maker decides that the reasons given by one's attitudes and subjective norms show that a prospective goal is desirable and that it is more desirable than other goals in competition with the focal goal or more desirable than not embracing the focal goal at all. This is the essence of a volitive desire (or of choices made amongst competing appetitive desires, for that matter).

The preactional phase and action initiation were modelled in the present study as trying. Trying is an omnibus term for the volitional processes needed to achieve a goal. These volitional processes comprise implementation intentions, decisions regarding means (i.e., self-efficacy, instrumentality, and affective appraisals of means), plans for executing the means, monitoring of progress toward goal attainment, guidance and control of instrumental acts, maintenance of commitment in the face of external impediments and weakness of will, and resumption of interrupted or stalled efforts.

An interesting finding in the actional phase of the model in Figure 12.2 is the dependence of dieting behaviours on will power, self-discipline, and time devoted for planning, but the independence of dieting from physical energy expended in trying to reach one's body weight goals. Apparently volitional processes in dieting are experienced primarily as mental activities with strong self-awareness of the need for vigilance and resoluteness, but physical energy is not a large part of self-consciousness. By contrast, the execution of exercise behaviours was preceded by a strong self-awareness of physical energy needed in trying to initiate these behaviours but not mental efforts at trying. Perhaps for the sample of respondents studied herein, exercising exhibits some routinised characteristics, and the kinematic properties of trying drive the behaviour more than extensive cognitive processing, per se. The repetitive nature of most exercise regimens seems to lead to volitional processes such as these. Moreover, as shown in Figure 12.2, attitude toward the process had an indirect, as well as a direct, impact on physical trying. The direct path might reflect some automatic or learned reaction to exercising and its initiation, as a function of one's feelings about the processes involved.

It thus appears that the operation and efficacy of self-regulatory strategies differs for cognitive and physical modes, depending on the qualities of the goal-directed actions at hand. Self-regulatory strategies involved in mental trying (i.e., in planning, monitoring, and control of implementation intentions and their execution) may be most functional when temptations are faced (e.g., being offered an attractive, but rich, dessert), on-going commitments must be adhered to (e.g., regular intake of pharmacological agents), and the motivation needed for action initiation is relatively low (e.g., reducing the amount of food eaten at a sitting). On the other hand, self-regulatory strategies associated with physical trying (which obviously also involve cognitive activity) may be most efficacious when the activities are aversive or effortful (e.g., exercising outdoors when the weather is cold or having to change one's work and social schedule to accommodate an exercise regimen) or require persistence at a high level (e.g., when one's metabolic rate is such that intense, sustained activity is needed to lose or maintain body weight).

PART II: GOAL SETTING

As shown in Figure 12.1, the predecisional phase in the self-regulation of body weight hypothesises that desires to lose or maintain one's weight are a function of goal efficacy; attitudes toward success, failure and the process of goal pursuit; and subjective norms. Each of these variables is a subjective summary or integration of specific information concerning one's appraisals of the consequences of goal achievement/failure or its evaluative or emotional significance.

The actual bases for goal setting, upon which the variables in the predecisional phase rest, are typically modelled as functions of expectancies and incentives. For example, contemporary theories of attitudes maintain that $A = \Sigma b_i e_i$, where A = attitude, b_i = belief about the likelihood of consequence i occurring, e_i = evaluation of consequence i, and n_i consequences are considered. Similarly, subjective norms are claimed to be functions of expectations and evaluations: $SN = \Sigma(NB)_j(MC)_j$, where SN = subjective norm, NB_j = normative belief of referent j, MC_j = motivation to comply with referent j, and n_j referents are taken into account. Finally, we might represent the antecedents of goal efficacy through $GE = \Sigma(IB)_k(SC)_k$, where GE = goal efficacy, IB_k = instrumental belief that if one performs goal-directed behaviour k, the goal will be achieved, SC_k = self-confidence that one can perform behaviour k, and n_k goal-directed behaviours are appraised.

There are at least four problems with expectancy-value approaches to goal setting that we wish to overcome in the present study. The first two, and most serious, concern conceptual issues. One drawback with expectancy-value representations is that they fail to capture the underlying structure, if any, amongst cognitions or beliefs. Instead, expectancy-value models assume that a single number, the sum of products of expectations and evaluations, represents people's reactions. Secondly and related to this, expectancy-value models do not permit the representation of relationships amongst beliefs, such as reflected in inferences, causal dependencies, or hierarchical arrangements.

Two operational problems with expectancy-value models should also be mentioned. Because measures of beliefs and evaluations are typically ordinal, or at best interval, scaled, a fundamental indeterminancy exists that can only be overcome by modelling appropriate additive and interaction effects (Evans, 1991). However for complex models with many dependent variables and interactions, this is difficult to accomplish, whether one uses regression or structural equation analyses. The second operational problem relates to the domain of beliefs to which one responds. In the usual procedure, beliefs are determined in a pretest, and a fixed list is presented to respondents in the main study. To the extent that people differ in the criteria taken into account in decision making (relying on more or less beliefs than found in the set of beliefs presented to them), an incomplete picture of goal setting will result.

To overcome the problems noted above, we represent the bases for a focal goal in terms of cognitive schemas and use a methodology for eliciting and testing these schemas that exhibits desirable properties. Consider first the notion of a cognitive schema for the bases of a focal goal. A schema is a person's knowledge structure about an object, person, or situation and consists of thoughts or ideas, based on experience, and connections amongst these thoughts or ideas (Anderson, 1980; Fiske & Taylor, 1991). The basic units of the cognitive schemas we investigate are goals to which the focal goal of losing or maintaining one's body weight is connected. By 'goal', we mean 'a mental image or other end point representation associated with affect toward which action may be directed' (Pervin, 1989, p. 474). Such cognitive units have been termed 'declarative knowledge' (Anderson, 1983), and reflect factual information, as well as abstract concepts. If we take 'losing or maintaining body weight' as our focal goal, we can specify a hierarchy of self-regulation based upon a three-fold classification of goals. Our focal goal can be viewed at the centre of the hierarchy and answers the question, '*What* is it that I strive for?'. Subordinate goals constitute the means for achieving the focal goal and answer the question, '*How* can I achieve my body weight goal?'. In our study, various modes of dieting and exercising are the specific subordinate goals leading to weight loss or maintenance. At the top of the hierarchy are superordinate goals, which answer the question, '*Why* do I want to lose or maintain my weight?'. For example, the central goals of losing or maintaining body weight might be linked to such superordinate goals as 'increased self-esteem', 'happiness', and 'enhanced health and longevity'. We can think of the superordinate goals that comprise a cognitive schema as supplying motives for pursuing the focal goal. This conceptualisation of a hierarchy of self-regulation is somewhat similar to control theory perspectives on action (e.g., Carver & Scheier, 1990; Pieters, 1993; Vallacher & Wagner, 1987). We hypothesise that the many abstract superordinate goals and their interconnections become summarised in, or transformed by, the global psychological responses comprising the predecisional phase of the theory of self-regulation (see Figure 12.1).

In our study we hypothesise that superordinate goals provide reasons for acting and exist in a hierarchy with relatively more concrete goals at the bottom and abstract goals at the top. Goals in the middle function in a central manner by channelling the effects of more concrete goals onto more abstract goals. To summarise an example later described under Results, the intermediate goal of 'good feelings' transforms more concrete reactions, such as 'looking good' and 'fitting into clothes', into more abstract reactions, such as 'social acceptance' and 'happiness'. The central goal, 'good feelings', shares some features attributed to basic-level categories (Rosch, 1978; Mervis & Rosch, 1981); namely, it functions as a basis for communication, making inferences, or cueing a cognitive schema. Of course, all these goals are superordinate in relation to the focal goal of losing or maintaining body weight.

The connections amongst goals have been termed 'procedural knowledge' in the literature (Anderson, 1983). These resemble if-then propositions. To illustrate, two inferences based on cognitive schemas discussed under Results below are 'if I look good as a result of losing weight, I shall be accepted socially' and 'if I fit into my clothes as a result of maintaining my body weight, I shall save money'.

For researchers, the value of representing the bases for a focal goal in a cognitive schema of superordinate goals is that it provides testable predictions for how information is integrated in memory, how inferences are made, how new information will be processed, and how these processes will affect the predecisional phase in the theory of self-regulation, and hence indirectly influence goal intentions and goal pursuit. For persons holding a cognitive schema of the bases for a focal goal, at least three functions of the schemas result: they help one understand and interpret new information, retrieve schema-relevant facts, and go beyond the data, so to speak, to make inferences.

Current methods for generating cognitive schemas have the disadvantages of yielding relatively flat structures and categories organised by semantic similarity, rather than inferential or causal processes (e.g., Andersen & Klatzky, 1987). This is a consequence of the procedures employed, which typically are based on measures of empirical association (e.g., correlational, cluster, or multidimensional scaling analyses). To produce more meaningful cognitive schemas, we use an approach that directly elicits cognitions and relationships amongst cognitions. The procedure furnishes means-end chains and has been used to study value structures (e.g., Bagozzi & Dabholkar, forthcoming) and goal structures (Bagozzi & Dabholkar, 1994; Pieters, Baumgartner, & Allen, 1995). The foundation of the methodology resides in ideas proposed by philosophers (e.g., Toulmin, 1958; Toulmin, Rieke, & Janik, 1979) on logic.

Briefly, a person's goal schema is uncovered by first asking him or her to provide personal reasons for why they hold their particular body weight goals. Given the set of self-generated reasons, respondents are next asked to explain why the reasons initially given were important to them. Then further justifications for the explanations are solicited, and the process continues until the possibilities are exhausted and no further backing can be given. By use of principles from network analysis, maps of hierarchical cognitive schemas are constructed based on the content and sequence of justifications supplied for respondents' goals. The result is a structured network comprised of sequences of reasons (i.e., superordinate goals) explaining why one holds a particular body weight goal. Regression analysis is employed to test the dependence of goal efficacy, attitudes, subjective norms, and desires on both individual superordinate goals and linkages between goals.

METHOD

A total of 206 undergraduate students was asked to respond to a questionnaire, for which 197 complete responses were obtained. Respondents first indicated whether their personal goal 'during the next four weeks' was to 'lose weight', 'maintain my current weight', 'gain weight', or 'I have no goal one way or the other with respect to my weight'. Then, depending on which goal was indicated, questions were asked to measure goal efficacy, attitudes, subjective norm, and desires. The same formats described above in part 1 of this chapter were used.

The elicitation of superordinate goals for wanting to lose or maintain weight was next conducted as follows (see Appendix for questions pertaining to losing weight). People were first asked to list five personal reasons for wanting to lose [maintain current] weight and to enter these separately in the left most column of boxes on a page in the questionnaire. Next, they were instructed to consider the first reason they provided, think about why it was important to them, and place their answer in the first box in column 2, which corresponded with the box for reason 1 in column 1. Respondents were then asked to address this second-level justification and explain why it was, in turn, important to them. The response was recorded as a third-level explanation in box 1, column 3. The process was repeated for the second initial reason expressed in row 2, column 1, and so on, until all first-level reasons were explained up to three levels. The net result was a table of 5 rows and 3 columns of ordered goals. The 15 goals consist of 5 strings of explanations provided in support of why one wants to loose or maintain his or her body weight. In sum, each subject could indicate up to 15 goals and 10 linkages.

RESULTS

The 197 respondents mentioned a total of 2236 superordinate goals as explanations for wanting to lose or maintain their body weights and 879 linkages amongst goals, for an average of 11.4 goals and 4.5 linkages, respectively, per respondent.

The idiosyncratic responses were then content analysed so as to categorise the goals into a smaller number of meaningful groupings. Two independent judges coded the 197 goal protocols by use of terms summarising like meanings. Coders were instructed to place named goals into classifications maintaining maximal within group similarity and between group dissimilarity. For example, 'accomplishment', 'achieve goals', 'performance', 'success in school or work', 'get better job' were all coded under the label, 'achievement'. The coders demonstrated 85 per cent agreement, and disagreements were subsequently resolved by discussion so that all responses were classified. A total of 19 categories of goals resulted (e.g., 'look good', 'enhance self-esteem', 'live longer'; see Table 12.1 for full list).

A first step in the analysis of the structure of goals was to construct an implication matrix. The implication matrix displays the number of times each goal leads to each other goal for respondents. It is a square matrix Z whose elements (z_{ij}) reflect how often goal i leads to goal j, where this is based on an aggregation across respondents. Table 12.2 shows the implication matrix for the 19 goals identified in the content analysis. Notice that each goal is mentioned twice, once in the rows and once in the columns. The numbers in the table indicate how frequently goal i leads to goal j. For example, 'looking good' as a result of losing or maintaining body weight leads to enhanced 'self-esteem' in 50 instances. The goals are arranged in the table by degree of abstractness (see column 1). Abstractness is computed as the ratio of in-degrees to the sum of in-degrees plus out-degrees. In-degrees show how often a goal is the object or end of a relation, whereas out-degrees indicate how often a goal is a source or origin. The abstractness ratio is a number from 0 to 1, inclusive, and measures the proportion of times a goal serves as a destination in a linkage, as opposed to a source. The assumption is that the more abstract a goal, the more likely it will be an end.

The implication matrix can be used to produce a visual representation or map of the hierarchical arrangement among superordinate goals, but before this can be done it is necessary to choose a cut-off level for the occurrence of linkages that makes the map interpretable. The objective is to make the cut-off level as low as possible so as to achieve as comprehensive a representation as possible, yet not yield a map so large and cluttered as to be incomprehensible. A rule of thumb used in the network literature is to choose a cut-off producing a map accounting for a large proportion of the total number of connections amongst goals with a relatively small number of cells in the implication matrix. A cut-off of 10 gave this result.

Figure 3 presents the hierarchical goal structure derived from the implication matrix, with a cut-off level of 10 applied. It was obtained from the information in Table 12.2 by graphing all linkages that equalled or exceeded the cut-off level. The placement of goals in a vertical direction follows the relative

Table 12.1   Prominence indices derived from goal structure

Goal	Abstractness	Centrality	Prestige
Fit in clothes	0.23	0.18	0.04
Don't want gain	0.25	0.03	0.01
Exercise	0.26	0.05	0.01
Upcoming events	0.27	0.02	0.01
Look good	0.27	0.29	0.08
Health	0.31	0.16	0.05
Recreation	0.44	0.01	0.00
Feel good	0.49	0.29	0.14
Energy	0.52	0.09	0.05
Endurance	0.54	0.04	0.02
Sex	0.59	0.01	0.01
Avoid embarrassment	0.61	0.01	0.01
Achievement	0.62	0.12	0.08
Self-esteem	0.65	0.25	0.16
Social acceptance	0.66	0.17	0.12
Live longer	0.69	0.10	0.07
Happiness	0.74	0.05	0.04
Enjoy life	0.84	0.05	0.04
Save money	0.84	0.08	0.06

ordering implied by the abstractness ratios. For example, 'fit in clothes' is the lowest-order goal and 'enjoy life' and 'save money' are the highest-order goals. Arrows go from goals that function as sources of motivation to goals that serve as intermediary or end-state objectives. The number attached to each arrow signifies the frequency that the designated linkage was mentioned, given the cut-off level chosen.

It can be seen in Figure 12.3 that three goals comprise high level motivations for losing or maintaining body weight: 'enjoy life', 'happiness', and 'save money'. Moreover, three general orientations toward the focal goal can be discerned. One of these is existential concerns and is reflected in the desire to be healthy, live longer, and enjoy life. A second orientation focuses upon utilitarian outcomes: fitting into one's clothes and saving money. The third and most extensive orientation deals with subjective well-being and includes such concrete instances as looking and feeling good, as well as more abstract ends such as self-esteem, achievement, social acceptance, and happiness.

An indication of the importance of goals can be obtained by examining the degree to which a goal serves as a source and/or object in the goal hierarchy. Such a measure has been termed 'prominence' in the network literature (Faust & Wasserman, 1992) and strives to depict the relative salience of a goal to all other goals. Table 12.1 summarises two indices of importance for each goal. *Prestige* is computed as the ratio of in-degrees of a specific goal to the total number of cell-entries in the implication matrix. It represents the extent to which a particular goal is the target of other goals. As shown in Table 12.1, 'self-esteem' is the most important goal in this sense, with 'feel good' a close second (see also Figure 12.3). *Centrality* is computed as the ratio of the sum of in-degrees plus out-degrees for a particular goal to the total number of cell-entries in the implication matrix. It reflects how frequently a particular goal is involved in linkages with other goals. It can be seen, in Table 12.1, that 'look good' and 'feel good' are the most central goals, with 'self-esteem' close behind (see also Figure 12.3).

One indication of the degree of organisation of goals in a map can be obtained by examination of what has come to be known as centralisation in the network literature (e.g., Faust and Wasserman, 1992; Freeman, 1979). The general formula for computing centralisation can be written as

$$C = \frac{\sum_{i=1}^{n} |C(g^*) - C(g_i)|}{\max \sum_{i=1}^{n} |C(g^*) - C(g_i)|}$$

where $C(g^*)$ = largest centrality for any goal in a map, $C(g_i)$ = centrality of goal i, and n = number of goals. This index equals 1 when one goal is connected to all other goals but none of the other goals is connected to any other. In other words, one goal overshadows or dominates the others. The index equals 0 when all goals have exactly the same centrality index; that is, each goal is linked to the other goals to the same degree and no goal dominates. Overall the centralisation index measures the extent to which one goal in a map is central and the remaining goals are peripheral. Although centralisation can be computed separately for in-degrees and for out-degrees, we focus on centralisation for in-degrees plus out-degrees for simplicity and further examine linkages unweighted by frequency. As recommended by Faust and Wasserman (1992), the denominator of the centralisation index in this case is simply $(n - 1)(n - 2)$. For Figure 12.3, 'feel good' is the most central goal and the centralisation index is 0.71, which suggests a relatively, tightly organised goal hierarchy with 'feel good' channelling the flow of goals and functioning to bind goals together in the network.

Do men and women exhibit different motives for wanting to lose or maintain their body weights? To address this question, we investigated cognitive schemas separately by gender. Figures 4 and 5 summarise the findings. The first thing to note is that in many respects the goal hierarchies are similar for men and women. Men and women both evidence 12 goals, and indeed 11 of these are in common (only women disclose 'happiness' as a goal, and only men display 'don't want to gain weight' as a goal, but the latter is rather a restatement of the focal goal). Likewise, men and women manifest the same three general motivational orientations toward losing or maintaining their body weights: existential concerns, utilitarian outcomes, and subjective well-being. Finally, many linkages between goals are similar for men and women, and most goals are located and function in the hierarchy in comparable ways. For example, 'look good', 'feel good', 'self-esteem', 'social acceptance', and 'achievement' are central goals; 'enjoy life' and 'save money' are end-state goals; and 'health', 'look good', and 'fit in clothes' are concrete goals, while 'enjoy life', 'self-esteem', 'social acceptance', and 'save money' are abstract goals for both men and women.

Despite the great similarity between men and women in their goal structures, a number of striking differences should be mentioned. Although men and

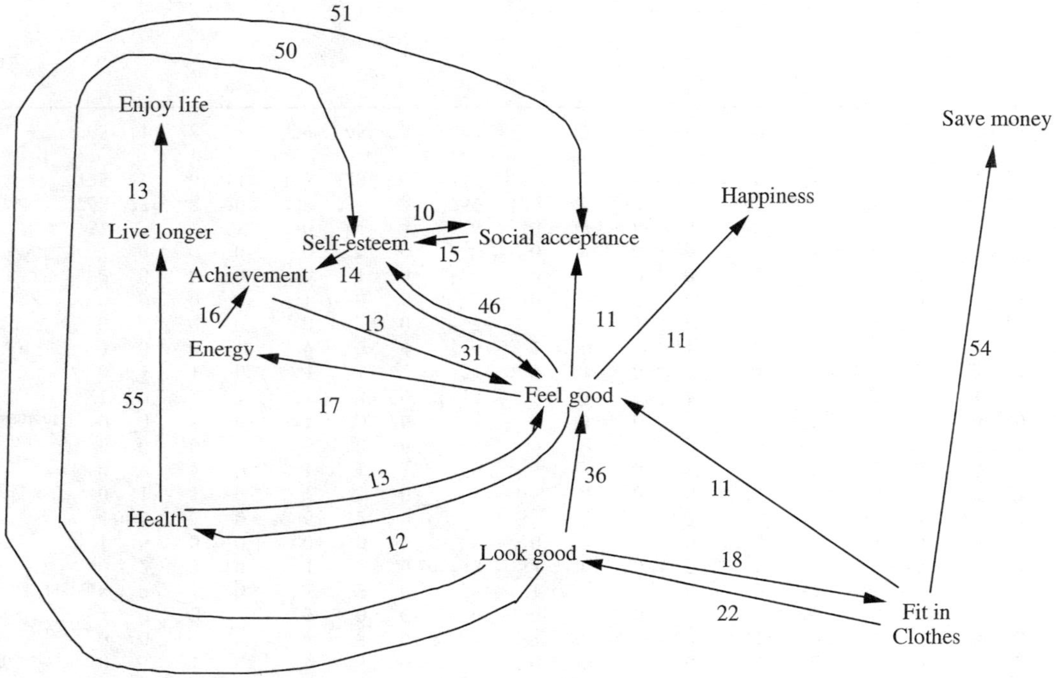

Figure 12.3 Hierarchical goal structure for reasons for losing or maintaining body weight (Men and Women, N = 197).

Table 12.2   Implication matrix for goals associated with losing and maintaining body weight (men and women)

Abstract ratio	#	Goal	1	2	3	4	5	6	7	8	9	10	11	12	13	14	15	16	17	18	19	Out deg's
0.23	1	Fit in clothes		1	0	3	22	0	1	11	0	0	1	1	6	9	8	0	2	0	54	119
0.25	2	Don't want gain	0		1	0	9	5	0	1	0	0	0	0	2	2	0	0	0	0	0	20
0.26	3	Exercise	0	0		0	4	8	0	4	7	4	0	0	1	2	0	1	0	0	0	31
0.27	4	Upcoming events	4	1	0		3	0	0	0	0	0	0	0	0	0	5	0	1	0	0	13
0.27	5	Look good	18	2	1	0		3	0	36	1	3	0	0	9	50	51	0	6	0	1	181
0.31	6	Health	0	2	2	0	4		0	13	4	1	1	0	5	2	2	55	1	4	0	94
0.44	7	Recreation	1	0	0	0	0	0		0	0	1	0	0	0	0	1	4	0	1	0	5
0.49	8	Feel good	4	0	2	0	6	12	0		17	1	1	3	6	46	11	4	11	4	0	128
0.52	9	Energy	0	1	1	0	1	1	0	4		4	0	0	16	0	3	0	2	3	0	36
0.54	10	Endurance	0	0	1	0	1	1	3	0	3		0	1	1	0	1	0	0	2	0	14
0.59	11	Sex	0	0	0	0	0	0	0	1	0	0		0	0	0	3	0	0	0	0	4
0.61	12	Avoid embarrassment	0	0	0	0	1	0	0	1	0	1	0		0	2	0	0	1	1	1	5
0.62	13	Achievement	1	0	2	1	5	3	0	13	1	0	0	1		6	3	0	2	3	0	40
0.65	14	Self-esteem	0	1	1	0	4	1	0	31	5	1	0	1	14		10	0	4	2	0	74
0.66	15	Social acceptance	2	0	0	1	9	2	0	6	1	0	2	1	5	15		0	1	13	0	50
0.69	16	Live longer	0	0	0	0	0	7	0	3	1	0	1	0	0	0	1		0	3	0	27
0.74	17	Happiness	0	0	0	0	1	0	0	2	0	0	0	0	1	3	1	0		0	0	11
0.84	18	Enjoy life	0	0	0	0	0	1	0	0	0	1	0	0	1	2	1	1	1		0	7
0.84	19	Save money	7	0	0	0	0	0	0	0	0	0	0	0	1	0	0	0	0	1		10
		In degrees	37	7	11	5	70	44	4	126	40	17	6	8	68	139	101	61	32	37	56	869
		Mentions per goal	255	27	48	20	298	235	7	259	120	45	17	14	142	227	275	73	44	43	87	
		Number people mentioning goal ≥ 1	128	21	36	14	155	128	6	162	69	25	10	12	76	125	164	63	34	32	59	
		Percent	65	11	18	7	79	65	3	82	35	13	5	6	39	63	83	32	17	16	30	

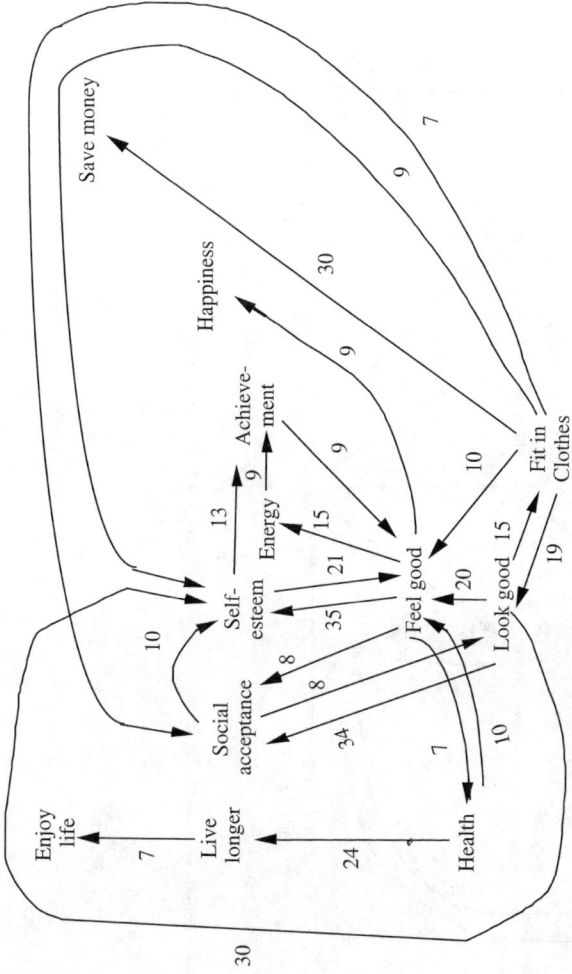

Figure 12.4 Hierarchical goal structure for reasons for losing or maintaining body weight (Women, *N* = 125).

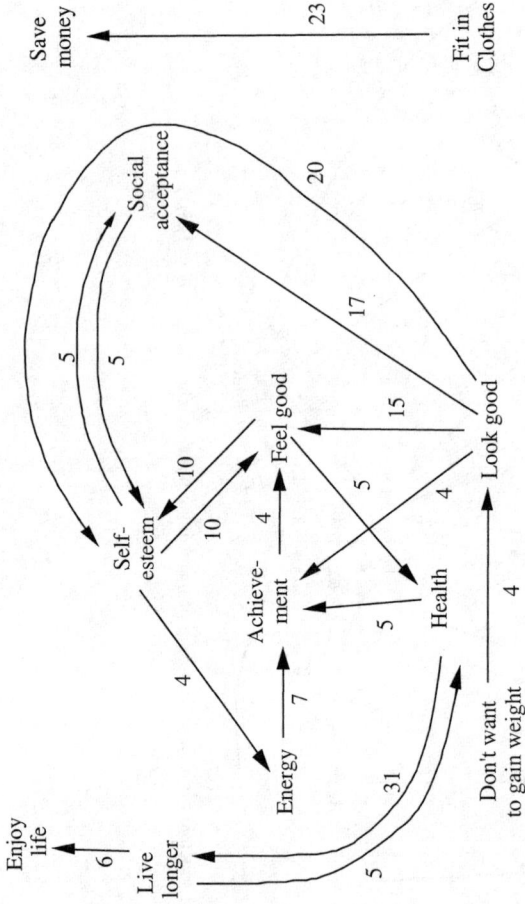

Figure 12.5   Hierarchical goal structure for reasons for losing or maintaining body weight (Men, *N* = 71).

women both demonstrate a link from 'fit in clothes' to 'save money', and indeed this link is amongst the most frequently mentioned by men and women, the role of 'fit in clothes' differs across gender. For men, the 'fit in clothes' to 'save money' link is completely isolated from the remainder of the goal structure. Apparently men view these consequences in strictly utilitarian ways. Women concur in this interpretation of the consequences of losing and maintaining body weight but at the same time recognise many other implications of fitting into one's clothes. Thus fitting into one's clothes is seen by women also as making one feel and look good and enhancing self-esteem and social acceptance (see Figure 12.4). Notice, too, the reciprocal feedback relationships between 'look good' and 'fit in clothes' for women, which points to added synergy between these goals.

The goal hierarchy for women is also more complex than that for men. This can be seen intuitively by noticing the greater number of linkages and greater number of direct and indirect feedback loops for women than men (see Figures 4 and 5). Women exhibit 23 linkages, while men show only 18. Women evidence 13 feedback loops (4 reciprocal, 9 indirect), while men demonstrate only 5 (3 reciprocal, 2 indirect). The total length of the feedback loops (i.e., the sum of links) for women is 40 but only 13 for men.

Finally the goal hierarchy for women is much more integrated than the hierarchy for men. For women, 'feel good' is the most central goal, and centralisation for the map in Figure 12.4 is 0.67. For men by contrast, 'self-esteem' is most central, but centralisation reaches only 0.34 (see Figure 12.5).

Up to this point, we have relied on descriptive information for characterising the cognitive schemas represented by the goal hierarchies. Now we wish to gain insight into the implications of schemas for the global, summary reactions found in the predecisional phase of the theory of self-regulation (see Figure 12.1).

To more formally ascertain how goal efficacy, attitudes, subjective norms, and desires are motivated, we regressed each of these onto the frequency with which respondents mentioned each goal and the frequency with which respondents mentioned each of the linkages between goals. Because information contained in the goals is correlated with information contained in linkages between goals, we followed the procedure developed by Appelbaum and Cramer (1974) for the evaluation of non-orthogonal designs.

Table 12.3 presents the findings. The first two rows in the table show the explained variances in attitude toward success, attitude toward failure, attitude toward process, subjective norms, goal efficacy, and desires as a function of goals and linkages, respectively. The third row shows the explained variances in the same set of variables as a function of both goals and linkages. The results summarised in the first three rows can be used to test for the significance of linkages and goals, since Models 1 and 2 are nested in Model 3. The test for linkages (Model 4 in Table 12.3) involves comparing Models 1 and 3: if adding linkages to Model 1 improves fit significantly, we can conclude that the specific linkages found to be significant are valid determinants of the dependent variable in question. The appropriate F–test is $\dfrac{(R_2^2 - R_1^2)h}{(1 - R_2^2)/(n - k - 1)}$, where R_2^2 and R_1^2 are the explained variances for the full model (Model 3) and nested model (either Models 1 or 2), h is the difference in degrees of freedom between Model 3 and the nested model, n is the sample size, and k is the number of independent variables in Model 3. Parallel comparisons are made between Models 2 and 3 to test for the effects of goals (Model 5 in Table 12.3).

Models 1 and 2 are based on stepwise regressions wherein independent variables that express the frequency with which a goal or linkage between goals was mentioned, respectively, were entered in a stepwise manner until the addition of the final variable failed to improve model fit significantly. Model 3 was run directly with the variables found from Models 1 and 2 by use of standard multiple regression procedures.

The results in Table 12.3 show that 6 goals and 9 linkages account for 24 per cent of the variance in attitude toward success, 3 goals and 7 linkages account for 29 per cent of the variance in attitude toward failure, 4 goals and 12 linkages account for 29 per cent of the variance in attitude toward process, 1 goal and 13 linkages account for 30 per cent of the variance in subjective norms, 5 goals and 2 linkages account for 17 per cent of the variance in goal efficacy, and 3 goals and 8 linkages account for 26 per cent of the variance in desires. With one exception, the model comparisons indicate that linkages and goals both predict attitudes, subjective norms, goal efficacy, and desires significantly, as hypothesised (see findings for Models 4 and 5 in Table 12.3). The lone exception occurs for attitude toward process, where only linkages were significant predictors.

The analyses presented in Table 12.3 show the effects of the set of goals and the set of linkages between goals as a whole on attitudes, subjective norms, goal efficacy, and desires. To gain an indication of which specific goals and linkages are the bases for information processing in the predecisional phase, we can inspect the findings for individual coefficients in the regressions.

For attitudes toward success, the only significant goal was 'social acceptance', while three linkages were significant: 'look good' → 'feel good', 'social acceptance' → 'happiness', and 'self-esteem' → 'feel good'. For attitudes toward failure, the significant goals were 'social acceptance' and 'self-esteem', while four linkages were significant: 'health' → 'live longer', 'health' → 'achievement', 'health' → 'energy', and 'fit in clothes' → 'feel good'. For attitudes toward the process, no goals were significant but six linkages were: 'look good' → 'social acceptance', 'look good' → 'fit in clothes', 'self-esteem' → 'look good', 'feel good' → 'live longer', 'don't want to gain weight' → 'look good', and 'feel good' → 'happiness'. For subjective norms, one goal, 'social acceptance', was significant, as were eleven linkages: 'look good' → 'happiness', 'achievement' → 'health', → 'energy' → 'social acceptance', 'energy' → 'endurance', 'energy' → 'feel good', 'energy' → 'achievement', 'fit in clothes' → 'social acceptance', 'fit in clothes' → 'save money', 'fit in clothes' → 'look good', 'fit in clothes' → 'self-esteem', and 'feel good' → 'achievement'. For goal efficacy, the significant goals were 'achievement', 'endurance', 'exercise', and 'don't want to gain weight', while two linkages were significant: 'exercise' → 'health' and 'feel good' → 'enjoy life'. Finally for desires, the significant goals were 'social acceptance' and 'self-esteem', while five linkages were significant: 'look good' → 'feel good', 'self-esteem' → 'feel good', 'social acceptance' → 'happiness', 'energy' → 'enjoy life', and 'feel good' → 'enjoy life'.

Table 12.3 Tests of model comparisons

Model		Attitude toward success	Attitude toward failure	Attitude toward process	Subjective norm	Goal efficacy	Desire
1.	Goals						
	R^2	0.14	0.11	0.11	0.02	0.12	0.11
	df	(6,176)	(3,181)	(4,181)	(1,198)	(5,196)	(3,197)
2.	Linkages						
	R^2	0.18	0.22	0.26	0.28	0.05	0.19
	df	(9,169)	(7,173)	(12,169)	(13,180)	(2,193)	(8,186)
3.	Goals plus linkages						
	R^2	0.24	0.29	0.29	0.30	0.17	0.26
	df	(15,163)	(10,170)	(16,165)	(14,179)	(7,188)	(11,183)
4.	Test of linkages						
	F-value	2.44[c]	6.16[a]	3.49[a]	5.51[a]	5.66[b]	4.64[a]
	df	(9,163)	(7,170)	(12,165)	(13,179)	(2,188)	(8,183)
5.	Test of goals						
	F-value	2.14[c]	5.59[b]	1.74	5.11[c]	5.44[a]	5.77[a]
	df	(6,163)	(3,170)	(4,165)	(1,179)	(5,188)	(3,183)

Dependent variables

[a] $p < 0.001$
[b] $p < 0.01$
[c] $p < 0.05$

Multiple regression analyses could also be applied separately by gender. However the sample size for men ($N = 71$) is rather low for these analyses, and therefore they were not conducted.

DISCUSSION

The purpose of the study reported in part 2 of this chapter was twofold. First, our aim was to uncover the key superordinate goals motivating the decision to lose or maintain one's body weight and to represent the structure of these goals in memory. Twelve salient goals were identified and found to function in the hierarchical pattern shown in Figure 12.3. Second, our objective was to investigate goal setting by testing the dependence of attitudes, subjective norms, goal efficacy, and desires on the superordinate goals and connections between goals represented in respondent's cognitive schemas. Multiple regression was used to test hypotheses. A number of goals and linkages between goals proved to be efficacious.

The 12 superordinate goals shown in Figure 12.3 traverse a wide range of motives for losing or maintaining one's body weight. Lower level goals – such as 'health', 'look good', and 'fit in clothes' – constitute subjective reactions with strong physical overtones. The higher level goals – 'enjoy life', 'live longer', 'achievement', 'self-esteem', 'social acceptance', 'happiness', and 'save money' – are ends dealing with abstract personal values or ideals. We can think of lower level goals as stimulating higher level goals, which in turn are the ultimate motives for wanting to lose or maintain one's body weight.

The intermediate goal, 'feel good', appears to perform a pivotal role in the pathway between lower level and end-state goals (see Figure 12.3). Indeed, 'feel good' channels the effects of the lower order goals on nearly all upper level goals and has the richest amount of associations of all goals. To the extent that 'feel good' is a basic level category, it may serve as a central criterion for people in interpreting new information related to the focal goal, making inferences and decisions, retrieving schema-relevant information, and communicating with others. In sum, the hierarchical goal structure represents a person's self-knowledge of motives for wanting a focal goal.

In addition to declarative knowledge, the goal structure conveys procedural knowledge through the ordered connections amongst goals. These connections provide information on *how* goal setting and goal pursuit might be stimulated. That is, the connections suggest means-end relations that could be targeted in change strategies, whether self-initiated or part of public or commercial influence campaigns. The goals in the hierarchy identify *what* needs to be targeted. Together, the goals and their interrelationships answer the question, *why* one wants to (or should) lose or maintain body weight.

Both individual goals and linkages between goals influenced attitudes, subjective norms, goal efficacies, and desires in the current study. However, as shown by the R^2 values in Table 12.3 and by specific regression coefficients, linkages amongst goals were generally more important determinants than goals. For the 6 dependent variables listed at top of Table 12.3, only 6 goals functioned as independent variables: i.e., significant predictions occurred for 'social acceptance' (on attitudes toward success and failure, subjective norms, and desires), 'self-esteem' (on attitude toward failure and desires), and 'achievement', 'endurance', 'exercise', and 'don't want to gain weight' (on goal efficacy). Attitude toward the process was not a direct function of any goals. In sum, 'social acceptance' has wide-spread influence, but the dependent variables are direct functions of only a limited number of other goals. The importance of 'social acceptance' is even more evident when we compare women with men (see Figures 12.4 and 12.5), a finding consistent with research showing that women are more concerned than men about body weight, physical appearance, the effects of eating, and self-esteem in relation to these issues (e.g., Pliner, Chaiken, & Flett, 1990; Tiggemann, 1992). This conclusion is also supported by the finding in the current study of a more integrated and tightly organised cognitive schema for women than men.

By contrast, a total of 28 linkages served to significantly predict the dependent variables. As only three of these linkages predicted more than one dependent variable (i.e., attitude toward success and desires were both predicted by 'social acceptance' → 'happiness' and by 'self-esteem' → 'feel good'; goal efficacy and desires were both predicted by 'feel good' → 'enjoy life'), the impact of inference-based influence spans a wide spectrum of paired goals across the dependent variables. In this sense, 'feel good' and 'look good' are the most pervasive goals in that they appear in 9 and 8 linkages, respectively. This suggests that people first experience the implications of the self-regulation of body weight in relatively concrete, personal terms, and these reactions then lead to the conclusion or inference that abstract ends and enduring values can be reached by controlling one's weight.

The hierarchical structure of superordinate goals constitutes a fundamentally different representation of the consequences of goal pursuit and goal achievement than expectancy-value models. Unlike the point-form summation of products of beliefs and evaluations, the hierarchical goal structure models the pattern and interdependence amongst goals. This potentially gives a richer explanation of goal formation and indicates which antecedents should be targeted in any change efforts. At the same time, empirical tests of the impact of any goal structure can be performed with traditional statistical procedures (e.g., *t*-tests multiple regression, structural equation models) and thus avoid the scaling problems and unwieldiness of tests of expectancy-value models (e.g., Evans, 1991).

Expectancy-value models and hierarchical goal structures can both be used to explore goal setting, but it is important to recognise that they rest on different assumptions concerning how people process information. Expectancy-value models presume piece-meal processing of consequences (e.g., Fiske & Pavelchak, 1986) and the integration of the information by use of an additive rule (e.g., Anderson, 1981). The processing is presumed to be bottom-up (i.e., data-driven) and memory based (Hastie & Park, 1986). Hierarchical goal structures, in contrast, are cognitive schemas which represent a person's knowledge of a particular domain. Processing of new information is performed on-line (Hastie & Park, 1986) but interpreted holistically in relation to an existing schema, rather than being combined according to a particular atomistic rule. Under schema-based processing, new information is first categorised, and then a schema is activated, if it exists (Fiske & Neuberg, 1990). The perception, remembrance, later retrieval, and subsequent inferences based on new information tend to be schema-consistent, although a number of factors moderate the relationships such as schema strength, expertise, time for processing, and situational complexity (Fiske & Taylor, 1991). More research is needed into the conditions under which piece-meal versus schema-based processing takes places in goal setting.

Research is needed as well into the processes behind the influence of cognitive schemas on the predecisional phase of self-regulation. It seems reasonable to expect that superordinate goals provide reasons for goal setting and these serve as input to attitude and subjective norm formation. Superordinate goals also resemble values in that they constitute specific standards of the desirable that people seek. Thus attitudes and subjective norms may serve value-expressive functions, as well as providing reasons for goal setting (e.g., McGuire, 1983). The dependence of goal efficacy on superordinate goals might follow a different process. Analogous to cognitive consistency theory and self-perception theory, we might hypothesise that people bring their self-efficacy and response efficacy judgements concerning a focal goal in line with their superordinate goals.

We have found considerable support for the processes of goal setting and goal pursuit outlined in Figure 12.1 in our field investigation of the self-regulation of body weight. Goal intentions to lose or maintain one's body weight were found to be primarily under the direct influence of desires and the indirect influence of goal efficacy judgements, subjective normative pressure, and attitudes toward success and the process of goal pursuit. Goal intentions next simulated trying (i.e., will power, self-discipline, time devoted to planning, and physical energy expended), which, in turn, initiated the goal-directed behaviours of exercising and dieting. Actual goal achievement was found to be affected by the extent of exercising and dieting.

Two distinctions are in need of further investigation with regard to the self-regulation of health related behaviours. One is the distinction between one-time and over-time goal pursuit processes, the other is the distinction between all or nothing and gradient goals. Some goals are achieved in a one-shot manner, such as getting an eye examination on a certain date. Other goals require repetitive attempts and entail an accumulation of sub-goals over time, such as losing one or two pounds a week enroute to a final goal of 5 pounds by the end of the month. Likewise, some goals are achieved in full, such as cessation of smoking, whereas others are only partially realised, such as the achievement of only 80 per cent of a planned reduction in one's blood sugar levels by a diabetic. The modelling of self-regulatory behaviours is difficult in any field context but is especially challenging for repetitive and gradient goals. In these situations, the ebb and flow of motivational and volitional processes, in conjunction with goal-directed behaviours and varying levels of goal attainment, create complex phenomena for study for those concerned about the external and ecological validity of basic research.

A new direction for research initiated by the current study is the investigation of the bases for goal setting. We attempted to show that the cognitive and motivational foundation for goal setting is more complex than currently depicted in leading theories. The motivation for a goal intention was found to be dependent on cognitive schemas people hold with respect to superordinate goals that a focal goal fulfils. The cognitive schemas consisted of a network of superordinate goals built upon if-then propositions amongst goals. A new procedure for the modelling of cognitive schemas was introduced to elicit such schemas, and multiple regression was used to test the dependency of attitudes, subjective norms, and goal efficacy on individual goals and linkages amongst goals represented in cognitive schemas.

Comments on Elicitation Procedure

Three issues with respect to the goal elicitation procedure developed herein should be pointed out. One concerns the binary recording of goals and linkages between goals, which limits the ability to detect effects on decisions with the use of conventional statistical procedures. We are now testing an extension of the goal elicitation procedure which first asks respondents to provide their reasons and linkages between reasons for pursuing a goal (according to the framework presented in the Appendix) and then requires respondents to indicate (a) the likelihood that each reason leads to the reason provided in justification for it and (b) how important each reason is personally to respondents. By measuring likelihoods and importances on quantitative scales, it is possible to employ more powerful statistical methods than done herein.

A second limitation of the elicitation procedure might be its focus only on reasons for choosing a goal to the exclusion of consideration of reasons for not choosing the goal. For example, when choosing to exercise or not, do people weigh the pros and cons before making a choice? Or is that choice to exercise predicated on a comparison of consequences for exercising to consequences for doing an alternative activity? These are unresolved issues that entail complex behavioural as well as philosophical questions. We are currently studying how people make decisions by investigating decision criteria respondents use and how they use these criteria. Two competing paradigms are under investigation: the traditional rational model where people estimate pros and cons and make a choice, and an alternative model where people are asked to consider their reasons for choosing one goal and reasons for not choosing an alternative goal. The latter approach is operationalised by requiring respondents to perform the elicitation task outlined in the Appendix two times: once for justifying the goal they have chosen and once for justifying why they have not chosen an alternative goal. The rationale for this programme of research builds upon the recent perspective proposed by Billig (1996, p. 2) in his rhetorical approach to social psychology, where he maintained that 'An argument for an issue of controversy is also an argument *against* counterviews... affirmation and negation are intertwined...' (emphasis in original).

A final issue with the goal elicitation procedure used herein is its ontological foundation. It might be argued that the goals and linkages represented in such a map as shown in Figure 12.3 capture internal mental processes. Such a point of view would be consistent with the philosophical tradition known as cognitivism but seems at odds with research questioning the self-awareness

(Nisbett & Wilson, 1977) and accessibility (Quattrone, 1985) of, and the ability to make causal inferences amongst (White, 1987), mental events. An alternative interpretation of cognitive maps is to regard them as mental constructions made within the context of a person's larger world view and his/her need to convey a particular image of the self and/or influence or convince others of one's rationale for a goal choice (Bagozzi & Dabholkar, forthcoming, Bagozzi, Bergami, & Leone, 1999). Following Wittgenstein (1953) and Harré (1998), we might conceive of the goal elicitation task proposed herein as a dialogue between researcher and respondent where cognitive processes are represented as discursive activities and thinking is manifest in one's use of language as constituted through public and private discourses. That is, the premise is that 'thinking is a form of internal argument, modelled on outward dialogue' (Billig, 1996, p. 2). The reasons given in the elicitation procedure and their interconnections serve expressive, defensive, and other functions for the self-concept. In this sense, they are windows into people's motives for acting the way they do.

Practical Implications

The research presented herein suggests different avenues for interventions. Broadly speaking, interventions can be targeted at either the motivation for acting (goal setting) or the steps needed to achieve a goal (goal striving).

Contemporary approaches for studying motives (i.e., 'content-general' theories) specify general motives presumed to apply universally across settings (e.g., Ford & Nichols, 1987; Novacek & Lazarus, 1990). Their main drawback lies in their inability to account for specific actions and to point to particular interventions to change behaviour. In contrast, the approach to goal setting proposed herein is a 'context-specific' way of dealing with reasons for acting that recognises the situational variability of behaviour and identities respondents' idiosyncratic motives for behaving in their particular situations. Thus although we expect that many health behaviours will exhibit similar existential, utilitarian, and subjective well-being concerns as found in the present study, the express range, articulation, and importance of concerns will vary form context to context and person to person. As a result, policies implied by the current research apply only to American university students of approximately 21 years of age who are concerned about their body weight.

For these individuals, the findings suggest the following policies with regard to motivation for losing or maintaining one's body weight. The desire to lose or maintain weight, a central determinant of goal intentions, was found to be a function of self-esteem and social acceptance. These abstract superordinate goals, in turn, can be reached through the linkages to more concrete motives revealed by the regressions. Thus in terms of message content to feature in educational brochures, advertisements, and face-to-face interactions with change agents, the findings suggest that two consequences of the abstract goals should be emphasised: feeling good and happiness. Likewise, the following means-end relations should be stressed: looking good will make one feel good, and more energy and feeling good will lead to greater enjoyment with life. These themes can be conveyed vicariously in dramatic interactions, communicated in narratives, explored in discussion groups, and practised through role playing exercises. The above comments refer to interventions intended to change desires as an objective. Different interventions would be required to change attitudes, subjective norms, and other aims, where the content of change efforts can be informed by specific goals and linkages between goals uncovered by the elicitation procedure proposed herein and the results of the regression analyses. As implied by the findings summarised in Figures 12.4 and 12.5, gender differences should also be taken account in the design of any intervention. For instance, the concrete goal, fitting into one's clothes, is limited to a pecuniary motive for men but stimulates such motives as feeling good, looking good, social acceptance, and self-esteem in women, in addition to saving money by controlling one's body weight.

Interventions aimed at goal striving might follow a number of strategies. In an effort to prepare effective persuasive communications and educative material, it is often wise to identify segments of a target population with different needs and design message content accordingly. Research by use of focus groups or pilot studies can be employed in this regard to uncover different target groups (based for example on opinions, media habits, socio-economic indicators, and other correlates of the target groups) and discover which groups are most vulnerable to different appeals. For example, research may reveal that some groups of individuals are more concerned with the costs of being overweight, others with the gains, and still others with the means needed to achieve weight loss. By measuring attitudes towards failure, success, and the process of weight maintenance, respectively, and validating their differential impact on desires in a pilot study, a basis can be found for using different persuasive strategies to reach target groups with these different requisites. Again guidelines for message content can be discovered by use of the goal elicitation procedure discussed herein.

A final and very important objective for intervention efforts is the transformation of goal intentions into goal-directed behaviours. In addition to getting people to plan when, where, and how they might engage in acts designed to control body weight, emphasis might be placed upon the choice of means from among alternative goal-directed behaviours. Here self-efficacies, outcome expectancies, and affect towards each instrumental behaviour need to be appraised (Bagozzi & Edwards, 1999).

APPENDIX

Finally, we would like to express *your personal reasons for wanting to lose weight*. For the questions below, plese follow this sequence: 1. List five reasons you have wanting to lose weight and place these in the boxes in column #1 under REASONS. 2. Then take your first reason and think of why this is important to you. Place your answer in the box adjacent to your first reason in Column #2 (If you have difficulty identifying why the reason is important to you, think about how you would feel if the reason was thwarted or did not take place). 3. After answering why your first reason is important, think about why the answer given is, in turn, important and put your respnse in the box in column #3 (again, if you have difficulty, think about how you would feel if the answer in the box Column #2 did not happen). 4. Repeat steps 2 and 3 for each remaining reason in Column #1. We have placed numbers in the upper left corners of each box to remind you of the sequence to follow. If you really can not list five reasons, leave one blank. But try your best.

REASONS	*WHY-1*	*WHY-2*
Reason 1 for losing weight	Why is it important to you?	Why is it important to you?

Reason 2 for losing weight	Why is it important to you?	Why is it important to you?

Reason 3 for losing weight	Why is it important to you?	Why is it important to you?

Reason 4 for losing weight	Why is it important to you?	Why is it important to you?

Reason 5 for losing weight	Why is it important to you?	Why is it important to you?

REFERENCES

Ajzen, I. (1985). From intentions to actions: A theory of planned behavior. In J. Kuhl and J. Beckmann (eds.) *Action Control: From Cognition to Behavior* (pp. 11–39). New York: Springer-Verlag.

Ajzen, I. (1991). The theory of planned behavior: Some unresolved issues. *Organizational Behavior and Human Decision Processes, 50,* 179–211.

Ajzen, I. & Fishbein, M. (1980). *Understanding attitudes and predicting social behavior.* Englewood Cliffs, NJ: Prentice-Hall.

Andersen, S. M. & Klatzky, R. L. (1987). Traits and social stereotypes: Levels of categorization in person perception. *Journal of Personality and Social Psychology, 53,* 235–246.

Anderson, J. R. (1980). *Cognitive Psychology and its Implications.* San Francisco, CA: Freeman.

Anderson, J. R. (1983). *The architecture of cognition.* Cambridge: Harvard University Press.

Anderson, N. H. (1981). *Foundations of Information Integration Theory.* New York: Academic Press.

Appelbaum, M. I. & Cramer, E. M. (1974). Some problems on the nonorthogonal analysis of variance. *Psychological Bulletin, 81,* 335–343.

Bagozzi, R. P. (1992). The self-regulation of attitudes, intentions, and behavior. *Social Psychology Quarterly, 55,* 178–204.

Bagozzi, R. P. & Dabholkar, P. A. (1994). Consumer recycling goals and their effect on decisions to recycle: A means-end chain analysis. *Psychology and Marketing, 11,* 313–340.

Bagozzi, R. P. & Dabholkar, P. A. (forthcoming). Discursive psychology and means-end chain theory: Application to perceptions of political candidates. *Psychology and Marketing.*

Bagozzi, R. P. & Edwards, E. A. (1999). Goal-striving and the implementation of goal intentions in the regulation of body weight. *Psychology and Health, 13,* 593–621.

Bagozzi, R. P. & Kimmel, S. K. (1995). A comparison of leading theories for the prediction of goal-directed behaviours. *British Journal of Social Psychology, 34,* 437–461.

Bagozzi, R. P. & Warshaw, P. R. (1990). Trying to consume. *Journal of Consumer Research, 17,* 127–140.

Bagozzi, R. P., Baumgartner, H., & Pieters, R. (1998). Goal-directed emotions. *Cognition and Emotion, 12,* 1–26.

Bagozzi, R. P., Baumgartner, H., & Yi, Y. (1992). Appraisal processes in the enactment of intentions to use coupons. *Psychology and Marketing, 9,* 469–486.

Bagozzi, R. P., Bergami, M., & Leone, L. (1999). Hierarchical representation of motives in goal-setting. Manuscript submitted for publication.

Bandura, A. (1991). Social cognitive theory of self-regulation. *Organizational Behavior and Human Decision Processes, 50,* 248–287.

Bentler, P. M. (1990). Comparative fit indexes in structural models. *Psychological Bulletin, 107,* 238–246.

Billig, M. (1996). *Arguing and Thinking.* New edition. Cambridge: Cambridge University Press.

Browne, M. W. & Cudeck, R. (1993). Alternative ways of assessing model fit. In K. A. Bollen & J. S. Long (eds.) *Testing Structural Equation Models* (pp. 136–162). Newbury Park, CA: Sage.

Carver, C. S. & Scheier, M. F. (1990). Principles of self-regulation: Action and emotion. In R. Sorrentino & E. T. Higgins (Eds.), *Handbook of Motivation and Cognition* (Vol. 2, pp. 3–52). New York: Guilford.

Conner, M. & Norman, P. (1996). Body weight and shape control: Examining component behaviours. Unpublished working paper. University of Leeds, United Kingdom.

Conner, M. & Sparks, P. (1996). The theory of planned behaviour and health behaviours. In M. Conner and P. Norman (eds.). Predicting Health Behaviour (pp. 121–162). Buckingham, England: Open University Press.

Davis, W. A. (1984). The two senses of desire. Philosophical Studies, 45, 181–195.

Evans, M. G. (1991). The problem of analyzing multiple composites. American Psychologist, 46, 6–15.

Faust, K. & Wasserman, S. (1992). Centrality and prestige: A review and synthesis. Journal of Quantitative Anthropology, 4, 23–78.

Fishbein, M. & Stasson, M. (1990). The role of desires, self-predictions, and perceived control in the prediction of training session attendance. Journal of Applied Social Psychology, 20, 173–198.

Fiske, S. T. & Neuberg, S. L. (1990). A continuum of impression formation, for category-based to individuating processes: Influences of information and motivation on attention and interpretation. In M. P. Zanna (ed.) Advances in Experimental Social Psychology (Vol. 23, pp. 1–74). New York: Academic Press.

Fiske, S. T. & Pavelchak, M. A. (1986). Category-based versus piecemeal-based affective responses: Developments in schema-triggered affect. In R. M. Sorrentino & E. T. Higgins (eds.), Handbook of Motivation and Cognition: Foundations of Social Behavior (pp. 167–203). New York: Guilford Press.

Fiske, S. T. & Taylor, S. E. (1991). Social Cognition, 2nd ed. New York: McGraw Hill.

Ford, M. E. & Nichols, C. W. (1987). A taxonomy of human goals and some possible applications. In M. E. Ford and D. H. Ford (eds.), Humans as Self-Constructing Giving Systems: Putting the Framework to Work (289–311). Hillsdale, NJ: Erlbaum.

Freeman, L. C. (1979). Centrality in social networks: Conceptual clarification. Social Network, 1, 215–239.

Godin, G. (1993). The theories of reasoned action and planned behavior: Overview of findings, emerging research problems and usefulness for exercise promotion. Journal of Applied Sport Psychology, 5, 141–157.

Gollwitzer, P. M. (1990). Action phases and mind-sets. In E. T. Higgins and R. M. Sorrentino (eds.), Handbook of Motivation and Cognition: Foundations of Social Behavior (Vol. 2, pp. 53–92). New York: Guilford Press.

Gollwitzer, P. M. (1993). Goal achievement: The role of intentions. European Review of Social Psychology, 4, 141–185.

Gollwitzer, P. M. (1996). The volitional benefits of planning. In P. M. Gollwitzer and J.A. Bargh (eds.), The Psychology of Action (pp. 287–312). New York: Guilford.

Gollwitzer, P. M., Heckhausen, H., & Ratajczak, H. (1990). From weighing to willing: Approaching a change decision through pre- or postdecisional mentation. Organizational Behavior and Human Decision Processes, 45, 41–65.

Harré, R. (1998). The Singular Self. London: Sage.

Hastie, R. & Park, B. (1986). The relationship between memory and judgment depends on whether the judgment task is memory-based or on-line. Psychological Review, 93, 258–268.

Heckhausen, H. (1991). Motivation and Action. Berlin: Springer-Verlag.

Heckhausen, H. & Gollwitzer, P. M. (1987). Thought contents and cognitive functioning in motivational versus volitional states of mind. Motivation and Emotion, 11, 101–120.

Jöreskog, K. G. & Sörbom, D. (1989). LISREL7A Guide to the Program and Applications, 2nd ed. Chicago: SPSS.

Kuhl, J. (1992). A theory of self regulation: A new theory for old applications. Applied Psychology: An International Review, 41, 97–130.

McGuire, W. J. (1983). A contextualist theory of knowledge: Its implications for innovation and reform in psychological research. In L. Berkowitz (ed.), *Advances in Experimental Social Psychology* (Vol. 16, pp. 1–47). San Diego, CA: Academic Press.

Mervis, C. B. & Rosch, E. (1981). Categorization of natural objects. In M. R. Rosenzweig & L. W. Porter (eds.) *Annual Review of Psychology* (Vol. 32, pp. 89–115). Palo Alto, CA: Annual reviews.

Nagel, T. (1970). *The Possibility of Altruism*. Oxford: Oxford University Press.

Netemeyer, R. G., Burton, S., & Johnston, M. (1991). A comparison of two models for the prediction of volitional and goal-directed behaviors: A confirmatory analysis approach. *Social Psychology Quarterly, 54*, 87–100.

Nisbett, R. E. & Wilson, T. D. (1977). Telling more than we can know: Verbal reports on mental processes. *Psychological Review, 84*, 231–259.

Novacek, J. & Lazarus, R. (1990). The structure and measurement of personal commitments. *Journal of personality, 58*, 693–715.

Pervin, L. A. (1989). Goal concepts: Themes issues and questions. In L. A. Pervin (ed.), *Goal Concepts in Personality and Social Psychology* (pp. 473–479). Hillsdale, NJ: Erlbaum.

Pieters, R. (1993). A control view on the behaviour of consumers: Turning the triangle. In G. J. Bamossy and W. F. van Raaij (Eds.) *European Advances in Consumer Research* (Vol. 1, pp. 507–512).

Pieters, R., Baumgartner, H., & Allen, D. (1995). A means-end chain approach to consumer goal structures. *International Journal of Research in Marketing, 12*, 227–244.

Pliner, P., Chaiken, S. & Flett, G. L. (1990). Gender differences in concern with body weight and physical appearance over the life span. *Personality and Social Psychology Bulletin, 16*, 263–273.

Rosch, E. (1978). Principles of categorization. In E. Rosch and B. B. Lloyd (Eds.) *Cognition and Categorization* (pp. 27–48). Hillsdale, NJ: Erlbaum.

Schifter, D. E. & Ajzen, I. (1985). Intention, perceived control, and weight loss: An application of the theory of planned behavior. *Journal of Personality and Social Psychology, 49*, 843–851.

Tiggemann, M. (1992). Body-size dissatisfaction: Individual differences in age and gender, and relationship with self-esteem. *Personality and Individual Differences, 13*, 39–43.

Toulmin, S. (1958). *The Uses of Argument*. Cambridge: Cambridge University Press.

Toulmin, S., Rieke, R., and Janik, A. (1979). *An Introduction to Reasoning*. New York: Macmillan.

White, P. A. (1987). Causal report accuracy: Retrospect and prospect. *Journal of Experimental Social Psychology, 23*, 311–315.

Wittgenstein, L. (1953). *Philosophical Investigations*. Translated by G. E. M. Anscombe. Oxford: Blackwell.

CHAPTER THIRTEEN

Health Promotion from the Perspective of Social Cognitive Theory

Albert BANDURA

The recent years have witnessed major changes in the conception of human health and illness from a *disease model*, to a *health model*. It is just as meaningful to speak of levels of vitality as of degrees of impairment. The health model, therefore, focuses on health promotion as well as disease prevention. Lifestyle habits exert a major impact on the quality of human health. Current health practices focus mainly on the supply side by reducing, rationing, and curtailing access to health care services to contain health costs. The social cognitive approach works on the demand side by helping people to stay healthy through good self-management of health habits. By exercising control over several health habits people can live longer, healthier, and slow the process of biological ageing (Bandura, 1997; Bortz, 1982; Fries, et al., 1993; Fries, 1997). As health economists amply document, medical care cannot substitute for healthful habits and environmental conditions (Fuchs, 1974; Lindsay, 1980). Self-management of habits that enhance health and reduction of those that impair it is good medicine. Indeed, if the huge benefits of a few key lifestyle habits were put into a pill, it would be declared a spectacular breakthrough in the field of medicine.

Research guided by various psychosocial theories of health behaviour have added to our understanding of how cognitive and social factors contribute to human health and disease. Among these various approaches are the health belief model (Becker, 1974; Rosenstock, 1974), social cognitive theory (Bandura, 1986, 1997), the theories of reasoned action (Ajzen & Fishbein, 1980), planned behaviour (Ajzen, 1991) and protection motivation (Rogers, 1983).

Proliferation of conceptual models of health behaviour tends to spawn cafeteria style research. Constructs are picked from various theories and strung together in the name of theoretical integration. This practice multiplies predictors needlessly in several ways. Similar factors, but given different names, are included in new conglomerates as though they were entirely different determinants. Facets of a higher-order construct are split into seemingly different determinants, as when different forms of anticipated outcomes of behavioural change are included as different constructs under the names of attitudes, normative influences, and outcome expectations. Following the timeless dictum that, the more the better, some researchers overload their studies with a host of factors that contribute only trivially to health habits because of redundancy. There is a marked difference between expanding the scope of an integrative theory and creating conglomerates from different theories with problems of redundancy and fractionation of predictors and theoretical disconnectedness.

The present chapter examines health promotion and disease prevention from the perspective of social cognitive theory. This theory posits a multifaceted causal structure in which self-efficacy beliefs operate in concert with cognized goals, outcome expectations, and perceived environmental impediments and facilitators in the regulation of human motivation, action, and well-being. This approach addresses the sociostructural determinants of health as well as the personal determinants. The factors singled out in the various theories overlap with subsets of determinants in social cognitive theory. Figure 13.1 presents the areas of overlap of the main set of sociocognitive determinants with those of some of the widely applied psychosocial theories of health behaviour. It is acknowledged that these theories differ in their specified range of application. However, they are applied to a variety of health behaviours and will be considered briefly in relation to such applications. Social cognitive theory in its totality specifies factors governing the acquisition of competencies that can profoundly affect physical and emotional well-being as well as the self-regulation of health habits.

SOCIOCOGNITIVE CAUSAL STRUCTURE

If people lack awareness of how their lifestyle habits affect their health, they have little reason to put themselves through the misery of changing the bad habits they enjoy. They are lectured more than they want to hear about their unhealthy practices. Applications of theories of health behaviour have tended to assume adequate knowledge of health risks. It is usually high. Knowledge creates the precondition for change. But additional self-influences are needed to overcome the impediments to adopting new lifestyle habits and maintaining them.

Beliefs of personal efficacy occupy a pivotal regulative role in the causal structure of social cognitive theory (Bandura, 1997). Perceived self-efficacy refers to beliefs in one's capabilities to organise and execute the courses of action required to produce given levels of attainments. Although a sense of personal efficacy is concerned with perceived capabilities to produce effects, the events over which personal influence is exercised varies widely. It may entail regulating of one's own motivation, thought processes, affective states and behaviour patterns, or changing environmental conditions, depending on which aspects of life one seeks to manage.

Efficacy belief is a major basis of action. Unless people believe they can produce desired effects by their actions, they have little incentive to act or to persevere in the face of difficulties and setbacks. Whatever else may serve as motivators, they must be founded on the belief that one has the power to produce desired changes by one's actions.

THEORIES	PSYCHOSOCIAL DETERMINANTS OF HEALTH BEHAVIOR							
	SELF-EFFICACY	OUTCOME EXPECTATIONS			GOALS		IMPEDIMENTS	
		Physical	Social	Self-Evaluative	Proximal	Distal	Personal & Situational	Health System
Social Cognitive Theory	✓	✓	✓	✓	✓	✓	✓	✓
Health Belief Model		✓	✓				✓	✓
Theory of Reasoned Action		✓	✓		✓			
Theory of Planned Behavior	✓	✓	✓		✓			
Protection Motivation Theory	✓	✓						

Figure 13.1 Summary of the main sociocognitive determinants and their areas of overlap in different conceptual models of health behaviour.

Exercise of control requires not only skills, but a strong sense of efficacy to use them effectively and consistently under difficult circumstances. Efficacy beliefs not only operate in their own right. They act on other determinants in the regulation of behaviour (Bandura, 1997). Beliefs in one's learning efficacy and efficient deployment of effort enhance acquisition of knowledge and skills for managing the demands of everyday life. Efficacy beliefs also regulate motivation by determining the goals people set for themselves, the strength of commitment to them and the outcomes they expect for their efforts. Belief in the power to produce effects determines how long people will persevere in the face of obstacles and failure experiences, their resilience to adversity, whether their thought patterns are self-hindering or self-aiding, and how much stress and depression they experience in coping with taxing environmental demands. The beliefs that people hold about their capabilities, therefore, affect whether they make good or poor use of the skills they possess. Self-doubts can easily overrule the best of skills.

People's beliefs in their personal efficacy can be developed by four main sources of influence. The most effective way of creating a strong sense of efficacy is through mastery experiences. Successes build a robust belief in one's personal efficacy. Failures undermine it, especially if failures occur before some sense of self-assurance has been established. If people experience only easy successes they come to expect quick results and are easily discouraged by failure. A resilient sense of efficacy requires experience in overcoming obstacles through perseverant effort.

The second way of creating and strengthening self-beliefs of efficacy is through the vicarious experiences provided by social models. Seeing people similar to oneself succeed by sustained effort raises observers' beliefs that they too possess the capabilities master comparable activities to succeed. Modelling influences do more than provide a social standard against which to judge one's own capabilities. Through their behaviour and expressed ways of thinking, competent models transmit knowledge and teach observers effective skills and strategies for managing environmental demands.

Social persuasion is a third way of strengthening people's beliefs that they have what it takes to succeed. People who are persuaded verbally that they possess the capabilities to master given activities are likely to mobilise greater effort and sustain it than if they harbour self-doubts and dwell on personal deficiencies when problems arise. Successful efficacy builders do more than convey positive appraisals of capabilities, however. They structure situations for people in ways that bring success and avoid placing them in situations prematurely where they are likely to fail often. They encourage people to measure success in terms of self-improvement.

People also rely partly on their somatic and emotional states in judging their capabilities. They interpret their stress reactions and tension as signs of inefficacy. In activities involving strength and stamina, people judge their fatigue, aches and pains as signs of physical debility. Mood also affects judgements of their personal efficacy. Positive mood enhances perceived self-efficacy, despondent mood diminishes it. The fourth way of modifying self-beliefs of efficacy is to reduce people's stress reactions, alter their negative emotional proclivities and correct misinterpretations of their physical states.

Most models of health behaviour now include an efficacy determinant (see Figure 13.1). Those that do not, sacrifice explanatory and predictive power. For example, when added to the variables in the theory of reasoned action, a sense of efficacy to exercise control promotes health behaviour both directly and by its influence on intention (Ajzen & Madden, 1986; deVries & Backbier, 1994; deVries, Dijkstra, & Kuhlman, 1988; Dzewaltowski, Noble, & Shaw, 1990; Kok, deVries, Mudde, & Strecher, 1991; Van Ryn, Lytte, & Kirscht, 1996; Schwarzer, 1992). Attitudes are usually predictive, especially of intention, but normative influences vary widely in their contribution across different types of health behaviour. Efficacy beliefs are consistently predictive.

There are two levels at which a sense of personal efficacy plays an influential role in human health (Bandura, 1992a, 1997). At the more basic level, people's beliefs in their capability to cope with stressors activate biological systems that mediate health and disease. Social cognitive theory views stress reactions in terms of perceived inefficacy to exercise control over threats and taxing environmental demands. If people believe they can deal effectively with potential stressors they are not perturbed by them. But if they believe they cannot control aversive events they distress themselves and impair their level of functioning. The impact of beliefs of coping efficacy on biological stress reactions is verified in experimental studies in which people are exposed to stressors under perceived inefficacy and after their beliefs of coping efficacy are raised to high levels through guided mastery experiences (Bandura, 1992; O'Leary & Brown, 1995). Exposure to stressors without perceived efficacy to control them activates autonomic, catecholamine and endogenous opioid systems. After people's perceived coping efficacy is strengthened they manage the same stressors without experiencing any distress, visceral agitation or activation of stress-related hormones. The types of biochemical reactions that have been shown to accompany a weak sense of coping efficacy are involved in the regulation of the immune system. Hence, exposure to uncontrollable stressors tends to impair the function of the immune system in ways that can increase susceptibility to illness (Herbert & Cohen, 1993b).

Most human stress is activated while learning how to exercise control over environmental demands and during the process of developing and expanding competencies. Stress aroused while gaining coping mastery over threatening situations can enhance different components of the immune system (Wiedenfeld, et al., 1990). Providing people with the means for managing acute and chronic stressors increases immunologic functioning (Antoni, et al., 1990; Gruber, Hall, Hersh, & Dubois, 1988; Kiecolt-Glaser, et al., 1986). The field of health has been heavily preoccupied with the physiologically debilitating effects of stressors. Self-efficacy theory also acknowledges the physiologically strengthening effects of mastery over stressors. A growing number of studies are providing empirical support for physiological toughening by successful coping (Dienstbier, 1989).

Depression is another affective pathway through which perceived self-efficacy can affect health functioning. Depression has been shown to reduce immune function, and to heighten susceptibility to disease. The more severe the depression, the greater the reduction in immunity (Herbert & Cohen, 1993a). A low sense of efficacy to exercise control over things one values highly produces depression in several ways. One route is through unfulfilled aspirations. People who impose on themselves standards of self-worth they judge they cannot attain drive themselves to bouts of depression (Bandura, 1991, Kanfer & Zeiss, 1983).

A second route to depression is through a low sense of social efficacy to develop social relationships that bring satisfaction to one's life, and cushion the adverse effects of chronic stressors. Social support reduces vulnerability to stress, depression, and physical illness. But social support is not a self-forming entity waiting around to buffer harried people against stressors. People have to go out and find, and create, supportive relationships for themselves. This requires a strong sense of social efficacy. The Holahans have shown that a low sense of social efficacy contributes to depression both directly, and by curtailing development of social supports (Holahan & Holahan, 1987a, b). Perceived self-efficacy and social support strengthen each other bidirectionally. Perceived social efficacy builds supportive relationships and social support enhances personal efficacy. Mediational analyses show that social support alleviates depression and physical dysfunction and fosters health-promoting behaviour only indirectly to the extent that it raises perceived coping efficacy (Cutrona & Troutman, 1986; Duncan & McAuley, 1993; Major, Mueller, & Hildebradt, 1985).

The second level at which beliefs of personal efficacy affect health is concerned with direct control over health habits and over the progression of biological ageing. People's beliefs in their efficacy to regulate their own motivation and behaviour affect every phase of personal change. They determine whether people even consider changing their health habits; whether they enlist the motivation and perseverance needed to succeed, should they choose to do so; how well they maintain the habit changes they have achieved; their vulnerability to relapse; and their success in restoring control after a setback.

A vast body of evidence reveals that belief in one's efficacy to exercise control over health-related behaviour plays an influential role in health status and functioning. The self-efficacy belief system operates as a common mechanism through which diverse modes of interventions affect different types of health outcomes. The stronger the instilled perceived self-efficacy, the more likely are people to enlist and sustain the effort needed to adopt and maintain health-promoting behaviour. These beneficial effects have been shown in such diverse areas of health as level of postcoronary recovery (Ewart, Taylor, Reese, & DeBusk, 1983; Schröder, Schwarzer, & Endler, 1997; Taylor, Bandura, Ewart, Miller, & DeBusk, 1985); recovery from coronary artery surgery (Allen, Becker, & Swant, 1990; Bastone & Kerns, 1995; Jensen et al., 1993; Mahler & Kulik, 1998; Oka, Gortner, Stotts, & Haskell, 1996; Sullivan, Andrea, LaCroix, Russo, & Katon, 1998); coping with cancer (Beckham et al., 1997; Cunningham, Lockwood, & Cunningham, 1991; Merluzzi & Sanchez, 1997) and end-stage renal disease (Devins, et al., 1982); adherence to immunosuppressive medication in renal transplantation and other prescribed medications (Brus, vandeLaar, Taal, Rasker, & Wiegman; DeGeest, et al., 1995); coping with oral surgery (Litt, Nye, & Shafer, 1995) and gastrointestinal endoscopy (Gattuso, Litt, & Fitzgerald, 1992); enhancing pulmonary function in patients suffering from chronic pulmonary disease (Kaplan, Atkins, & Reinsch, 1984); countering the debilitating and distressing effects of chronic fatigue syndrome (Findley, Kerns, Weinberg, & Rosenberg, 1998); decreasing the risk of osteoporosis through physical activity and calcium intake (Haran, Kim, Gendler, Froman, & Patel, 1998); reducing pain and dysfunction in rheumatoid arthritis (Holman & Lorig, 1992; Schiaffino, Revenson, & Gibofsky, 1991); reducing the pain of childbirth and electing vaginal over repeat cesarean delivery (Dilles & Beal, 1997; Manning & Wright, 1983); eliminating tension headaches (Holroyd et al., 1984; Martin, Holroyd, & Rokicki, 1993); managing chronic low back, neck and leg pain and impairment (Council, Ahern, Follick, & Kline, 1988; Dolce, 1987; Kaivanto, Estlander, Moneta, & Vanharanta, 1995); modifying eating habits and disorders (Desmond & Price, 1988; Glynn & Ruderman, 1986; Love, Ollendick, Johnson, & Schlezinger, 1985; Schneider, O'Leary, & Agras, 1987); reducing cholesterol through dietary means (McCann, et al., 1995); adhering to prescribed rehabilitative activities (Ewart et al., 1986); adopting and adhering to programs of physical exercise (Desharnais, Bouillon, & Godin, 1986; McAuley, 1992; Sallis et al., 1986); self-management of diabetes (Grossman, Brink, & Hauser, 1987; Hurley & Shea, 1992); exercise of control over sexual coercion and sexual practices that pose high risk for transmission of AIDS (Bengel, Beltz-Merk, & Farin, 1996; McKusick, Coates, & Morin, 1989; Walsh & Foshee, 1998; Witte, 1992); and controlling alcohol and drug abuse that impair health (DiClemente, Fairhurst & Piotrouski, 1995; Marlatt, Baer & Quigley, 1995; Stevens, Wertz, & Roffman, 1995).

That self-efficacy beliefs yield functional dividends in other spheres of adaptation and change is verified by meta-analytic studies (Holden, Moncher, Schinke, & Barker, 1990; Stajkovic & Luthans, 1998). Meta-analyses similarly confirm the influential role of self-efficacy beliefs across diverse domains of health functioning (Gilles, 1993; Holden, 1991). In studies applying multiple controls, efficacy beliefs retain their predictiveness after the influence of baseline function, sociodemographic characteristics, affective states, and other relevant factors are removed.

In social cognitive theory, efficacy beliefs operate as one of many determinants that regulate motivation, affect, and behaviour. Studies comparing the predictiveness of different theoretical models should, therefore, measure the full set of determinants posited by social cognitive theory rather than only the efficacy component. Outcome expectations about the effects of different lifestyle habits also contribute to health behaviour. Outcome expectations can take three major forms (Figure 13.2). Within each form, the anticipated positive outcomes serve as incentives, the negative outcomes as disincentives. One class of outcomes includes the physical effects that accompany the behaviour. They include pleasant sensory experiences and physical pleasures in the positive forms, and aversive sensory experiences, pain, and physical discomfort in the negative forms. Behaviour is also partly regulated by the social reactions it evokes. The positive and negative social sanctions constitute the second class of outcomes.

People do not behave like weathervanes, constantly shifting to whatever social influences happen to impinge on them at the moment. They adopt

PERSON ──────────▶ BEHAVIOR ──────────▶ OUTCOME

```
┌─────────────────────────┐       ┌─────────────────────────┐
│    EFFICACY BELIEFS      │       │  OUTCOME EXPECTANCIES   │
│         Level            │       │        Physical         │
│        Strength          │       │         Social          │
│       Generality         │       │     Self-Evaluative     │
└─────────────────────────┘       └─────────────────────────┘
```

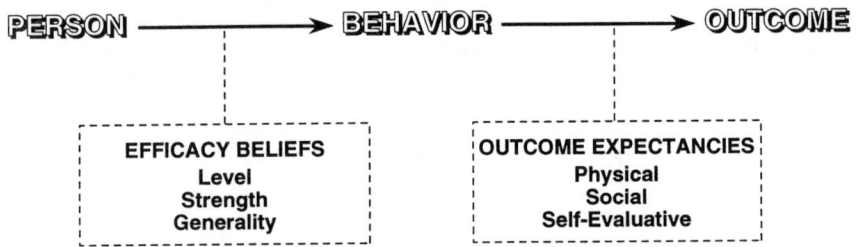

Figure 13.2   Diagrammatic representation of the conditional relations between efficacy beliefs and outcome expectancies. In given domains of functioning, efficacy beliefs vary in level, strength and generality. The outcomes that flow from a given course of action can take the form of positive or negative physical, social, and self-evaluative effects.

personal standards and regulate their behaviour by their self-sanctions. They do things that give them self-satisfaction and self-worth, and refrain from behaving in ways that breed self-dissatisfaction. This third class of outcomes concerns the positive and negative self-evaluative reactions to one's behaviour. Evaluative self-sanction is one of the more influential regulators of human behaviour but is typically ignored in models of personal change.

Most of the factors included in the different conceptual models correspond to these various types of outcome expectations. Perceived severity and susceptibility to disease in the health belief model represents the expected negative physical outcomes (Becker, 1974). The perceived benefits of preventive action represent the positive outcome expectations.

In the theories of reasoned action and planned behaviour, the intention to engage in a behaviour is governed by attitudes toward the behaviour and by subjective norms (Ajzen, 1991; Ajzen & Fishbein, 1980). These determinants correspond to different classes of outcome expectations. Attitude is measured in terms of perceived outcomes and the value placed on those outcomes. Norms are measured by perceived social pressures by significant others and one's motivation to comply with their expectations. Norms correspond to expected social outcomes for given styles of behaviour.

In social cognitive theory, normative influences regulate actions through two control processes. These include social sanctions and self-sanctions. Norms influence behaviour anticipatorily by the social consequences they provide. Behaviour that fulfils social norms gains positive social reactions. Behaviour that violates social norms brings social censure. In addition, social norms convey behavioural standards. Adoption of standards creates a self-regulatory system that operates through self-sanctions. In this process, people regulate their behaviour by self-evaluative reactions. Some researchers report that normative pressures have little impact on health behaviour (deVries, Kok, & Dykstra, 1992; Kok, et al., 1991; Lechner & deVries,1995). This raises the question of whether normative influences are ineffectual, which seems highly unlikely, or whether they need to be measured more comprehensively as different forms of social outcome expectations.

In social cognitive theory, cognised goals, rooted in a value system, provide further self-incentives and guides to health behaviour (Bandura, 1986). Goals may be distal ones that serve an orienting function, or proximal ones that regulate effort and guide action in the here and now. Intentions are essentially proximal goals. Both '*I aim to do x*' and '*I intend to do x*' refer to what a person proposes to do. Goals are an interlinked facet of a motivational mechanism, not simply a discrete predictor to be tacked on a conceptual model (Bandura, 1991). In self-motivation through goal setting, people monitor their behaviour and react positively or negatively to their attainments depending on how they compare to their goal aspirations. Efficacy beliefs affect goal setting and whether substandard performances spark greater effort or are demoralising. But goals make independent contribution to performance.

Personal change would be trivially easy if there were no impediments or barriers to surmount. Hence, perceived barriers are an important factor in the health belief model and in elaborated versions of it. Social cognitive theory distinguishes between different types of barriers. Some of them are personal impediments that impede performance of the health behaviour itself. They form an integral part of self-efficacy assessment. Efficacy beliefs must be measured against gradations of challenges or impediments to successful performance. For example, in assessing personal efficacy to stick to an exercise routine, individuals judge the strength of their efficacy to get themselves to exercise regularly when they are under pressure from work, are tired, depressed, have more interesting things to do and face foul weather. If there are no impediments to surmount, the behaviour is easily performable and everyone is totally efficacious.

The regulation of behaviour is not solely a personal matter. Some of the impediments to healthful living reside in health systems rather than in personal or situational impediments. Unavailability of health resources presents a second class of barriers to healthful behavior. These impediments are rooted in how health services are structured socially and economically. We shall consider the sociostructural determinants of health in a later section of this chapter.

TESTS FOR REDUNDANCY OF PREDICTORS

Figure 13.3 provides one example of how similar determinants bearing different labels influence health behaviour through different postulated causal structures. In the top causal model, perceived self-efficacy has been severed from social cognitive theory and grafted on the theory of reasoned action. We saw earlier that it adds incremental prediction. In the bottom causal model, perceived self-efficacy remains integrated with its conceptual brethren in the causal structure of social cognitive theory. The redundancy of predictors under different names in different models of health behaviour is an issue of both theoretical and empirical interest.

Some researchers have tested whether factors in other models add incremental prediction over and above the determinants in social cognitive theory. For example, Dzewaltowski, Noble and Shaw (1990) included efficacy beliefs, expected physical health benefits and self-sanctions for healthful behaviour in the sociocognitive subset. They found that efficacy beliefs and

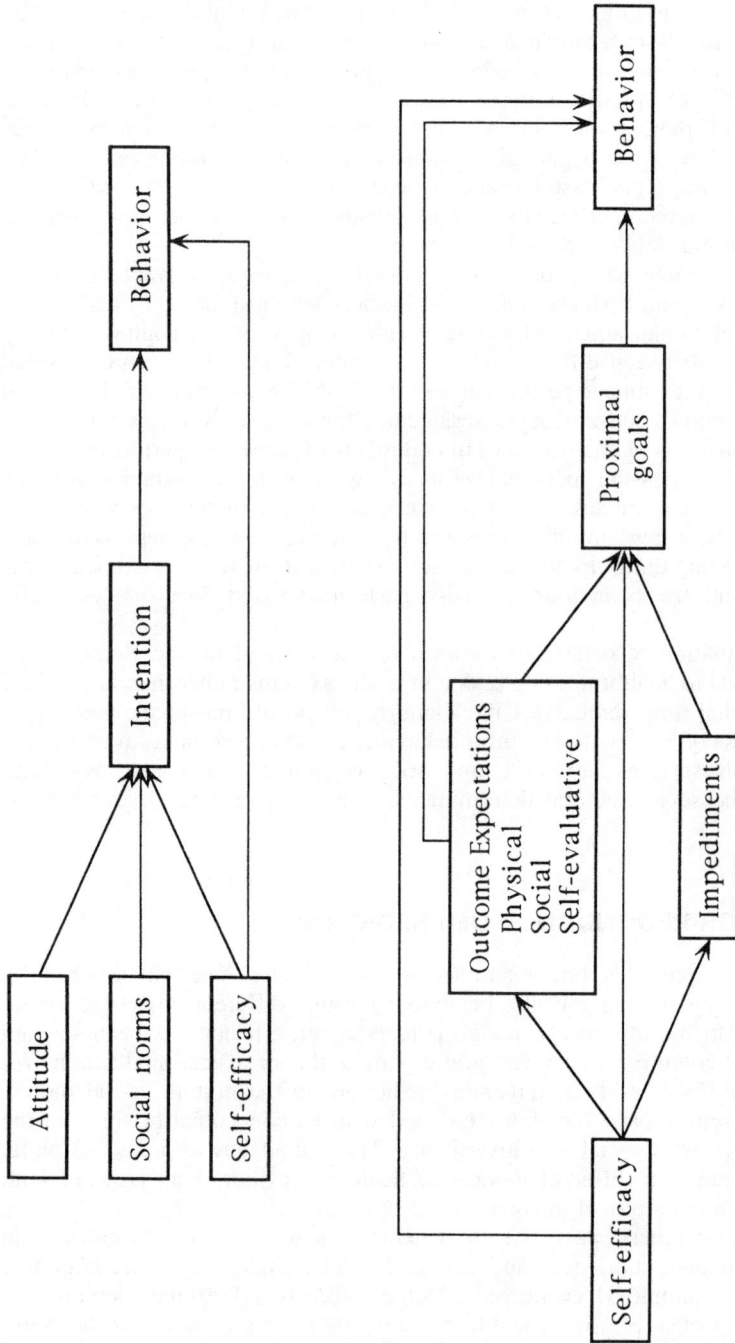

Figure 13.3   Contrasting theoretical schemes when the self-efficacy determinants is appended to the theory of reasoned action or embedded in the integrated causal structure of social cognitive theory.

self-sanctions contribute to adherence to healthful behaviour. Attitudes and perceived social pressure also account for healthful behaviour. But they do not improve prediction when added to the subset of sociocognitive determinants. These findings suggest redundancy of similar determinants under different names rather than dissimilar determinants. However, the generality of construct redundancy needs to be tested further across different types of health behaviour.

We seek theories of human behaviour with integrative principles of broad applicability. The same set of determinants and mechanisms posited by social cognitive theory operate in markedly diverse areas of functioning as they do in health behaviour (Bandura, 1997). The value of a psychological theory is judged not only by its explanatory and predictive power, but by its operational power to effect change. Most of the models of health behaviour are concerned mainly with predicting health habits, but they offer little guidance on how to change them. In addition to providing a unified conceptual framework, social cognitive theory embeds its determinants in a large body of knowledge that specifies the mechanisms through which they operate and how to enlist them to enhance human health (Bandura, 1986; 1997). It provides guidelines on how to structure goals and incentive systems to heighten motivation for personal change. It supplies a body of knowledge on how to build resilience to the demoralising effects of difficulties and setbacks. The variables that form the prediction model are the same ones that inform the intervention model.

STAGES OF CHANGE

Stage theories are undergoing a dignified burial in psychology (Flavell, 1978). Human functioning is too multifaceted and multidetermined to be shrunk to a few discrete categories. Yet many health researchers are adopting the stages-of-change notion as their guiding scheme (Prochaska & DiClemente, 1992). According to this view, in adopting new patterns of behaviour people presumably move through a sequence of stages from precontemplators with no intention to change, to contemplators who intend to change, to actors who adopt the behaviour but not yet regularly, and to maintainers who perform it regularly. A genuine stage theory is rooted in three basic assumptions: Qualitative transformations across discrete stages, invariant sequence of change, and nonreversibility. The stages-of-change scheme violates each of these requirements.

To begin with, the categories in the stages-of-change scheme are arbitrary pseudo-stages rather than genuine stages. In a genuine stage theory, the characteristics at one stage are transformed into qualitatively different ones at the next stage. For example, in stage progression in biological change a caterpillar gets transformed into a butterfly. In Piaget's stage progression of cognitive change, preoperational thinking is transformed into qualitatively different operational thinking. In the stages-of-change scheme, differences in degree are arbitrarily subdivided into discrete categories called 'stages.' The first two stages are differences in degree of intention. Noncontemplators have no intention to change. Contemplators have some intention to change. The subsequent stages are gradations of the very behaviour to be explained. The action and maintenance stages are arbitrary subdivisions of degree of duration of adopted behaviour rather than differences in kind. Thus, performing the behaviour less than 6 months is the action stage. Doing it for more than 6 months is the maintenance stage. At the upper levels of this stage view, one can continue doing the same thing but be propelled from one stage (action) to the next one (maintenance) simply with the passage of time. This conceptual scheme creates circularity of explanation and prediction. To ask whether high stage status foretells enduring change, is to ask whether good maintainers (the maintenance stage) are good maintainers. In short, these are not stages. Sectioning behaviour at 6 months into different stages is arbitrary rather than grounded in a transformational change. One can split the behaviour anywhere, at 1 month, 3 months, 6 months or a year.

In a genuine stage theory, the stages constitute a fixed sequence that everyone must pass through. One cannot skip any of them along the way. One cannot become a butterfly without first being a caterpillar or an operational thinker by skipping the preoperational stage. For smokers who abruptly quit smoking and remain abstinent, there is no progression through stages. Most participants do not exhibit a stable progression through the postulated sequence (Sutton, 1996). Where stages differ in gradation rather than in kind, the notion of stage progression is stripped of meaning or simply acknowledges the logical necessity that a brief adoptive duration precedes a longer one. And finally genuine stage progression does not permit recycling through stages. A butterfly cannot revert to a caterpillar, nor can an operational thinker go back again to a low mode of thinking.

Even genuine stage theories lead into a thicket of problems. That is why they are being abandoned. People do not fit neatly into prefixed categories. As a result, substages or transitional ones have to be created. So, predictably, an intermediate stage of preparing for action has now been inserted to the stages-of-change scheme.

The stage view substitutes a categorical approach for a process model of human adaptation and change. Contrary to claims, shift from one descriptive category of intention to another, or from a short duration of behaviour to a longer duration does not make the stage approach a 'dynamic process model.' Even a genuine stage theory is at best a descriptive device rather than an explanatory one. For example, categorising individuals as 'precontemplators' provides no explanation for why they do not consider making changes that could benefit them. They may be disinclined to change because they are uninformed about the risks of their current habits or the benefits of alternative habits. They may know the potential risks and benefits but are convinced they lack the efficacy to alter their health habits. Or they may have little incentive to change because they view the aversiveness of change worse than its potential benefits. These various determinants of inaction – risk perception, efficacy belief, outcome expectations – call for different strategies to get so-called noncontemplators to seriously consider altering their detrimental habits.

People do not recycle through discrete stages. They fluctuate in their struggle to exercise control over their health behaviour. Their successes are a product of a triadic reciprocal interaction of personal factors, behaviour, and environmental facilitators and impediments. In these fluctuations, which can occur over very brief periods, people are varying in their self- regulatory command not undergoing repeated transformational changes. The basic processes of personal change have been identified and their determinants extensively researched (Bandura, 1986; O'Leary & Wilson, 1987). They include: The adoption of new styles of behaviour; their generalisation across situational contexts, response modalities, and social conditions; relapse and recovery; and maintenance over time.

The stage scheme converts these standard change processes to descriptive categories stripped from their extensive knowledge base. This recasting is regressive rather than progressive. The stage scheme reminds us that some people have no interest in changing their health habits. Others are riper for change. But this common knowledge hardly requires the encumbrance of stage theorising. Interventions must, of course, be tailored to the determinants governing the health habits of the individuals undergoing change and to their rate of progress.

Proponents of the stage view linked stages to sociocognitive determinants. They showed that self-regulatory efficacy and the balance of expected costs and benefits of change differentiate individuals cast into the various stages. Precontemplators believe they do not have what it takes to succeed. They expect the disadvantages of habit change to outweigh the expected benefits. In contrast, those who are confident they can effect change and expect to gain major benefits by doing so, become good adoptors and adherers to healthful habits.

The stage scheme comes with a host of interventions drawn from divergent theories on the assumption that the theories may be incompatible on aetiology but compatible on behaviour change. In point of fact, the behaviouristic, psychodynamic and existential theories, from which this 'transtheoretical' collection is forged, offer contradictory prescriptions on how to change human behaviour. This menagerie of interventions is not transtheoretical, which implies an over-reaching integration of seeming diversity. It is atheoretical. For example, counterconditioning and altering faulty beliefs would be regarded as incompatible strategies by the proponents of these alternative approaches. Conditioning theorists reject beliefs as causes of behaviour and, therefore, consider it pointless to change them. Cognitivists, in turn, construe conditioning operations as a laborious way of creating outcome expectations that serve as motivators rather than as automatic implanters of responses.

The stages mainly describe behaviour rather than specify determinants or operative mechanisms. Therefore, linkage of interventions to stages is rather loose and debatable rather than explicitly derivable from the stages. Effective interventions must target the constellation of determinants governing health habits in given individuals not contrived stages. For example, precontemplators forsake efforts to quit smoking because of low efficacy and negative outcome expectations. An effective intervention must persuade them of the benefits of quitting, instil beliefs that they have the capability to succeed, and enlist social supports to see them through tough times. Unlike the categorising approach, a process model specifies the determinants and intervening mechanisms governing different facets of change. Such knowledge provides guidelines for how to structure effective interventions to initiate, generalise, and maintain habit changes. Classifying behaviour by regularness or duration says nothing about its determinants that would aid selection of appropriate interventions.

Individualised interventions in general practice settings that tailor health messages to recipients' sociodemographic characteristics are more effective than uniform ones as Strecher and his colleagues have shown (Strecher, et al., 1994). Interactive computer systems can now provide personalised interventions effectively and economically to large numbers of people. However, the benefits of personalization will depend on whether weak or strong determinants are targeted. I will describe shortly one personalised system combining self-regulatory knowledge with computer assisted implementation for reducing health risk factors and promoting healthful habits. The interventions are tailored to the psychosocial determinants operating for given individuals rather than to categorical stages. The system is structured to build self-regulatory efficacy through progressive mastery experiences. Unlike the pseudo-stage approach, a self-regulatory model is a process model linked to explicit interventions.

GENERATIONAL CHANGES IN PSYCHOSOCIAL INTERVENTIONS

The models of disease prevention and health promotion have undergone several generational changes. The initial approaches tried to scare people into health by informing them about the grave health risks of detrimental habits and the benefits of healthful habits. It did not take long to discover the limitations of information about health risks alone. However, this judgement requires qualification. Our knowledge about the changeability of health habits is seriously biased by selective focus on the habitual losers who seek help. We do not see the vast number of self-changers who succeed on their own. For example, those depressing relapse curves for smoking cessation in American samples should be superimposed on the 40 million smokers who successfully quit on their own. As the Carey's have shown longitudinally, successful self-changers have a high sense of efficacy that they can regulate their motivation and behavior (Carey & Carey, 1993; Carey, Kalra, Carey, Halperin, & Richards, 1993). They are the ones who mobilise the effort needed to succeed. Granfield and Cloud (1996) put it well when they characterised the conspicuous inattention to the vast number of successful self-changers as, 'The elephant that no one sees.' Our theories grossly overpredict psychopathology and overstate the inability to effect personal changes because of the selective focus on hard-core cases (Bandura, 1999).

Faced with refractory cases the next approach tried to reward people into health by linking health habits to extrinsic rewards and penalties. The changes achieved by imposed incentive control were modest to begin with and usually dissipated after control was lifted. One-sided environmental determinism eventually gave way to models of interactive causation in which individuals operate as proactive agents with self-directing capabilities. Individuals continuously preside over their own behaviour. Therefore, they are in the best position to exercise control over it. This next generational change focused on development of self-regulatory capabilities. People were equipped with motivational and self-management skills and resilient beliefs in their efficacy to exercise control over their health habits. Efficacy in self-management enhances adoption and maintenance of health habits (Bandura, 1997; Holroyd & Creer, 1986).

The further evolution of the health promotion model treats personal change as occurring within a network of social influences. It adds socially-oriented interventions designed to provide social supports for personal change and to alter the practices of social systems that impair health and to foster those that enhance it. A socially-oriented approach is especially important in high risk behavioural practices that are subjected to strong social influences (Bandura, 1994). Depending on their nature, social influences can aid, retard or undermine efforts at personal change. Viewed from this broad perspective, health is the product of the complex interplay of self-regulatory influence, biological endowment, and sociostructural influences.

STRUCTURE OF SELF-REGULATORY FUNCTIONS

Habit change is not achieved through an act of will. It requires development of self-regulatory skills. Self-regulation operates through a set of psychological subfunctions that must be developed and mobilised for self-directed change (Bandura, 1986). Neither intention nor desire alone has much effect if people lack the capability for exercising influence over their own motivation and behaviour (Bandura & Simon, 1977). The constituent subfunctions in the exercise of self-regulation through self-reactive influence are summarised in Figure 13.4.

People cannot influence their own motivation and actions very well if they do not pay adequate attention to their own performances, the conditions under which they occur, and to the immediate and distal effects they produce. Therefore, success in self-regulation partly depends on the fidelity, consistency, and temporal proximity of self-monitoring. Activities vary on a number of evaluative dimensions, some of which are listed in Figure 13.4. Self-observation serves at least two important functions in the process of self-regulation. It provides the information needed for setting realistic goals and for evaluating one's progress toward them. In addition, paying close attention to one's thought patterns and actions in different social contexts can contribute to self-directed change. When people attend closely to their performances they are inclined to set themselves goals of progressive improvement. Goal setting enlists evaluative self-reactions that mobilise efforts toward goal attainment.

Observing one's behaviour is the first step toward doing something to affect it, but, in itself, such information provides little basis for self-directed reactions. Actions give rise to regulatory self-reactions through a judgmental function that includes several subsidiary processes. Personal standards for judging and guiding one's actions play a major role in the exercise of self-directedness. Whether a given performance is regarded favourably or negatively will depend upon the goals or personal standards against which it is evaluated.

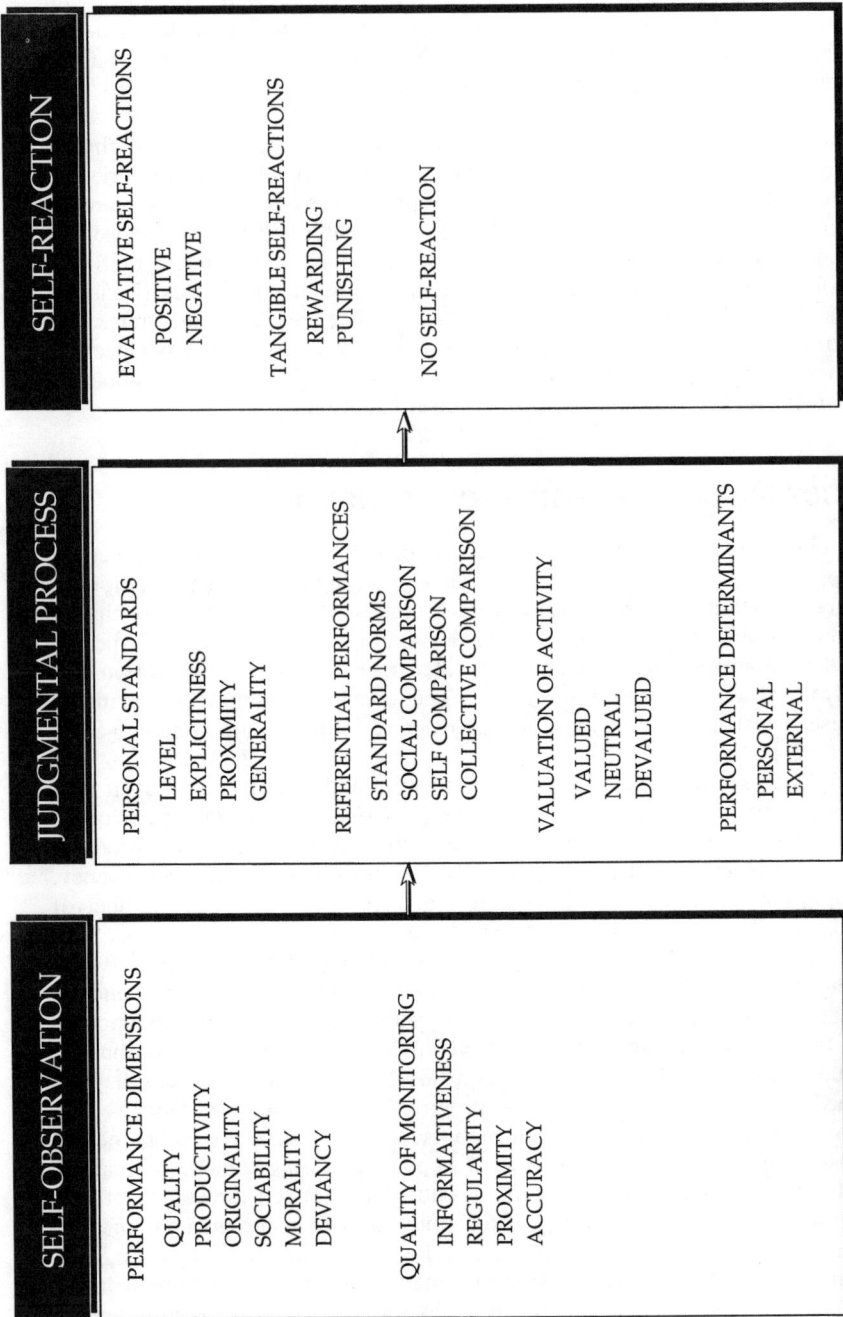

SELF-OBSERVATION	JUDGMENTAL PROCESS	SELF-REACTION
PERFORMANCE DIMENSIONS	PERSONAL STANDARDS	EVALUATIVE SELF-REACTIONS
QUALITY	LEVEL	POSITIVE
PRODUCTIVITY	EXPLICITNESS	NEGATIVE
ORIGINALITY	PROXIMITY	
SOCIABILITY	GENERALITY	TANGIBLE SELF-REACTIONS
MORALITY		REWARDING
DEVIANCY	REFERENTIAL PERFORMANCES	PUNISHING
	STANDARD NORMS	
QUALITY OF MONITORING	SOCIAL COMPARISON	NO SELF-REACTION
INFORMATIVENESS	SELF COMPARISON	
REGULARITY	COLLECTIVE COMPARISON	
PROXIMITY		
ACCURACY	VALUATION OF ACTIVITY	
	VALUED	
	NEUTRAL	
	DEVALUED	
	PERFORMANCE DETERMINANTS	
	PERSONAL	
	EXTERNAL	

Figure 13.4   Structure of the system of self-regulation of motivation and action through internal standards and self-reactive influences.

Referential comparisons also enter into the judgement of personal attainments. In many activities people compare their performances to the achievement of others or to standard norms based on representative groups. In health behaviour, self-comparison with one's prior attainments supplies the measure of adequacy. Past attainments affect self-management mainly through their effects on perceived self-efficacy and goal setting. Subgoal attainments provide markers of increasing mastery that enhance belief of self-regulatory efficacy. Hence, people generally try to surpass their past accomplishments. After a given level of performance has been attained, it is no longer challenging and people seek new self-satisfactions by striving for progressive improvements.

Another factor in the judgmental component of self-regulation concerns the valuation of activities. People do not care much how they do in activities that have little or no significance for them. They expend little effort on devalued activities. It is mainly in areas affecting their welfare and self-esteem that performance appraisals activate self-reactions. Self-reactions also vary depending on how people perceive the determinants of their behaviour. They are most likely to take pride in their accomplishments when they ascribe their successes to their abilities, strategies, and efforts. But they do not derive much self-satisfaction when they view their performances as heavily dependent on external aid or special situational supports.

Performance judgements set the occasion for self-reactive influence. Self-reactions provide the mechanism by which standards regulate courses of action. The self-regulatory control is achieved by creating incentives for one's own actions and by anticipative affective reactions to one's behaviour depending on how it measures up to an internal standard. When people make self-satisfaction or tangible benefits conditional upon certain accomplishments, they motivate themselves to expend the effort needed to attain the requisite performances. Both the anticipated satisfactions of desired accomplishments and the dissatisfactions with insufficient ones provide incentives for actions that increase the likelihood of performance attainments. In the case of tangible self-motivators, people get themselves to do things they would otherwise put off or avoid altogether by making tangible rewards dependent upon performance attainments. People who reward their own attainments accomplish more than those who perform the same activities without self incentives (Bandura, 1986).

Beliefs of personal efficacy partly determine how the various subfunctions of a self-regulatory system operate. Such beliefs affect the self-monitoring and cognitive processing of different aspects of one's performances and the outcomes expected to flow from them. People vary in their perceived efficacy to monitor their health-related activities consistently. Beliefs of personal efficacy influence the perceived causes of successes and failures (Bandura, 1997). Thus, people who regard themselves as highly efficacious tend to ascribe their failures to insufficient effort or deficient strategies, whereas those who regard themselves as inefficacious view the cause of their failures as stemming from low ability. Self-beliefs of efficacy also affect the goal-setting subfunction of self- regulation. The more capable people judge themselves to be, the higher the goals they set for themselves and the more firmly committed they remain to them. Whether negative discrepancies between personal standards and behavioural accomplishments are motivating or discouraging is partly determined by people's beliefs that they can attain the goals they set for themselves. Those who harbor self-doubts about their capabilities are easily dissuaded by obstacles or failures. Those who are assured of their capabilities intensify their efforts when they fail to achieve what they seek and they persist until they succeed.

COMPUTERIZED SELF-REGULATORY SYSTEM

The social impact of our knowledge of self-regulatory mechanisms has not been fully realised because of weak models of implementation. Advances in computer interactive technologies now enable us to promote self-regulatory efficacy in a personalised way to large numbers of people efficiently and inexpensively. Health promotion and risk reduction programs are often structured in ways that are costly, cumbersome, and minimally effective. The net result is minimal prevention and costly remediation. DeBusk and his colleagues have devised an efficacy-based system combining self-regulatory principles with computerised implementation that promotes habits conducive to health and reduces those that impair it (DeBusk, et al., 1994). The system is founded on knowledge of the major subfunctions of self-regulation and their self-efficacy underpinning.

This self-regulatory system equips participants with the skills and personal efficacy to exercise self-directed change. It includes exercise programs to build cardiovascular capacity. Nutrition programs to reduce risk of heart disease and cancer. Weight reduction programs. Smoking cessation programs. One can add stress management programs to reduce the wear and tear on the body. For each risk factor, individuals are provided with detailed guides on how to achieve and maintain behaviour conducive to health.

A single program implementor, assisted by the computerised system, can oversee the behavioural changes of hundreds of participants concurrently. Figure 13.5 portrays the structure of the self-management system. Participants monitor the behaviour they seek to change. They set short-range attainable subgoals to motivate and guide their efforts. They receive detailed feedback of progress as further motivators for self-directed change. The system is structured in this way based on knowledge that self-motivation requires both goal challenges and performance feedback. Neither goals without knowing how one is doing, nor knowing how one is doing without any goals has any motivational impact.

At selected intervals, the computer generates and mails to participants individually-tailored guides for self-directed change. These guides provide attainable subgoals for progressive change. The participants mail performance cards to the implementor on the changes they have achieved and their perceived efficacy for the next cycle of self-directed change. Efficacy ratings identify areas of vulnerability and difficulties and foretell likely relapse. The computer-generated feedback portrays graphically the progress patients are making toward each of their subgoals, their month-to-month changes, and also suggests strategies on how to surmount the identified difficulties. The program

SELF-REGULATORY DELIVERY SYSTEM

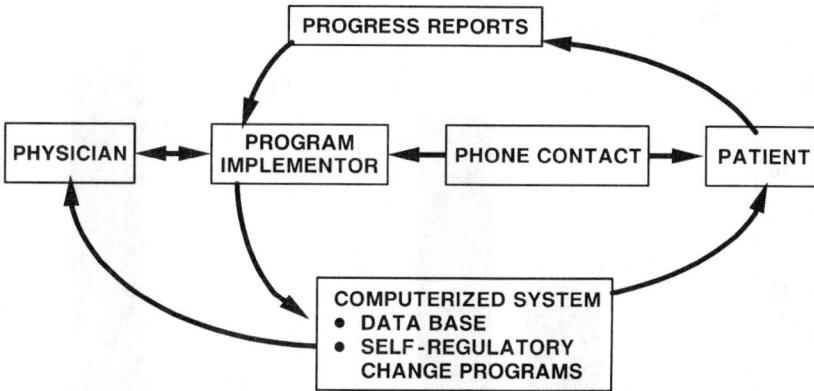

Figure 13.5 Computer-assisted self-regulatory system for altering health habits.

implementor maintains telephone contact with the participants, if necessary, and is available to provide them extra guidance and support should they run into difficulties. The implementor also serves as the liaison to medical personnel who are called upon when their expertise is needed.

The effectiveness of this system was initially tested in a cholesterol reduction program conducted with employees with elevated cholesterol levels drawn from work sites. One nutritionist ran the computer-assisted system for many participants. They reduced their consumption of saturated fat and lowered their serum cholesterol (Figure 13.6). They achieved an even larger risk reduction if their spouses took part in the dietary change program as well. The more room for change in nutritional habits, the greater the cholesterol reduction.

Further studies attest to the efficacy of the self-management system in reducing plasma cholesterol (Clark, et al., 1997). Adding counselling by a dietitian to the self-regulatory system does not produce any further treatment gains (DeBusk, et al., 1999). The achieved cholesterol reductions are sustained. This approach can thus provide health-promoting services to large numbers of people at low cost. The self-monitoring component of the self-management system also provides an effective means for differentiating patients most likely to benefit from dietary treatment because of unhealthy eating habits, from those with hyperlipidemia despite a healthy diet, and thus require lipid-lowering drug therapy.

APPLICATION OF THE SELF-REGULATORY MODEL TO HYPERTENSION

People consume a lot of foods high in sodium. Sodium intake is linked to hypertension in people who are sensitive to this mineral, a sensitivity that increases with age as the body loses some of its efficiency. Left unchecked,

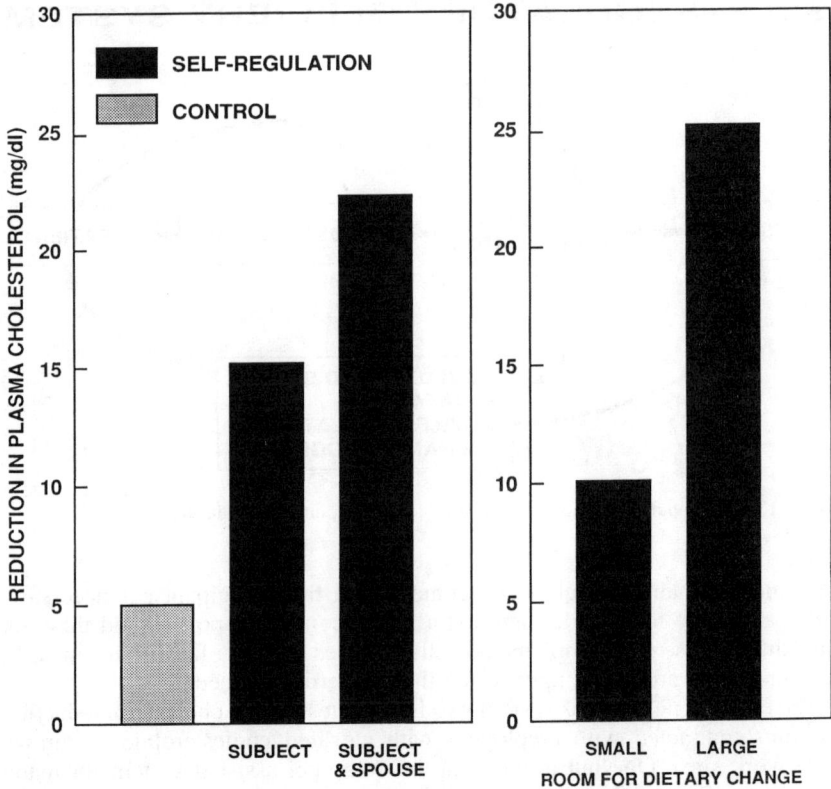

Figure 13.6 Levels of reduction in plasma cholesterol achieved with the computerised self-regulation system. The panel on the left summarises the mean cholesterol reductions achieved in applications in the workplace by participants who used the system either by themselves, along with their spouses, or did not receive the system to provide a control baseline. The right panel presents the mean cholesterol reductions achieved with the self-regulative system by patients whose daily cholesterol and fat intake was high or relatively low at the outset of the program.

hypertension increases risk of stroke, heart disease, and kidney failure. Sodium-reduction programs can lower blood pressure sufficiently to reduce the need for antihypertensive medication or to discontinue it altogether (Whelton, et al., 1998), especially if combined with other lifestyle changes (Reid, et al., 1994).

West and his colleagues demonstrated the effectiveness of the self-management system in helping patients with heart disease to cut back on their level of sodium intake (West, et al., 1999). Foods high in sodium content were targeted for the dietary change. As can be seen in Figure 13.7, training in self-management enhanced patients' perceived self-efficacy to adopt a low sodium diet. They not only reduced their sodium intake to the recommended target level, but maintained the dietary change stably over time. At each

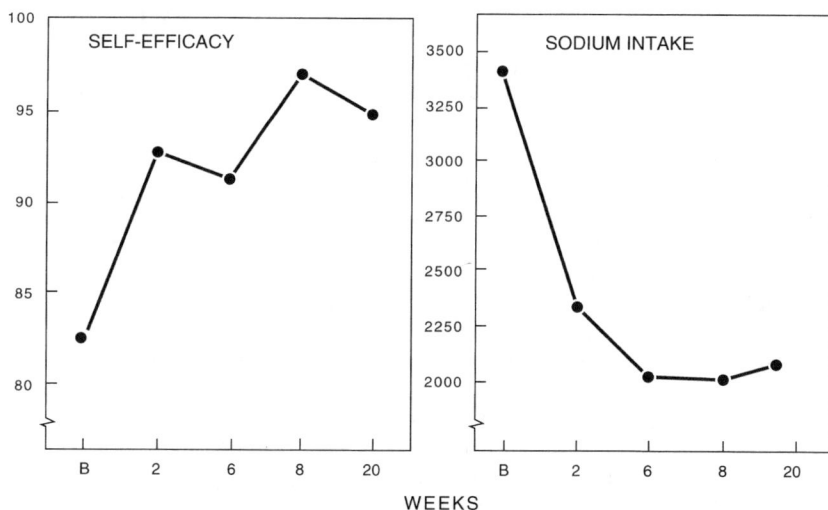

Figure 13.7 Enhancement of perceived self-regulatory efficacy and reduction of sodium intake through the aid of the self-management system (West, et al., 1999).

successive point in the self-change program, the stronger the perceived self-regulatory efficacy, the greater the reduction in sodium intake.

Some patients cannot achieve sufficient control over their blood pressure solely by dietary and other lifestyle habit changes. They require antihypertensive medication. Controlling blood pressure with drugs presents major challenges because nonadherence with prescribed medications is an endemic problem (Rudd, 1997). This is doubly so with nonsymptomatic disorders where neither the benefits of taking medication regularly, nor the detrimental health effects of nonadherence are noticeable. People are reluctant to stick to bothersome drug routines that have no easily noticeable health benefits, but cause some unpleasant side effects. Medical nonadherence not only poses health risks, but may lead physicians to prescribe stronger medications or more drastic interventions in response to the seeming failure of the prescribed treatment.

Building adherence requires feedback systems that make unnoticeable effects observably conditional. In research in progress on compliance with anti-hypertension medication, participants measure their blood pressure daily at designated times at home, keep track of their pill taking with a microchip record, and receive feedback that enables them to link their blood pressure to the regularity of their self-medication. In this self-persuasary arrangement, the participants are essentially engaged in self-experimentation in the exercise of personal control. Seeing how their blood pressure covaries with level of adherence to medications provides them with evidence that it is within their power to lower their blood pressure. If enabled to do so, successes can build and strengthen self-regulatory efficacy, and positive outcome expectations can provide incentives to stick to the self-medication routine.

SELF-REGULATORY IMPACT ON CORONARY ARTERY DISEASE

Haskell used this self-regulatory system to promote lifestyle changes in patients suffering from coronary artery disease (Haskell, et al., 1994). The targeted risk factors included smoking, exercise, weight, nutrition and, if necessary, lipid-lowering drug treatment. At the end of four years, those receiving the usual medical care by their physicians showed no change or a worsening of their condition. In contrast, those aided in self-management of health habits achieved substantial reductions in risk factors (Figure 13.8). They lowered their intake of dietary fat, lost weight, lowered their bad cholesterol, and raised their good cholesterol, exercised more, and increased their cardiovascular capacity.

The program also altered the physical progression of the disease. Those receiving the self- management program had 47% less build up of plaque on artery walls, a higher rate of reversal of arteriosclerosis, and fewer hospitalisations for coronary heart problems and cardiac deaths (Figure 13.9).

The self-regulatory system combines the high individualisation of the clinical approach with the large-scale applicability of the public health approach. The system is well received by patients for several reasons. It is individually tailored to their needs. It provides them with continuing personalised guidance and informative feedback that enables them to exercise considerable control over their own change. It is a home-based program that does not require any special facilities, equipment, or attendance at group meetings that usually have high drop-out rates. It is not constrained by time and place. It can serve large numbers of people simultaneously. It provides valuable health-promoting services at low cost.

In the present application the computer is used mainly as a tool to guide self-directed change through goal setting and feedback of progress. Linking the interactive aspects of this self-management model to the Internet can vastly expand its reach and availability, and boost its health promotive power by providing a ready means for enlisting social support and strategic guidance when needed. The amount and form of personalised guidance can be tailored to recipients needs. Much needed productivity gains in risk reduction and health promotion can be realised by creative coupling of self-regulatory knowledge with the disseminative and instructive power of computer-assisted implementation.

SELF-REGULATORY SYSTEM IN POST-CORONARY CARE

Most patients who suffer heart attacks have the bad health habits that put them at risk for another one. They receive intensive treatment in the hospital but little help following discharge in changing behavioural risk factors. The success of the self-regulatory system is being compared against the standard medical post-coronary care to reduce morbidity and mortality in post-coronary patients (DeBusk, et al., 1994). The project includes nearly 600 post-coronary patients from five hospitals. The risk factors include cholesterol, smoking and physical exercise. The differences in cardiovascular risk factors after the first year of post-coronary care are summarised in Figure 13.10. The self-regulatory system is more effective in reducing risk factors and increasing functional

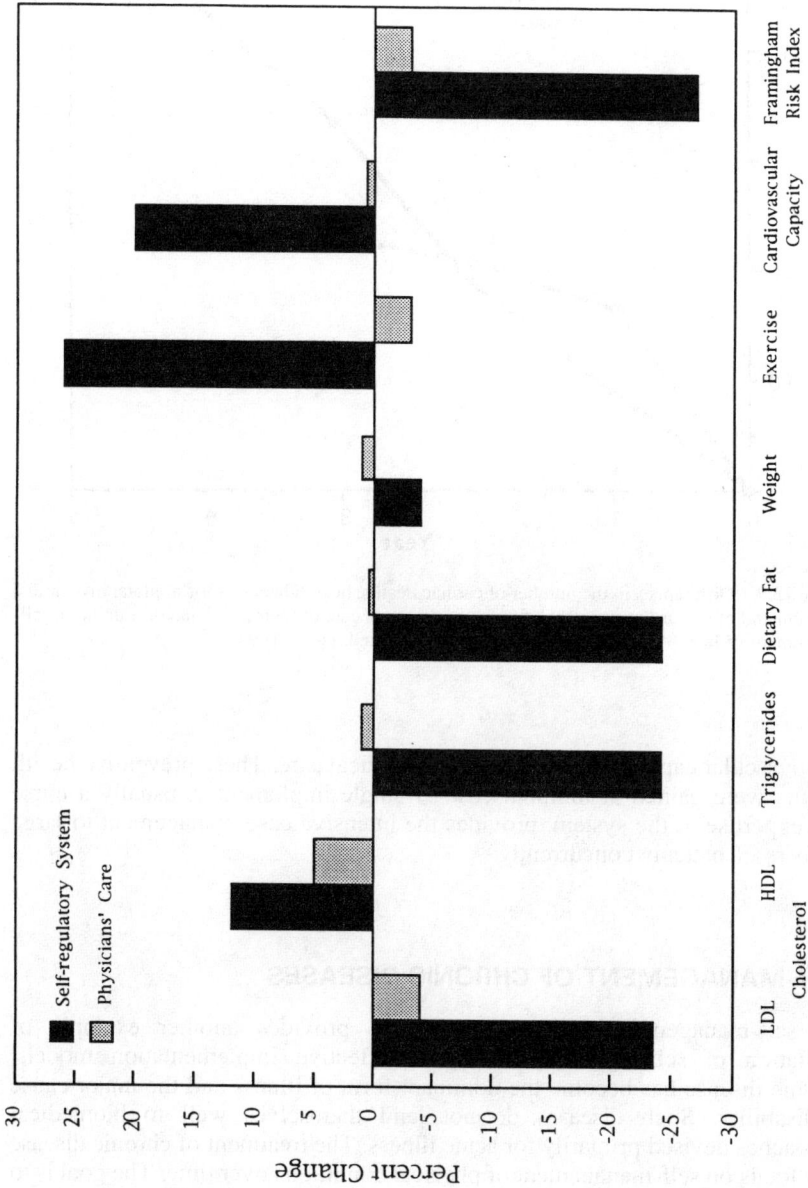

Figure 13.8 Reduction in multiple risk factors by patients with coronary atherosclerosis depending on whether they received the usual care of their physician or training in self-management of health habits. Plotted from data of Haskell, et al., 1994.

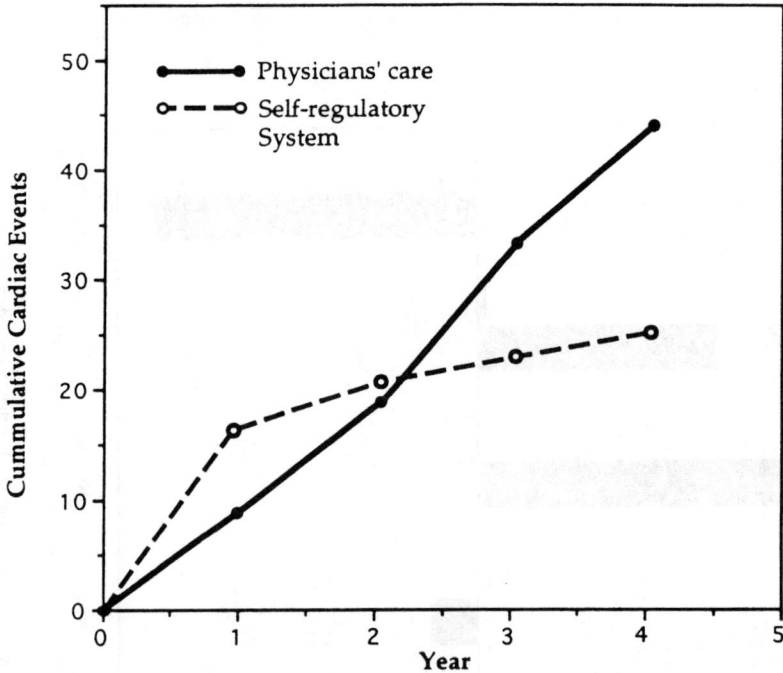

Figure 13.9   Differences in the number of cardiac deaths, hospitalizations for nonfatal myocardial infarction and other cardiac events who received the usual care of their physician or training in self-management of health habits. Plotted from data of Haskell, et al., 1994.

cardiovascular capacity than the standard medical care. These preventive health benefits were gained at minimal cost. A single implementor, usually a nurse with expertise in the system, provides the intensive case management to large numbers of patients concurrently.

SELF-MANAGEMENT OF CHRONIC DISEASES

The self-management of chronic diseases provides another example of translation of self-regulatory theory to effective implementation models. Chronic disease has become the dominant form of illness and the major cause of disability. Such diseases do not lend themselves well to biomedical approaches devised primarily for acute illness. The treatment of chronic disease must focus on self-management of physical conditions over time. The goal is to retard the biological progression of impairment to disability and to improve the quality of life of people with chronic disease. Holman and Lorig (1992) devised a prototypic model for the self-management of chronic diseases.

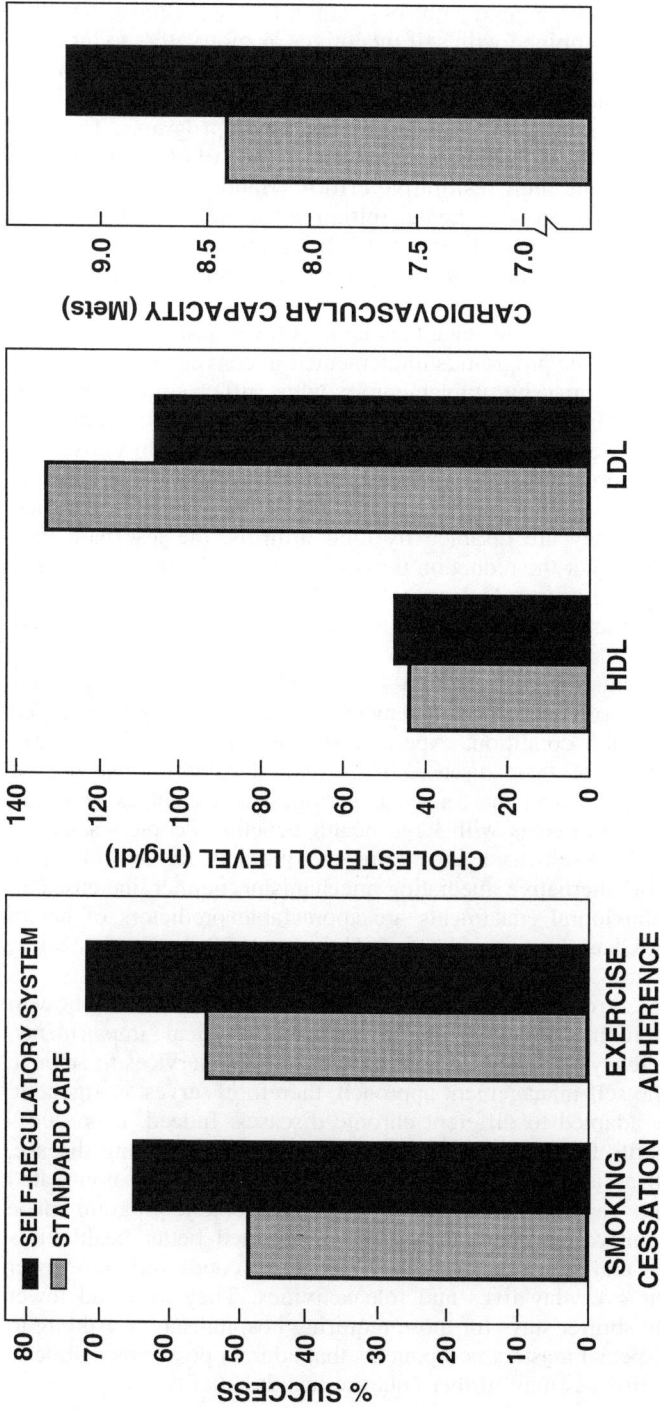

Figure 13.10 Changes in coronary risk factors by patients during the first year after acute myocardial infarction depending on whether they received the usual medical care or training in self-management of health habits. Plotted from data of DeBusk, et al., 1994.

People are taught cognitive pain control techniques, self-relaxation, and proximal goal setting combined with self incentives as motivators to increase level of activity. They are also taught problem solving and self-diagnostic skills for monitoring and interpreting changes in one's health status, skills in locating community resources and managing medication programs. The way health care systems deal with clients can alter their sense of efficacy in ways that support or undermine their restorative efforts (Bandura, 2000). Clients are, therefore, taught how to take greater initiative for their health care and dealings with health personnel. These capabilities are developed through modelling of self-management skills, guided mastery practice, and informative feedback.

The effectiveness of this self-management approach was tested with patients suffering from arthritis. The program is implemented in convenient community settings in a group format by implementors who suffer similar physical impairments but surmount them. Their modelled successes in prevailing over physical debility provide participants with instructive guides and incentives for personal change. The program greatly increases patients' efficacy that they can exercise some control over their physical condition. The higher their perceived self-efficacy the less they are disabled by their arthritis, the less pain they experience, and the greater the reduction they achieve in inflammation in their joints (O'Leary, Shoor, Lorig, & Holman, 1988). Patients who believe they can do something about their physical condition are also less depressed and less stressed.

Figure 13.11 presents the changes in a 4-year follow-up. Arthritic patients who had the benefit of the self-management program displayed increased efficacy to manage their condition, experienced reduced pain, and a slower biological progression of their disease. They also decreased their use of medical services by 43% over the four-year period. These changes represent huge reductions in health costs with large health benefits. People's sense of efficacy at the end of the self-management program predicts the level of health benefits. In tests of alternative mediating mechanisms neither increases in knowledge nor behavioural enactments are appreciable predictors of health functioning (Lorig, Chastain, Ung, Shoor, & Holman, 1989; Lorig, Seleznick, et al., 1989).

Different types of chronic diseases present many similar problems on how to manage pain, overcome impediments created by physical impairments, maintain self-sufficiency and exercise control over medical services to achieve the best results. The self-management approach, therefore, serves as a generic model that can be adapted to different chronic diseases. Indeed, it produces similar health benefits for people suffering from heart disease, lung disease, and stroke as well as arthritis (Lorig et al., 1999). Compared to nontreated controls, those who had the benefit of the self-management program made greater use of cognitive symptom management, reported better health, less fatigue, disability, and distress over their physical condition and fewer limitations on their everyday lives and role activities. They also had fewer hospitalisations and shorter stays for those requiring hospitalisation. Adding to the generic model special mastery components that address problems unique to particular chronic diseases may further enhance health benefits.

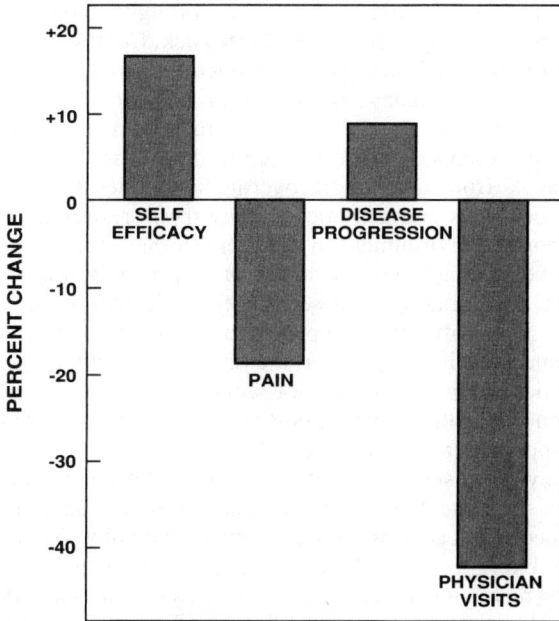

Figure 13.11 Enduring healthful changes achieved by training in self-management of arthritis as revealed in a follow-up assessment four years later. The 9% biological progression of the disease is much less than the 20% disease progression one would normally expect over four years for this age group. Plotted from data of Lorig, 1990.

SOCIALLY-ORIENTED INTERVENTIONS

Human agency operates within a broad network of social structural influences. Many health habits are deeply embedded in people's social lives. Social inducements and constraints strain self-regulatory capabilities. The newest generation of interventions requires an expanded social perspective to human adaptation and change. Because of individualistic bias, our knowledge base and models for effecting social change leave much to be desired. Psychological programs that increase success rates by creating social structural supports for personal change are rarely adopted despite their success. They are troublesome to create and their management requires attention to the mundane hassles of everyday life. Unlike drug treatments, a beneficial social technology is not a merchandisable product that is readily prescribable, demands little effort, and requires repeated purchase and use to sustain its profitable production.

Self-help groups who suffer the problems are more likely to create beneficial social systems than are professional health providers. The outstanding Delancy program for hard-core drug abusers is one example (Silbert, 1984). It is built on a enablement model that provides the sociostructural means for transforming addicted criminal lives into prosocial productive ones. The substantial reductions in HIV infections in San Francisco were achieved largely by the unprecedented social and behavioural changes brought about by the self-empowering efforts of the gay community (McKusick, Coates, Morin, Pollack, Hoff, 1990). The longitudinal predictors of reduction in risky sexual practices were a strong sense of efficacy in exercising self-protective control and association with groups that adopted safer sex practices as the norm.

The benefits of an expanded perspective are further illustrated in alcoholism. In making the break from alcohol, recovering alcoholics face a bleak life stripped of their social ties and activities as they try to restructure their lives. They need a supportive environment to see them through the tough transition and help them develop a new way of life. Not surprisingly, the treatment of alcoholism yields discouraging relapse curves. Self-help groups, such as Alcoholic's Anonymous, offer many supports for a new life without alcohol for those who become deeply committed members. Unfortunately, adding a referral to Alcoholics Anonymous does not seem to help many people because of the high attrition rate. Alternative supportive subcommunities are needed for rebuilding and supporting an alcohol-free life.

Azrin (1976) devised a self-governed social group for recovered alcoholics and their families to serve the supportive and enabling function. A social system that is embedded in a multifaceted treatment and tailored to the needs of the participants is likely to be used well. Indeed, it improves familial, social, occupational and recreational functioning in ways that support sobriety. Recovering alcoholics who have the benefit of such a social system achieve greater improvements in health, family life and employment than do recovering alcoholics without the supportive group (Hunt & Azrin, 1973). Despite the substantial benefits of this system, I have yet to find an adoption of it. We are incredibly slow on the uptake of needed social extensions for successful interventions. In the biological field, pharmaceutical and medical industries quickly translate new knowledge into saleable products in areas that promise vast consumership. In the psychosocial field, we have few, if any, serviceable social mechanisms for diffusing effective programs.

CHILDHOOD HEALTH PROMOTION MODELS

As noted earlier, health promotion and disease prevention has evolved into a multifaceted model that addresses the reciprocal interplay between personal and environmental determinants of health behaviour. Health knowledge, incentive systems, self-regulatory capabilities and sociostructural supports all have a role to play in the successful pursuit of health. Many of the lifelong habits that jeopardise health are formed during childhood and adolescence. It is easier to prevent detrimental health habits, than to try to change them after they have become deeply entrenched as part of a lifestyle.

Health habits are rooted in familial practices. However, schools have a vital role to play in promoting the health of a nation. This is the only place where all children can be easily reached. However, beleaguered educators do not want the additional responsibilities of health promotion and disease prevention. Nor are they equipped to do so even if they were willing to undertake this role. They have enough problems fulfilling their basic academic mission. Moreover, schools are reluctant to get embroiled in societal controversies regarding sexuality, drug use and other social morbidities that place youth at risk. Many educators rightfully argue that it is not their responsibility to remedy societies' social ills. Like other professionals, educators devote their efforts to the activities on which they are evaluated. As long as health promotion is regarded as tangential to the central mission of schools, it will continue to be slighted and resisted.

Researchers are applying promising prevention models in school settings under severe constraints well suited to undermine their effectiveness. The general conclusion is that these approaches work in the short run, but their effects dissipate over time. There are several problems with this indiscriminate verdict. Informative evaluation research requires assessment of quality of implementation. Otherwise, there is no way of knowing whether weak results reflect a deficient model or deficient application of a good one. Outcome studies of school-based programs rarely provide data on adequacy of implementation. Journal editors should insist that outcome studies include sound data on quality of implementation.

School-based applications are long on didactics but short on personal enablement. By enablement I do not mean a stock set of refusal tactics. Rather, it involves equipping children with skills and efficacy beliefs that enable them to regulate their own behaviour and manage the diverse pressures in interpersonal relationships for detrimental conduct. Meta-analyses show that the more children practice exercising regulatory control, the more successful they are in resisting detrimental health habits (Bruvold, 1993; Murray, Pirie, Luepker, & Pallonen, 1989). The more intensive the program and the better the implementation the stronger the impact (Connell, Turner, & Mason, 1985). Comprehensive approaches that integrate school-based health programs with familial and community efforts are more successful in promoting health than if schools try to do it alone (Perry, Kelder, Murray, & Klepp, 1992).

Schools provide a good setting for health promotion and early intervention. But this does not mean that educators should be the standard-bearers for the health mission. Health promotion must be structured as part of a societal commitment that makes children's health a matter of high priority. A serious commitment must provide the multidisciplinary personnel and the resources needed to foster the health of its youth. This requires creating new school-based models of health promotion that operate in concert with the home, community and the society at large. The programs are in school but not of the school. The implementors must have the operational control needed to do the job well. Otherwise, promotive efforts do more to discredit psychosocial approaches through deficient implementation than to advance health.

COLLECTIVE EFFICACY FOR POLICY INITIATIVES

The quality of health of a nation is a social matter not just a personal one. Health depends heavily on behavioural, sociostructural, and economic factors. While individuals play an important role in their own health, it is the product of the interplay of personal and sociostructural determinants. Therefore, a comprehensive approach to health promotion requires changing the practices of social systems that affect health rather than only changing the habits of individuals. It takes a great deal of united effort to dislodge entrenched detrimental practices of industries that wield sociopolitical power. People's beliefs in their collective efficacy to accomplish social change, therefore, play a key role in the policy and public health perspective to health promotion and disease prevention.

Billions of dollars are spent annually on lobbying and advertising campaigns to promote the very products that jeopardise health. They are influential contributors to lifestyle habits. The tobacco industry is a notable example. Cigarette smoking is the single most personally preventable cause of death. About 3,000 children in the United States take up smoking each day, a third of whom will die of tobacco related diseases (Pierce, Fiore, Novotny, Hatziandreu, & Davis, 1989). Policy remedies that raise tobacco taxes, limit juvenile access to tobacco products, and ban smoking in public places and the workplace to remove the health hazard of secondhand smoke, lower the smoking rates in a society (Lynch & Bonnie, 1994). Regulating the nicotine dosage in cigarettes below addictive levels would aid those struggling to quit the smoking habit. Smoking rates are exceedingly high in many countries. This widespread habit will incur a heavy toll of deaths and staggering medical costs from smoking-related diseases. As smoking rates decline in the United States the tobacco industry seeks lucrative markets abroad, especially in Eastern Europe, Asia, and the Middle East (Perlez, 1997). Aggressive marketing tactics recruit new smokers who foreshadow a global cancer epidemic.

We do not lack sound policy prescriptions in the field of health. What is lacking is the collective efficacy to realise them. There is growing disaffection and cynicism about our centralised public institutions. All too often what is good public policy is self-jeopardising politics for lawmakers. As a result, heavily-lobbied lawmakers block policy initiatives designed to protect human health. The tobacco industry provides an informative example of the changing social dynamics of health protection through collective social action. Despite the fact that tobacco products are the most toxic legalised substances and kill about 400,000 people annually in the United States (McGinnis & Foege, 1993), our lawmakers have exempted nicotine from any bill concerning drugs. Moreover, they federalised control with preemptive laws that ban states from regulating tobacco products and advertising. The power of tobacco money over the behaviour of federal lawmakers is graphically revealed in Figure 13.12. The more tobacco campaign money they receive, the more likely they are to fend off legislation to regulate tobacco products. Most of the proposed legislation is killed in committee. This legislative behaviour protects the reelection of lawmakers at the heavy cost of national health.

In addition to beholden legislators, the vast supporting cast contributing to the promotion of this noxious product include executives of the tobacco industry steadfastly disputing that nicotine is addictive and that smoking is a major contributor to lung cancer despite evidence to the contrary; talented chemists discovering ammonia as a means to increase the nicotine 'kick' by speeding the body's absorption of nicotine (Meier, 1998); inventive biotech researchers genetically engineering a tobacco seed that doubles the addictive

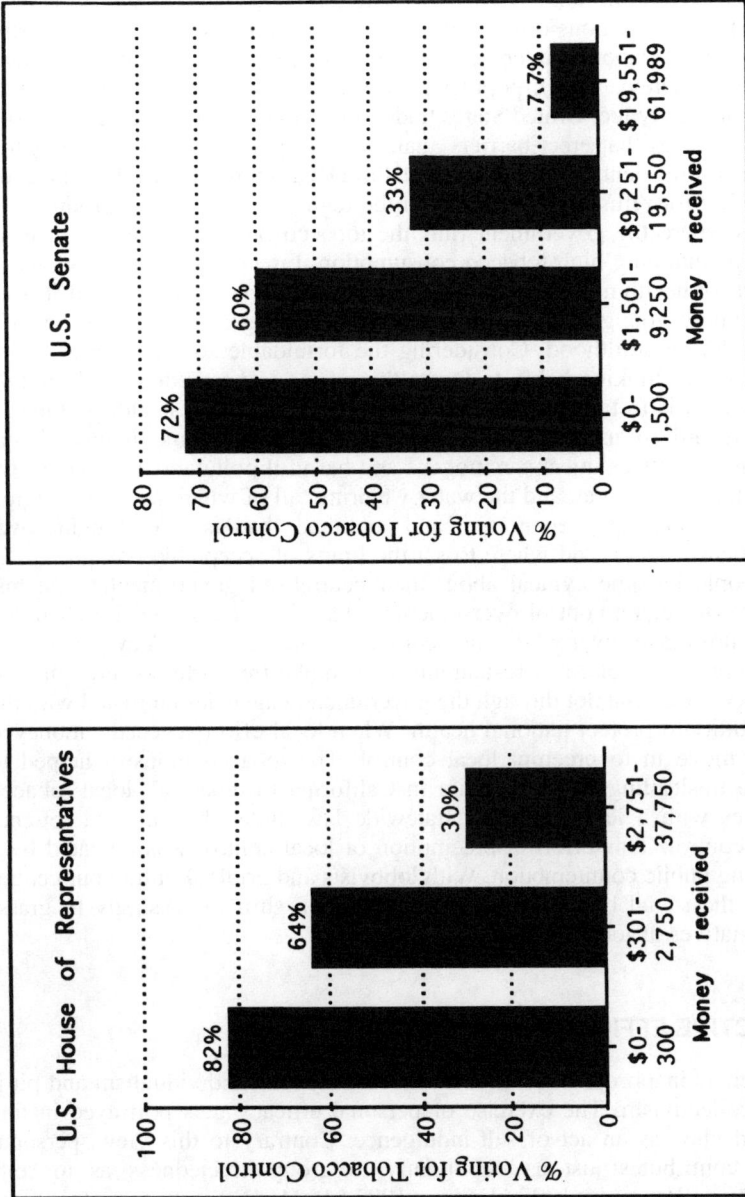

Figure 13.12   Relationship between the amount of campaign money legislators receive from the tobacco industry and their likelihood of voting against legislation to regulate tobacco products. Public Citizen Health Research Group, 1993.

nicotine content of tobacco plants (Meier, 1998); creative advertisers with multibillion dollar budgets targeting young age groups with merchandising and advertising schemes depicting smoking as a sign of youthful hipness, modernity, freedom, and women's liberation (Dedman, 1998; Lynch & Bonnie, 1994); ingenious officials in a subsidiary of a major tobacco company engaging in an elaborate international cigarette smuggling operation to evade excise taxes (Drew, 1998); popular movie actors agreeing to smoke in their movies for a hefty fee; United States trade representatives threatening sanctions against countries that erect barriers against the importation of U.S. cigarettes, and even a President firing his head of the Department of Health, Education and Welfare for refusing to back off on the regulation of tobacco products. In countries where the government runs the tobacco business it has a financial stake in maintaining high tobacco consumption. Finance ministries counteract the efforts of health ministries to reduce this major public health hazard (Efron, 1997). Unless youngsters take up smoking as teenagers they rarely become smokers during adulthood. Considering the formidable sociostructural forces promoting the smoking habit, to locate the causes and remedies solely within the individual is to take a conceptually myopic view of the health problem.

With regard to injurious environmental conditions, some industrial and agricultural practices inject carcinogens and harmful pollutants into the air we breathe, the food we eat, and the water we drink, all of which take a heavy toll on health. Vigorous economic and political battles are fought over environmental health and where to set the limits of acceptable risk.

As people become cynical about their centralised governmental systems, they strive to regain control over practices that affect their lives by changing local circumstances over which they command some control. They got smoke-free workplaces, smoke-free restaurants, and smoke-free airliners through their own collective action not through the governmental agencies entrusted with the responsibility to protect national health. When local effort succeeds, moneyed interests move in to preempt local control. The tobacco industry helped to finance a misleading ballot measure in California to repeal all local tobacco ordinances with a less restrictive statewide law under the guise of tougher tobacco control. This effort at preemption of local control was defeated by a resounding public counteraction. With lobbyists and gridlock ruling our central systems, the social battles over health protection shift increasingly to grass-roots initiatives at local levels.

COLLECTIVE EFFICACY

Some writers inappropriately equate self-efficacy with individualism and pit it against collectivism. The exercise of personal efficacy gets portrayed in this jaundiced view as an act of self-indulgence. Contrary to this view, personal efficacy contributes just as importantly to group-directedness as to self-directedness (Bandura, 1997; Earley, 1993, 1994). Efficacy is valued, not because of reverence for individualism, but because a strong sense of personal efficacy is vital for success regardless of whether it is achieved individually or by people working together.

A comprehensive approach to health must provide people with the knowledge, skills and sense of collective efficacy to mount social and policy initiatives that affect human health. Such social efforts are aimed at raising public awareness of health hazards, educating and influencing policymakers, mobilising public support for policy initiatives, and devising effective strategies for improving health conditions. Knowledge on how to develop and exercise collective efficacy can provide the guidelines for moving us further in the enhancement of human health.

We are gaining knowledge on how to frame policy issues strategically and how to use the media to enlist public support for policy changes that promote health (Bandura, 1997; Wallack, Dorfman, Jernigan, & Themba, 1993). Symbolic modelling in the broadcast media provides another means of altering detrimental normative practices and enabling people to achieve changes that have widespread societal impact. Basic research on modelling and self-regulatory mechanisms has provided guidelines for programs designed to achieve society-wide changes. These macrosocial applications address some of the growing global problems. The burgeoning population growth is the foremost and, by far, the most urgent global problem. The world population is doubling at an accelerated rate. Unless the explosive population growth is checked, we will destroy the interdependent ecosystems that sustain life. Sabido (1981), applied sociocognitive principles creatively in developing a highly effective media format to inform, enable and motivate people to reduce their rate of childbearing and to raise the status of women in societies where they have a subservient status with little or no say about family size. These lengthy dramatic serials model family planning, women's equality, beneficial health practices and a variety of effective life skills in familial, occupational and community relations. Applications of this creative format in Africa, Asia and South America are raising people's efficacy to exercise control over their family lives, raising the status of women and lowering the rates of childbearing (Rogers, Vaughan, Swalehe, Rao, & Sood, 1996; Singhal & Rogers, 1989; Westoff & Rodriquez, 1995). These macrosocial applications are also reducing sexual practices that pose risk of infection with the AIDS virus (Rogers, et al., 1996).

Achievement of structural changes is a slow, arduous process. In the metaphoric words of John Gardner, '*Getting things done socially is no sport for the short winded.*' While concerted efforts are made to produce structural changes, people need to improve their current life circumstances over which they command some control. We need to develop sociostructural principles and implementation models on how best to enable people to work together to change their lives for the better.

The approaches that work best promote community self-help through collective enablement (Bandura, 1997). Consider, by way of example, a community effort to reduce infant mortality resulting from unsanitary conditions in poor Latino neighbourhoods (McAlister, Puska, Orlandi, Bye, & Zbylot, 1991). The community was fully informed of the impact of unsanitary conditions on children's health through the local media, churches, schools and neighbourhood meetings conducted by influential persons in the community. The residents were taught how to install plumbing systems, sanitary sewerage facilities and refuse storage. They were advised how to secure the financing needed from different local and governmental sources. This enabling self-help program greatly improved the community's sanitation and markedly reduced infant mortality.

There is mass migration of people from rural to urban areas. As cities swell uncontrollably, centralised urban systems, especially in poor countries, fail to provide adequate human services. Through community enablement people can work together to improve problems of sanitation, safe water, health and public safety in their localities. However, many of these pandemic problems require some material resources if collective self-help is to achieve much success. People need to be given the necessary resources and enabling guidance to help themselves. Otherwise, simply to tell people to fend for themselves with intractable problems is an evasion of societal responsibility. Unsupported prescription of local self-help can be easily used as a political subterfuge for civic neglect. Adverse changes in living conditions in poor nations – burgeoning populations, poverty, malnutrition, environmental deterioration and toxification, desertification of productive land – will present major challenges to preservation of health in the coming years (Hancock & Garrett, 1995).

If we are to contribute significantly to the betterment of human health we must broaden our perspective on health promotion and disease prevention beyond the individualistic level. This calls for a more ambitious socially-oriented agenda of research and social practice. We can further amplify our impact on human health by making creative use of evolving technologies that enhance the scope and strength of health promotion efforts.

AUTHOR'S NOTE

Some sections of this chapter include revised and updated material from the book, *Self-Efficacy: The Exercise of Control*. Freeman, 1997.

REFERENCES

Ajzen, I. (1991). The theory of planned behavior. *Organizational Behavior and Human Decision Processes, 50*, 179–211.

Ajzen, I. & Fishbein, M. (1980). *Understanding Attitudes and Predicting Social Behavior*. Englewood Cliffs, NJ: Prentice-Hall.

Ajzen, I. & Madden, T. J. (1986). Prediction of goal-directed behavior: Attitudes, intentions, and perceived behavioral control. *Journal of Experimental Social Psychology, 22*, 453–474.

Allen, J. K., Becker, D. M., Swank, R. T. (1990). Factors related to functional status after coronary artery bypass surgery. *Heart Lung, 19*, 337–343.

Antoni, M. H., Schneiderman, N., Fletcher, M. A., Goldstein, D. A., Ironson, G., & Laperriere, A. (1990). Psychoneuroimmunology and HIV-1. *Journal of Consulting and Clinical Psychology, 58*, 38–49

Azrin, N. H. (1976). Improvements in the community-reinforcement approach to alcoholism. *Behaviour Research And Therapy, 14*, 339–348.

Bandura, A. & Simon, K. M. (1977). The role of proximal intentions in self-regulation of refractory behavior. *Cognitive Therapy And Research, 1,* 177–193.

Bandura, A. (1986). *Social Foundations Of Thought and Action: A Social Cognitive Theory.* Englewood Cliffs, NJ: Prentice-Hall.

Bandura, A. (1991). Self-regulation of motivation through anticipatory and self-regulatory mechanisms. In R. A. Dienstbier (ed.), *Perspectives On Motivation: Nebraska Symposium On Motivation* (Vol. 38, pp. 69–164). Lincoln: University of Nebraska Press.

Bandura, A. (1992). Self-efficacy mechanism in psychobiologic functioning. In R. Schwarzer (ed.), *Self-Efficacy: Thought Control Of Action* (pp. 355–394). Washington, D.C.: Hemisphere.

Bandura, A. (1994). Social cognitive theory and exercise of control over HIV infection. In R. J. DiClemente and J. L. Peterson (eds.), *Preventing AIDS: Theories and Methods of Behavioral Interventions* (pp. 25–59). New York: Plenum, 1994.

Bandura, A. (1997). *Self-Efficacy: The Exercise of Control.* New York: Freeman.

Bandura, A. (1999). A sociocognitive analysis of substance abuse: An agentic perspective. *Psychological Science, 10,* 214–217.

Bandura, A. (2000). Psychological aspects of prognostic judgments. In R. W. Evans, D. S. Baskin, & F. M. Yatsu (eds.), *Prognosis Of Neurological Disorders* (Vol. 2) (pp. 11–27). New York: Oxford University Press.

Bastone, E. C. & Kerns, R. D. (1995). Effects of self-efficacy and perceived social support on recovery-related behaviors after coronary artery bypass graft surgery. *Annals of Behavioral Medicine, 17,* 324–330.

Becker, M. H. (ed.). (1974). The health belief model and personal health behavior. *Health Education Monographs, 2,* 324–473.

Beckham, J. C., Burker, E. J., Lytle, B. L., Feldman, M. E., & Costakis, M. J. (1997). Self-efficacy and adjustment in cancer patients: A preliminary report. *Behavioral Medicine, 23,* 137–142.

Bengel, J., Belz-Merk, M., & Farin, E. (1996). The role of risk perception and efficacy cognitions in the prediction of HIV-related preventive behavior and condom use. *Psychology and Health, 11,* 505–525.

Bortz, W. M., II (1982). Disuse and aging. *Journal of the American Medical Association, 248,* 1203–1208.

Brus, H., vandeLaar, M., Taal, E., Rasker, J., & Wiegman, O. (1999). Determinants of compliance with medication in patients with rheumatoid arthritis: the importance of self-efficacy expectations. *Patient Education and Counseling, 36,* 57–64.

Bruvold, W. H. (1993). A meta-analysis of adolescent smoking prevention programs. *American Journal of Public Health, 83,* 872–880.

Carey, K. B. & Carey, M. P. (1993). Changes in self-efficacy resulting from unaided attempts to quit smoking. *Psychology of Addictive Behaviors, 7,* 219–224.

Carey, M. P, Kalra, D. L., Carey, K. B, Halperin, S., & Richards, C. S. (1993). Stress and unaided smoking cessation: A prospective investigation. *Journal of Consulting and Clinical Psychology, 61,* 831–838.

Clark, M., Ghandour, G., Miller, N. H., Taylor, C. B., Bandura, A., & DeBusk, R. F. (1997). Development and evaluation of a computer-based system for dietary management of hyperlipidemia. *Journal of the American Dietetic Association, 97,* 146–150.

Council, J. R., Ahern, D. K., Follick, M. J., & Kline, C. L. (1988). Expectancies and functional impairment in chronic low back pain. *Pain, 33,* 323–331.

Connell, D. B., Turner, R. R., & Mason, E. F. (1985). Summary of findings of the school health education evaluation: Health promotion effectiveness, implementation, and costs. *Journal of School Health, 55,* 316–321.

Cunningham, A. J., Lockwood, G. A., & Cunningham, J. A. (1991). A relationship between perceived self-efficacy and quality of life in cancer patients. *Patient Education and Counseling, 17,* 71–78.

Cutrona, C. E. & Troutman, B. R. (1986). Social support, infant temperament, and parenting self-efficacy: A mediational model of postpartum depression. *Child Development, 57*, 1507–1518.

DeBusk, R. F., Clark, M., Kraemer, H. C., Bandura, A., Miller, N. H., Fisher, L., Greenwald, M. D., & Jaffe, M. (1999). *Computer-assisted dietary intervention for hyperlipidemia: Results of a randomized trial and implications for clinical management.* Submitted for publication.

DeBusk, R. F., Miller, N. H., Superko, H. R., Dennis, C. A., Thomas, R. J., Lew, H. T., Berger III, W. E., Heller, R. S., Rompf, J., Gee, D., Kraemer, H. C., Bandura, A., Ghandour, G., Clark, M., Shah, R. V., Fisher, L., & Taylor, C. B. (1994). A case-management system for coronary risk factor modification after acute myocardial infarction. *Annals of Internal Medicine, 120*, 721–729.

Dedman, B. (1998, March 3). Executive says he's uncertain about tobacco harm. *New York Times*, p. A16.

DeGeest, S., Borgermans, L., Gemoets, H., Abraham, I., Vlaminck, H., Evers, G., & Vanrenterghem, Y. (1995). Incidence, determinants, and consequences of subclinical non-compliance with immunosuppressive therapy in renal transplant recipients. *Transplantation, 59*, 340–346.

Desharnais, R., Bouillon, J., & Godin, G. (1986). Self- efficacy and outcome expectations as determinants of exercise adherence. *Psychological Reports, 59*, 1155–1159.

Desmond, S. M. & Price, J. H. (1988). Self-efficacy and weight control. *Health Education, 19*, 12–18.

Devins, G. M., Binik, Y. M., Gorman, P., Dattel, M., McCloskey, B., Oscar, G., & Briggs, J. (1982). Perceived self- efficacy, outcome expectations, and negative mood states in end- stage renal disease. *Journal of Abnormal Psychology, 91*, 241– 244.

deVries, H. & Backbier, M. P. H. (1994). Self-efficacy as an important determinant of quitting among pregnant women who smoke: The Ø-pattern. *Preventive Medicine, 23*, 167–174.

deVries, H., Dijkstra, M., & Kuhlman, P. (1988). Self-efficacy: The third factor besides attitude and subjective norm as a predictor of behavioural intentions. *Health Education Research, 3*, 273–282.

deVries, H., Kok, G., & Dijkstra, M. (1990). Self-efficacy as a determinant of the onset of smoking and interventions to prevent smoking in adolescents. In R. J. Takens, et al. (eds.), *European Perspectives in Psychology* (Vol. 2, pp. 209–224). London: Wiley & Sons.

DiClemente, C. C., Fairhurst, S. K., & Piotrowski, N. A. (1995). Self-efficacy and addictive behaviors. In J. E. Maddux (ed.), *Self-Efficacy, Adaptation, and Adjustment: Theory, Research and Application* (pp. 109–141). New York: Plenum.

Dienstbier, R. A. (1989). Arousal and physiological toughness: Implications for mental and physical health. *Psychological Review, 96*, 84–100.

Dilles, F. M. & Beal, J. A. (1997). Role of self-efficacy in birth choice. *Journal of Perinatal and Neonatal Nursing, 11*, 1–9.

Dolce, J. J. (1987). Self-efficacy and disability beliefs in behavioral treatment of pain. *Behaviour Research and Therapy, 25*, 289–300.

Drew, C. (1998, December 23). RJR subsidiary pleads guilty to smuggling. *New York Times*, p. A1.

Duncan, T. E. & McAuley, E. (1993). Social support and efficacy cognitions in exercise adherence: A latent growth curve analysis. *Journal of Behavioral Medicine, 16*, 199–218.

Dzewaltowski, D. A., Noble, J. M., & Shaw, J. M. (1990). Physical activity participation: Social cognitive theory versus the theories of reasoned action and planned behavior. *Journal of Sport and Exercise Psychology, 12*, 388–405.

Earley, P. C. (1993). East meets West meets Mideast: Further explorations of collectivistic and individualistic work groups. *Academy Of Management Journal, 36*, 319–348.

Earley, P. C. (1994). Self or group? Cultural effects of training on self-efficacy and performance. *Administrative Science Quarterly, 39*, 89–117.

Efron, S. (1997, May 18). Japan slow to tell consumers tobacco is a health hazard. *San Francisco Examiner*, p. A-14.

Ewart, C. K., Taylor, C. B., Reese, L. B., & DeBusk, R. F. (1983). Effects of early post-myocardial infarction exercise testing on self-perception and subsequent physical activity. *American Journal of Cardiology, 51*, 1076–1080.

Ewart, C. K., Stewart, K. J., Gillilan, R. E., & Kelemen, M. H. (1986). Self-efficacy mediates strength gains during circuit weight training in men with coronary artery disease. *Medicine and Science in Sports and Exercise, 18*, 531–540.

Findley, J. C., Kerns, R., Weinberg, L. D., & Rosenberg, R. (1998). Self-efficacy as a psychological moderator of chronic fatigue syndrome. *Journal of Behavioral Medicine, 21*, 351–362.

Flavell, J. H. (1978). Developmental stage: Explanans or explanadum? *The Behavioral and Brain Sciences, 2*, 187–188.

Fries, J. F. (1997). Reducing the need and demand for medical care: Implications for quality management and outcome improvement. *Quality Management in Health Care, 6*, 34–44.

Fries, J. F., Koop, C. E., Beadle, C. E., Cooper, P. P., England, M. J., Greaves, R. F., Sokolov, J. J., Wright, D., & the Health Project Consortium (1993). Reducing health care costs by reducing the need and demand for medical services. *New England Journal of Medicine, 329*, 321–325.

Fuchs, V. (1974). *Who Shall Live? Health Economics and Social Choice*. New York: Basic Books.

Glynn, S. M. & Ruderman, A. J. (1986). The development and validation of an eating self-efficacy scale. *Cognitive Therapy and Research, 10*, 403–420.

Gattuso, S. M., Litt, M. D., & Fitzgerald, T. E. (1992). Coping with gastrointestinal endoscopy: Self-efficacy enhancement and coping style. *Journal of Consulting and Clinical Psychology, 60*, 133–139.

Granfield, R. & Cloud, W. (1996). The elephant that no one sees: Natural recovery among middle-class addicts. *Journal of Drug Issues, 26*, 45–61.

Gillis, A. J. (1993). Determinants of a health-promoting lifestyle: an integrative review. *Journal of Advanced Nursing, 18*, 345–353.

Grossman, H. Y., Brink, S., & Hauser, S. T. (1987). Self- efficacy in adolescent girls and boys with insulin-dependent diabetes mellitus. *Diabetes Care, 10*, 324–329.

Gruber, B., Hall, N. R., Hersh, S. P., & Dubois, P. (1988). Immune system and psychologic changes in metastatic cancer patients using relaxation and guided imagery: A pilot study. *Scandinavian Journal of Behaviour Therapy, 17*, 25–46.

Hancock, T. & Garrett, M. (1995). Beyond medicine: Health challenges and strategies in the 21st century. *Futures, 27*, 935–951.

Haskell, W. L., Alderman, E. L., Fair, J. M., Maron, D. J., Mackey, S. F., Superko, H. R., Williams, P. T., Johnstone, I. M., Champagne, M. A., Krauss, R. M., & Farquhar, J. W. (1994). Effects of intensive multiple risk factor reduction on coronary atherosclerosis and clinical cardiac events in men and women with coronary artery disease. *Circulation, 89*, 975–990.

Herbert, T. B. & Cohen, S. (1993a). Depression and immunity: A meta-analytic review. *Psychological Bulletin, 113*, 472–486.

Herbert, T. B. & Cohen, S. (1993b). Stress and immunity in humans: A meta-analytic review. *Psychosomatic Medicine, 55*, 364–379.

Holahan, C. K. & Holahan, C. J. (1987a). Self-efficacy, social support, and depression in aging: A longitudinal analysis. *Journal of Gerontology, 42*, 65–68.

Holahan, C. K. & Holahan, C. J. (1987b). Life stress, hassles, and self-efficacy in aging: A replication and extension. *Journal of Applied Social Psychology, 17*, 574–592.

Holden, G. (1991). The relationship of self-efficacy appraisals to subsequent health related outcomes: A meta-analysis. *Social Work in Health Care, 16*, 53–93.

Holden, G., Moncher, M. S., Schinke, S. P., & Barker, K. M. (1990). Self-efficacy of children and adolescents: A meta-analysis. *Psychological Reports, 66*, 1044–1046.

Holman, H. & Lorig, K. (1992). Perceived self-efficacy in self-management of chronic disease. In R. Schwarzer (ed.), *Self-Efficacy: Thought Control of Action* (pp. 305–323). Washington, D.C.: Hemisphere.

Holroyd, K. A. & Creer, T. L. (eds.). (1986). *Self-Management of Chronic Disease: Handbook of Clinical Interventions and Research.* New York: Academic Press.

Holroyd, K. A., Penzien, D. B., Hursey, K. G., Tobin, D. L., Rogers, L., Holm, J. E., Marcille, P. J., Hall, J. R., & Chila, A. G. (1984). Change mechanisms in EMG biofeedback training: Cognitive changes underlying improvements in tension headache. *Journal of Consulting and Clinical Psychology, 52*, 1039–1053.

Haran, M. L., Kim, K. K., Gendler, P., Froman, R. D., & Patel, M. D. (1998). Development and evaluation of the osteoporosis self-efficacy scale. *Research in Nursing & Health, 21*, 395–403.

Hunt, G. M. & Azrin, N. H. (1973). A community-reinforcement approach to alcoholism. *Behaviour Research and Therapy, 11*, 91–104.

Hurley, C. C. & Shea, C. A. (1992). Self-efficacy: Strategy for enhancing diabetes self-care. *The Diabetes Educator, 18*, 146–150.

Jensen, K., Banwart, L., Venhaus, R., Popkess-Vawter, S., & Perkins, S. B. (1993). Advanced rehabilitation nursing care of coronary angioplasty patients using self-efficacy theory. *Journal of Advanced Nursing, 18*, 926–931.

Kaivanto, K. K., Estlander, A-M., Moneta, G. B., & Vanharanta, H. (1995). Isokinetic performance in low back pain patients: The predictive power of the self-efficacy scale. *Journal of Occupational Rehabilitation, 5*:87–99.

Kanfer, R. & Zeiss, A. M. (1983). Depression, interpersonal standard-setting, and judgments of self-efficacy. *Journal of Abnormal Psychology, 92*, 319–329.

Kaplan, R. M., Atkins, C. J., & Reinsch, S. (1984). Specific efficacy expectations mediate exercise compliance in patients with COPD. *Health Psychology, 3*, 223–242.

Kiecolt-Glaser, J. K., Glaser, R., Strain, E. C., Stout, J. C., Tarr, K. L., Holliday, J. E., & Speicher, C. E. (1986). Modulation of cellular immunity in medical students. *Journal of Behavioral Medicine, 9*, 5–21.

Kok, G., deVries, H., Mudde, A. N., & Strecher, V. J. (1991). Planned health education and the role of self-efficacy: Dutch research. *Health Education Research, 6*, 231–238.

Lechner, L. & De Vries, H. (1995). Starting participation in an employee fitness program: Attitudes, social influence, and self-efficacy. *Preventive Medicine, 24*, 627–633.

Lindsay, C. M. (ed.). (1980). *New directions in public health care* (3rd ed.). San Francisco: Institute for Contemporary Studies.

Litt, M. D., Nye, C., & Shafer, D. (1995). Preparation for oral surgery: Evaluating elements of coping. *Journal of Behavioral Medicine, 18*, 435–459.

Lorig, K. (1990, April). *Self-efficacy: Its contributions to the four year beneficial outcome of the arthritis self-management course.* Paper presented at the meeting of the Society for Behavioral Medicine, Chicago, IL.

Lorig, K., Chastain, R. L., Ung, E., Shoor, S., & Holman, H. (1989). Development and evaluation of a scale to measure perceived self-efficacy in people with arthritis. *Arthritis And Rheumatism, 32*, 37–44.

Lorig, K., Seleznick, M., Lubeck, D., Ung, E., Chastain, R. L., & Holman, H. R. (1989). The beneficial outcomes of the arthritis self-management course are not adequately explained by behavior change. *Arthritis and Rheumatism, 32*, 91–95.

Lorig, K., Sobel, D. S., Stewart, A. L., Brown, B. W., Bandura, A., Ritter, P., Gonzalez, V. M., Laurent, D. D., & Holman, H. R. (2000). Evidence suggesting that a chronic disease self-management program can improve health status while reducing hospitalization: A randomized trial. Manuscript, Stanford University.

Love, S. Q., Ollendick, T. H., Johnson, C., & Schlezinger, S. E. (1985). A preliminary report of the prediction of bulimic behavior: A social learning analysis. *Bulletin of the Society of Psychologists in Addictive Behavior, 4*, 93–101.

Lynch, B. S. & Bonnie, R. J. (eds.)(1994). *Growing Up Tobacco Free: Preventing Nicotine Addiction in Children and Youths*. Washington, DC: National Academy Press.

Mahler, H. I. M. & Kulik, J. A. (1998). Effects of preparatory videotapes on self-efficacy beliefs and recovery from coronary bypass surgery. *Annals of Behavioral Medicine, 20*, 39–46.

Major, B., Mueller, P. & Hildebrandt, K. (1985). Attributions, expectations, and coping with abortion. *Journal of Personality and Social Psychology, 48*, 585–599.

Manning, M. M. & Wright, T. L. (1983). Self-efficacy expectancies, outcome expectancies, and the persistence of pain control in childbirth. *Journal of Personality and Social Psychology, 45*, 421–431.

Marlatt, G. A., Baer, J. S. & Quigley, L. A. (1995). Self-efficacy and addictive behavior. In A. Bandura (ed.), *Self-Efficacy in Changing Societies* (pp. 289–315). New York: Cambridge University Press.

Martin, N. J., Holroyd, K. A. & Rokicki, L. A. (1993). The headache self-efficacy scale: Adaptation to recurrent headaches. *Headache Journal, 33*, 244–248.

McAlister, A. L., Puska, P., Orlandi, M., Bye, L. L., & Zbylot, P. (1991). Behaviour modification: Principles and illustrations. In W. W. Holland, R. Detels, & E. G. Knox (eds.), *Oxford Textbook of Public Health: 2nd ed., Vol. 3. Applications in Public Health* (pp. 3–16). Oxford: Oxford University Press.

McAuley, E. (1992). Understanding exercise behavior: A self-efficacy perspective. In G. C. Roberts (ed.), *Motivation in Sport and Exercise.* (pp. 107–127). Champaign, IL: Human Kinetics

McCann, B. S., Bovbjerg, V. E., Brief, D. J., Turner, C., Follette, W. C., Fitzpatrick, V., Dowdy, A., Retzlaff, B., Walden, C. E., & Knopp, R. H. (1995). Relationship of self-efficacy to cholesterol lowering and dietary change in hyperlipidemia. *Annals of Behavioral Medicine, 17*, 221–226.

McGinnis, J. M. & Foege, W. H. (1993). Actual causes of death in the United States. *Journal of the American Medical Association, 270*, 2207–2212.

McKusick, L., Coates, T. J., & Morin, S. F. (1989). Longitudinal predictors of reductions in high risk sexual behaviors among gay men in San Francisco: The AIDS behavioral research project. *American Journal of Public Health, 80*, 978–983

McKusick, L., Coates, T. J., Morin, S. F., Pollack, L., & Hoff, C. (1990). Longitudinal predictors of reductions in unprotected anal intercourse among gay men in San Francisco: The AIDS behavioral research project. *American Public Health, 80*, 978–983.

Meier, B. (1998, January 8). U.S. brings its first charges in the tobacco investigation. *New York Times,* p. A17.

Meier, B. (1998, January 15). Files of R. J. Reynolds tobacco show effort on youths. *New York Times,* p. A10.

Meier, B. (1998, February 23). Cigarette maker manipulated nicotine, its records suggest. *New York Times,* p. 1, A16.

Merluzzi, T. V. & Martinez-Sanchez, M. A. (1997). Assessment of self-efficacy and coping with cancer: Development and validation of the cancer behavior inventory. *Health Psychology, 16*, 163–170.

Murray, D. M., Pirie, P., Luepker, R. V., & Pallonen, U. (1989). Five- and six-year follow-up results from four seventh- grade smoking prevention strategies. *Journal of Behavioral Medicine, 12*, 207–218.

Oka, R. K., Gortner, S. R., Stotts, N. A., & Haskell, W. L. (1996). Predictors of physical activity in patients with chronic heart failure secondary to either ischemic or idiopathic dilated cardiomyopathy. *American Journal of Cardiology, 77*, 159–163).

O'Leary, A. & Brown, S. (1995). Self-efficacy and the physiological stress response. In J. E. Maddux (ed.), *Self-Efficacy, Adaptation, and Adjustment.* (pp. 227–248). New York: Plenum Press.

O'Leary, A., Shoor, S., Lorig, K., & Holman, H. R. (1988). A cognitive-behavioral treatment for rheumatoid arthritis. *Health Psychology, 7*, 527–544.

O'Leary, K. D. & Wilson, G. T. (1987). *Behavior Therapy: Application and Outcome* (2nd ed.). Englewood Cliffs, NJ: Prentice-Hall.

Perlez, J. (1997, June, 24). Fenced in at home, Marlboro man looks abroad. *New York Times*, pp. A-1, A-9.

Perry, C. L., Kelder, S. H., Murray, D. M., & Klepp, K. (1992). Communitywide smoking prevention: Long-term outcomes of the Minnesota heart health program and the class of 1989 study. *American Journal of Public Health, 82*, 1210–1216.

Pierce, J., Fiore, M., Novotny, T., Hatziandreu, E., and Davis, R. (1989). Trends in cigarette smoking in the United States. *Journal of the American Medical Association, 261*, 56–61.

Prochaska, J. O. & DiClemente, C. C. (1992). Stages of change in the modification of problem behaviors. In M. Hersen, R. M. Eisler, & P. M. Miller (eds.), *Progress in behavior modification* (Vol. 28, pp. 184-218). Terre Haute, IN: Sycamore.

Reid, C. M., Murphy, B., Murphy, M., Maher, T., Ruth, D., & Jennings, G. (1994). Prescribing medication versus promoting behavioural change: A trial of the use of lifestyle management to replace drug treatment of hypertension in general practice. *Behaviour Change, 11*, 77–185.

Rogers, R. W. (1983). Cognitive and physiological processes in fear appeals and attitude change: A revised theory of protection motivation. In J. T. Cacioppo & R. E. Petty (eds.), *Social Psychophysiology* (pp. 153–176). New York: Guilford Press.

Rogers, E. J., Vaughan, P. W., Swalehe, R. M. A., Rao, N., & Sood, S. (1996). *Effects of an entertainment-education radio soap opera on family planning and HIV/AIDS prevention behavior in Tanzania*. Unpublished manuscript, Department of Communication and Journalism, University of New Mexico, Albuquerque.

Rosenstock, I. M. (1974). The health belief model and preventive health behavior. *Health Education Monographs, 2*, 354–386.

Rudd, P. J. (1997). Compliance with antihypertensive therapy: Raising the bar of expectations. *American Journal of Managed Care, 4*, 957–966.

Sabido, M. (1981). *Towards the Social Use of Soap Operas.* Mexico City, Mexico: Institute for Communication Research.

Sallis, J. F., Haskell, W. L., Fortmann, S. P., Vranizan, M. S., Taylor, C. B., & Solomon, D. S. (1986). Predictors of adoption and maintenance of physical activity in a community sample. *Preventive Medicine, 15*, 331–341.

Schiaffino, K. M., Revenson, T. A., & Gibofsky, A. (1991). Assessing the impact of self-efficacy beliefs on adaptation to rheumatoid arthritis. *Arthritis Care and Research, 4*, 150–157.

Schneider, J. A., O'Leary, A., & Agras, W. S. (1987). The role of perceived self-efficacy in recovery from bulimia: A preliminary examination. *Behaviour Research and Therapy, 25*, 429–432.

Schröder, K. E. E., Schwarzer, R., & Endler, N. S. (1997). Predicting cardiac patients' quality of life from the characteristics of their spouses. *Journal of Health Psychology, 2*, 231–244.

Schwarzer, R. (1992). Self-efficacy in the adoption and maintenance of health behaviors: Theoretical approaches and a new model. In R. Schwarzer (ed.), *Self-Efficacy: Thought Control of Action* (pp. 217–243). Washington, D.C.: Hemisphere.

Silbert, M. H. (1984). Delancy Street Foundation–Process of mutual restitution. In F. Riessman (ed.), *Community Psychology Series* (Vol. 10, pp. 41–52). New York: Human Sciences Press.

Singhal, A. & Rogers, E. M. (1989). Pro-social television for development in India. In R. E. Rice & C. K. Atkin (eds.), *Public Communication Campaigns* (2nd ed., pp. 331–350). Newbury Park, CA: Sage.

Stajkovic, A. D. & Luthans, F. (1998). Self-efficacy and work-related performance: A meta-analysis. *Psychological Bulletin, 124*, 240–261.

Stephens, R. S., Wertz, J. S., & Roffman, R. A. (1995. Self-efficacy and marijuana cessation: A construct validity analysis. *Journal of Consulting and Clinical Psychology, 63*, 1022–1031.

Strecher, V. J., Kreuter, M., Den Boer, Dirk-Jen, Kobrin, S., Hospers, H. J., & Skinner, C. S. (1994). The effects of computer-tailored smoking cessation messages in family practice settings. *The Journal of Family Practice, 39*, 262–268.

Sullivan, M. D., LaCroix, A. Z., Russo, J., & Katon. W. J. (1998). Self-efficacy and self-reported functional status in coronary heart disease: A six-month prospective study. *Psychosomatic Medicine, 60*, 473–478.

Sutton, S. (1996). Can "stages of change" provide guidance in the treatment of addictions?: A critical examination of Prochaska and DiClemente's model. In G. Edwards & C. Dare (eds.), *Psychotherapy, Psychological Treatments and the addictions* (pp. 189–205). Cambridge: Cambridge University Press.

Taylor, C. B., Bandura, A., Ewart, C. K., Miller, N. H., & DeBusk, R. F. (1985). Exercise testing to enhance wives' confidence in their husbands' cardiac capabilities soon after clinically uncomplicated acute myocardial infarction. *American Journal of Cardiology, 55*, 635–638.

Van Ryn, M., Lytle, L. A., & Kirscht, J. P. (1996). A test of the theory of planned behavior for two health-related practices. *Journal of Applied Social Psychology, 26*, 871–883.

Wallack, L., Dorfman, L., Jernigan, D., & Themba, M. (1993). *Media Advocacy and Public Health: Power for Prevention.* Newbury Park, CA: Sage.

Walsh, J. F. & Foshee, V. (1998). Self-efficacy, self-determination and victim blaming as predictors of adolescent sexual victimization. *Health Education Research, 13*, 139–144.

West, J. A., Bandura, A., Clark, E., Miller, N. H., Ahn, D., Greenwald, G., & DeBusk, R. F. (1999). *Self-efficacy predicts adherence to dietary sodium limitation in patients with heart failure.* Manuscript, Stanford University.

Westoff, C. F. & Rodriguez, G. (1995). The mass media and family planning in Kenya. *International Family Planning Perspectives, 21*, 26–31,36.

Whelton, P. K., Appel, L. J., Espeland, M. A., Applegate, W. B., Ettinger, W. H., Kostis, J. B., Kumanyika, S., Lacy, C. R., Johnson K. C., Folmar S., & Cutler, J. A. (1998). Sodium reduction and weight loss in the treatment of hypertension in older persons. *Journal of American Medical Association, 279*, 839–846.

Wiedenfeld, S. A., O'Leary, A., Bandura, A., Brown, S., Levine, S., & Raska, K. (1990). Impact of perceived self-efficacy in coping with stressors on components of the immune system. *Journal of Personality and Social Psychology, 59*, 1082–1094.

Witte, K. (1992). The role of threat and efficacy in AIDS prevention. *International Quarterly of Community Health Education, 12*, 225–249.

Section 6 –
Conclusions and Future Directions

CHAPTER FOURTEEN

Towards a Psychology of Health-Related Behaviour Change

Charles ABRAHAM, Paul NORMAN and Mark CONNER

In the introduction to this volume Abraham and Sheeran reviewed evidence showing that self-report cognition measures specified by motivational models such as the theory of planned behaviour (TPB, Ajzen, 1991) and social cognitive theory (see Bandura, Chapter 13; 1997) are useful predictors of health-related behaviour (e.g., Godin & Kok, 1996). Abraham and Sheeran also discuss extensions of these models which (i) specify postdecisional or volitional cognitive processes which distinguish between those who are more or less prepared to enact their intentions (see e.g., Gollwitzer & Oettingen, Chapter 11) and (ii) goal prioritisation processes which determine which goal will be pursued when conflicting goals are salient (e.g., Bagozzi & Edwards, Chapter 12).

Theoretical models combined with reliable measures of cognitive preparation for action have allowed researchers to specify cognitive changes that are likely to precede behaviour change. The applied importance of this work was established by early applications of the health belief model (e.g., Haefner & Kirscht, 1970) and continues to be demonstrated in recent interventions. For example, having shown that the TPB predicted cycle helmet use (see chapter 4), Quine, Arnold and Rutter (1999) have developed a TPB-based intervention which has been found to significantly increase helmet use. Moreover, there is evidence, in some behavioural domains, that interventions based on social cognitive models are more successful than other interventions. For example, while very few early HIV-preventive interventions were found to be effective (Fisher & Fisher, 1992; Oakley et al., 1995) interventions based on social cognitive models have been shown to effectively promote safer sexual behaviour (e.g., Bryan, Aiken & West, 1996; Kalichman, Carey & Johnson, 1996).

This success notwithstanding, important theoretical and practical questions arise when these models are applied to the promotion of behaviour change. For example, having identified potentially modifiable cognitions associated with target behaviours, how should these cognitions be changed and should particular persuasive techniques be directed towards particular people? The answer to such questions may, in part, depend upon how we conceptualise cognitive change. For example, does cognitive and behavioural change occur in a linear fashion or in stages with different change processes operating at different times? This latter question is addressed by a number of the chapters in this volume and we review the evidence and its implications for health promotion below.

A different question concerns the relationship between personality, modifiable cognitions and behaviour. For example, in Chapter 6, Trafimow discusses findings implying that the relationship between subjective norms and strength of intention is weak for most people across a range of behaviours but strong for a minority of people, that is 'normatively controlled' people (Trafimow & Finlay, 1996). This moderating effect is based on individual differences that persist across behavioural domains. As such it is suggestive of a personality trait rather than a cognition measure. It would be interesting, therefore, to establish whether being 'normatively controlled' is related to other dispositions such as self-monitoring and extraversion (see John, Cheek & Klohnen, 1996). Findings such as those of Trafimow and Finlay imply that different cognitive change processes may be responsible for behaviour change amongst people with different personality trait scores and suggest that intervention targets could be personality-specific. We explore this idea in more detail below.

Answers to the questions posed above can help target interventions so that people with particular beliefs or dispositions receive appropriate health promotion. However, other practical questions remain. For example, what kind of psychology of cognitive change can health promoters draw upon to effectively change beliefs about the consequences of health-related behaviour and are beliefs the best target for our persuasive efforts? How can we change intentions, implementation intentions or goal priorities? For example, in Chapter 8, Courneya, Nigg and Estabrooks recommend integrating cognition measures specified by the theory of planned behaviour and the 'processes of change' included in the transtheoretical model in order to focus on '*how*', rather than why, people change. In the third, and main, section of this chapter we shall explore the relationships between identification of cognitive antecedents of behaviour and the development of techniques which can successfully change behaviour. Work at this interface is required to develop health promotion practices that change behaviour by employing theoretically based procedures to change theoretically specified cognitive prerequisites of action.

In a concluding section we reflect on the need for experimental work which confirms the mediating effects of interventions on cognitions and consider some measurement problems which may arise in tracking cognitive change. Finally, we note the importance of the wider societal and political context both on the potential effectiveness of health promotion interventions and on the diffusion of effective interventions into routine practice in school and health care settings.

THE UTILITY OF DEFINING COGNITIVE CHANGE STAGES: ARE STAGE-SPECIFIC INTERVENTIONS MORE EFFECTIVE?

There has been some debate about whether cognitive assessment can identify discrete stages of preparedness for action that could be matched to stage-specific interventions across different behaviours. Prochaska and DiClemente's (1983) transtheoretical model (TTM) is the most widely applied stage model (but see also Weinstein, 1988; Weinstein & Sandman, 1992). The most common version of the TTM categorises people as precontemplators (who are not presently thinking about change), contemplators (who are considering action), those preparing for action, those taking action to change and those maintaining a previous change (Prochaska, DiClemente, & Norcross, 1992; Prochaska, DiClemente, Velicer & Rossi, 1993; Harlow et al., 1999). Finally, when relapse ceases to be a risk, people enter a termination phase in which no further change is necessary. The model proposes that particular change processes are involved in moving between stages and that interventions should be tailored to help people move from one stage to the next (Prochaska et al., 1993; Heather, Rollnick, Bell & Richmond, 1996). If people change in stages then those in the same stage will face common barriers to change (Weinstein, Rothman & Sutton, 1998). Therefore, not only will stage-specific interventions be more effective but interventions which are effective for people in one stage could, potentially, be counter productive for those in a different stage (see Sutton, Chapter 10).

As Weinstein (1998) and Sutton (1996; Chapter 10) note, stage models of change are conceptually distinct from social cognition models such as the TPB. The TPB implies that attitude change, for example, should always promote intention formation, which, in turn, should render action more likely. The theory does not state that attitude change will only be effective for those with weak intentions, although, since strength of intention is thought to mediate the effects of attitudes on behaviour, this would not be inconsistent with the theory (e.g., Ajzen, 1991). Nonetheless, in its current form, the TPB does not specify stages of cognitive change implying that different interventions would be suitable for recipients with different cognitions.

Bandura (Chapter 13) and others have argued that there is little evidence to support the TTM stage model and Sutton (1996; Chapter 10), has cast doubt on the validity of TTM stage definitions. For example, Sutton (1996) notes that previous studies (e.g., McConnaughy, DiClemente, Prochaska & Velicer, 1989) found that scores on stage-classifying questionnaires were as highly correlated between stages which did not follow directly from one another (e.g., between precontemplation and maintenance) as between adjacent stages. This suggests that individuals may simultaneously score highly on non-sequential stages, arguing against a series of staged of transitions. Inspecting stage definitions more closely (in Chapter 10) Sutton concludes that the stage distinctions are 'logically flawed and based on arbitrary time periods'. For example, he points out that, by definition, some smokers cannot move directly between sequential stages. Sutton has also noted that Prochaska and DiClemente's own data show that smokers do not typically progress through the TTM stages. For example, Prochaska et al. (1991) report that only 16% of participants progressed from one stage to the next without reversals over a two year period and that 12% moved backwards during this period. Similarly Budd and Rollnick (1996) found that a readiness-to-change questionnaire based on the TTM was only able to categorise 40% of heavy drinkers into a single stage and that factors based on items used to identify TTM stages were highly interdependent and lacking in discriminant validity. Their analysis suggested that one underlying factor provided a better description of the data, indicating that readiness to change amongst heavy drinkers corresponds more closely to a continuum than a series of stages. Collectively, this evidence suggests that TTM stage definitions are, at best, questionable.

More importantly, Sutton (Chapter 10) and Weinstein, Rothman and Sutton (1998) argue that there is little evidence supporting the use of TTM, stage-specific interventions. This is critical because the promise of stage models lies in their capacity to guide intervention design so that individuals receive health promotion corresponding their action-readiness state which has maximum impact on their health-related behaviour. Sutton (Chapter 10) argues that tests of the utility of stage models should compare the effectiveness of stage-specific interventions that are either matched or mismatched to participants' stage of change. He points out that there are few such studies and that available evidence either fails to demonstrate enhanced effectiveness of TTM stage-specific interventions or offers only very weak support. This is disappointing as it suggests that investment in TTM stage-specific interventions is unwarranted.

So how do continuous models of change, like the TPB, relate to stage models of change? In Chapter 8, Courneya, Nigg and Estabrooks demonstrate the utility of the TPB in predicting exercise behaviour over time and report that TPB measures, and especially measures of intention, were better predictors than TTM stage categorisations. De Vries and Mudde (in Chapter 9) used intention measures to define TTM stages. Precontemplators were defined as those who do not intend to stop smoking in the next six months. Contemplators intended to stop in the next six months but not the next month and preparers intended to stop in the next month. De Vries and Mudde found that only greater perceived benefits of quitting predicted whether precontemplators would become contemplators, preparers or actual quitters while only self-efficacy predicted whether those in preparation would quit. Since stage of change was defined by intentions concerning when to quit, these results suggest that attitude measures are useful predictors of the likelihood of developing immediate smoking cessation intentions while measures of perceived behavioural control (or self-efficacy) predict smoking cessation (but not the development of immediate cessation intentions). These findings emphasise the cognitive importance of intention formation and could be construed within an extended TPB model in which perceived control is seen to be especially important in the implementation of short-term intentions to quit (i.e., in the next month).

A number of theorists have distinguished between a motivational stage of action preparation which culminates in intention formation and a postdeci-sional or volitional stage involving cognitive regulation of the enactment of intentions (e.g., Gollwitzer, 1993; Heckhausen, 1991; Schwarzer, 1992). For example, Schwarzer's Health Action Process Approach (HAPA) proposes a motivation phase, leading to intention formation, followed by a volition phase during which the formation of 'action plans' is crucial. The importance of such volitional processes is emphasised by Gollwitzer and Oettingen (Chapter 13) who show that intentions are more likely to be enacted if they are translated into 'implementation intentions' specifying when and where a particular act is to be undertaken.

The utility of regarding motivational and volitional stages as discontinuous has also been supported experimentally. Employing the Precaution Adoption Process framework (Weinstein, 1988), Weinstein, Lyon, Sandman and Cuite (1998) distinguished between those who were 'undecided' and those who had 'decided to act' in relation to purchasing radon testing kits. They found that a video-based intervention emphasising the risk of finding unhealthy levels of radon in one's home had a greater effect on intentions to test amongst the undecided group than the decided group. Moreover, an intervention designed to make it easy to buy a test kit was three times more effective, than the risk-inducing intervention, in prompting purchases amongst those who were decided. This 'easy-to-buy' intervention also prompted three times as many purchases amongst those who had decided than amongst those who were undecided. These results support a two-stage model and suggest that those who have decided (i.e., those in the volitional stage) are likely benefit most from interventions designed to enhance perceived behavioural control (e.g., by reducing barriers to action). Such findings recommend investment in interventions designed to promote theory-derived action readiness, in terms of motivational or volitional stages. However, it should be noted that they do not clarify whether interventions which combine such theory-derived targets, e.g., including motivational and volitional targets, are less effective than those which only target one cognitive stage.

Stage-matched interventions involve stage categorisation of potential audiences in terms of theoretically defined stage transitions (Harlow, et al., 1999). For example, De Vries and Mudde (Chapter 9) operationalised TTM stages in terms of how soon people intended to take action and Weinstein et al. (1998) distinguished between people who were decided and undecided. These are usefully simple categorisations but it is unclear whether they are appropriate indicators of movement between motivational and volitional stages. The TPB suggests that measures of how strongly people intend to take action within a specified time indicate progress through the motivational stage. This approach would avoid defining stages on the basis of arbitrary time horizons but also implies degrees of having 'decided to act'. Similarly, measures of certainty of intention and stability of intentions over time have been shown to moderate the intention-behaviour relationship so that more certain (e.g., Bagozzi & Yi, 1989) and more stable (Conner, Sheeran, Norman & Armitage, in press; Sheeran, Orbell & Trafimow, 1999) intentions predict behaviour more accurately. Thus it is not clear whether 'having decided' means having an intention to act or having a strong intention that is held with certainty and consistently expressed over time. It may be relatively easy to identify prototypical 'motivational' individuals. For example, T. S. Elliot's Prufrock observed that there was 'time .. for a hundred indecisions before the taking of a toast and tea' (Elliot, 1974). However, it may be more difficult to define the cognitive boundaries between putative motivational and volitional stages. Stages may refer to cognitive states of action readiness which can be easily described within a continuous mutlidimensional model of beliefs, attitudes, intentions and plans.

Thus the utility of motivational and volitional stage-specific interventions may depend on pragmatic, rather than theoretical considerations. Investment in stage-specific interventions may be justified in some circumstances but not others. For example, stage-specific interventions may be appropriate when: (i) the identification of stage-defined (e.g., motivational and volitional) audiences is unproblematic and inexpensive; (ii) evidence suggests that administering stage-mismatched interventions is likely to be counter-productive, for example when motivational interventions are seen to weaken the resolve of those with strong intentions; (iii) the expense of administering combination interventions (e.g., those designed to promote greater cognitive preparedness for action amongst people in both motivational and volitional stages) is high. In such circumstances interventions designed specifically to raise awareness of a threat, or to change people's beliefs about the consequences of recommended actions, or alternatively, to reduce barriers to action should be directed towards particular audiences or launched in sequence as audiences move through predictable stages (Weinstein, 1988). However, at present, we conclude that there is little evidence suggesting that investment in stage-specific interventions is likely to be cost effective when compared to combination interventions which are designed to promote a variety of theoretically-specified cognitive changes and do not need to be precisely targeted in terms of audience preparedness for change.

PERSONALITY TRAITS, COGNITIONS AND HEALTH-RELATED BEHAVIOUR

Categorisations based on particular cognitions or groups of cognitions, constituting stages of change, describe transitory states. For example, people formulate intentions and generate specific plans to implement them and, in doing so, move between motivational and volitional stages. However, categorisations in terms of personality traits identify more stable personal characteristics (Costa & McCrae, 1994). Research in this area has focused on the 'big five' personality traits (i.e., openness, conscientiousness, extraversion, agreeableness and neuroticism) (McCrae & Costa, 1987) and an extensive literature links such traits to health outcomes (e.g., Marshall, Wortman, Vickers, Kusulas & Hervig, 1994; Vingerhoets, Croon, Jeninga & Menges, 1990), psychological wellbeing and coping (e.g., O'Brien & Delongis, 1996) and, health-related behaviour (e.g., Booth-Kewley & Vickers, 1994; Furnham & Heaven, 1999). Thus, these traits provide potentially important explanations of individual differences in health-related behaviour.

Personality traits may affect health outcomes through differences in emotional reactivity or because personality differences express underlying constitutional differences (Van Heck, 1997). More interesting in this context, however, is the possibility that personality affects individuals' selection of interpersonal situations and behaviours, through personality-related goal hierarchies, thereby shaping intention formation, intention implementation and health-related behaviour. Such relationships would be relevant to health promotion efforts because they might suggest that interventions would be more effective when matched to personality types or that some people are especially in need of particular types of interventions. In fact, few studies have explored links between personality traits, cognitions and health-related behaviour. There are, however, indications that future research in this area could be informative.

Booth-Kewley and Vickers (1994) suggest that personality traits may affect the extent to which people engage in general clusters of health-related behaviours such as 'wellness behaviours' (e.g., taking exercise), accident prevention/control behaviour (e.g., removing hazards in the home) and substance use risk behaviours (e.g., smoking and drinking alcohol). For example, in relation to substance use, both extraversion and neuroticism have been studied in relation to smoking and smoking initiation. However, the evidence is mixed. Overall, longitudinal studies have found little support for the importance of extraversion to becoming a smoker but do suggest that those with higher neuroticism scores are more likely to take up smoking and maintain the habit (Canals, Bladé & Domènech, 1997; Cherry & Kiernan, 1976; Stein, Newcomb & Bentler, 1996; but see also White, Hill & Hopper, 1996). Studies also suggest that these traits are related to cognition measures associated with health-related behaviours. For example, Tucker (1984) showed that adolescents who did and did not intend to smoke differed on various personality dimensions including neuroticism and Byrne, Byrne and Reinhart (1993) found that neuroticism correlated with smoking intentions in a similar aged sample.

Openness and agreeableness have been less widely studied in relation to health-related behaviour (Marshall et al., 1994; Booth-Kewley & Vickers, 1994) although low agreeableness, in the form of hostility, has been shown to be important in relation to coronary heart disease and type A categorisation (e.g., Matthews, 1988). By contrast, a number of studies have highlighted the importance of conscientiousness to health and health-related behaviour. Friedman, Tucker, Tomlinson-Keasay, Schwartz, Wingard and Criqui (1993) found that childhood conscientiousness predicted longevity and Friedman et al. (1995) showed that this was partly accounted for by its effect on smoking and alcohol usage; that is, conscientious children were less likely to become heavy smokers and drinkers. Booth-Kewley and Vickers (1994) found that conscientiousness was more strongly correlated with clusters of health-related behaviours than the other big five traits and especially with wellness and accident control behaviours. Finally, Mutén (1991) found that patients high in conscientiousness were more likely to show enhanced adherence following interventions directed towards learning self-regulation skills.

These findings can be readily understood because those who score highly on measures of conscientiousness are thought to be more organised, careful, dependable, self-disciplined and achievement-orientated than others (McCrae & Costa, 1987; McCrae & John, 1992). There is also evidence that more conscientious people tend to engage in problem-focused rather than emotion-focused coping, that they are more likely to employ positive reappraisal and support seeking strategies (Watson & Hubbard, 1996) and less likely to use escape-avoidance and self-blame strategies (O'Brien & Delongis, 1996). Thus conscientiousness may lead to the development of enhanced motivational, action control and self-regulation processing which, in turn, translates into more consistent health-related behaviour. There are, however, few direct tests of these relationships. Siegler, Feaganes and Rimer (1995) showed that regular mammography attendance was predicted by conscientiousness and extraversion and that these effects were mediated by reports of friends and relatives having breast cancer and by the perceived costs of seeking mammography. Results of this kind suggest that the relationship between conscientiousness and health-related behaviour may be mediated by traditional health belief measures, such as perceived susceptibility and perceived barriers. However, in a cross sectional study, Conner and Abraham (1999) found that, controlling for cognition measures derived from the health belief model and the TPB, conscientiousness, unlike neuroticism and extraversion, had an unmediated, direct relationship with strength of intention to care for one's health. This finding suggests that conscientiousness may have an effect on intention formation that is not explained by cognitive models of motivation. These relationships warrant further investigation.

One of the few researchers who has attempted to integrate work on cognition, personality, self-regulation and behaviour is Julius Kuhl (e.g., Kuhl, 1992). Kuhl has identified a series of affective and self-representational tendencies which inhibit volitional processes and, therefore, the enactment of intentions. He proposes that some people, 'state-orientated' individuals, have general action control and self-regulation difficulties. Such people tend to focus on their present state or on intended future states without adequately considering possible actions that would enable them to realise intended future states. They are more likely to become preoccupied by uncompleted goals and are less able to distinguish between self-chosen and other-directed goals. By contrast, 'action-orientated' individuals are better able to translate discrepancies between present states and intended future states into action plans and are, therefore, able to act on their intentions without undue hesitation, unwanted cognitive intrusions or rumination over past failures. Kuhl (1985) developed the Action Control Scale to measure dispositional differences in state versus action orientation.

Fuhrmann and Kuhl (1998) have applied these concepts to understanding how people maintain a healthy diet. They found that action-orientated individuals are likely to perform better if eating-related goals are perceived as self-chosen (rather than recommended), especially if they require impulse control, for example, avoiding eating unhealthy food. However, state-orientated individuals did not differ significantly in the performance of self-chosen and recommended goals. This suggests that health promotion interventions should combine recommended actions with encouragement to set positive, individual goals.

Kuhl's work highlights the complexity of integrated models of dispositional tendencies, cognitions and specific health-related behaviours. For example, Fuhrmann and Kuhl found that action-orientated individuals performed better when positive, efficacy-enhancing, success-focused strategies are used to monitor and acknowledge progress (as opposed to self-discipline strategies aimed at avoiding failure). However, state-orientated individuals performed better when encouraged to focus on avoiding failure. This suggests that detailed action control and self-regulation strategies may need to be tailored to dispositional differences if interventions are to be most effective. Fuhrmann and Kuhl also suggest that state-oriented people may benefit from longer-term training designed to develop meta-regulation skills. For example, by acknowledging both the short-term action-control benefits of failure-avoidance motivational strategies and the long-term self-regulation problems they generate, training programmes could seek to sharpen state-orientated individuals' awareness of the relationship between health goals and valued social identities, and encourage them to develop positive success-focused action-control strategies for self-congruent health goals. A number of interesting research questions arise in this context. For example, could such training involve tuition on implementation intention formation or employ positive fantasy versus negative reality contrasts as discussed by Gollwitzer and Oettingen (in Chapter 11). Additionally, how do the big five personality measures relate to Kuhl's dispositional measures? For example, are conscientious individuals more action orientated? Early evidence suggests that there may well be associations between these measures. For example, Beswick and Mann (1994) report that state orientation is associated with high levels of neuroticism.

Relating dispositional features to cognition models (such as the TPB) and behaviour is also likely to require complex models. For example, it follows from Kuhl's theory that 'state oriented' people should be less able to act on their intentions, that is, Action Control Scale scores should moderate intention-behaviour correlations. However, a series of studies have failed to find convincing evidence of this effect using both between-subjects (e.g., Bagozzi, Baumgartner & Yi, 1992; Kendzierski, 1990) and within-subjects (e.g., Norman, Sheeran & Orbell, 1997) analyses. Moreover, Kuhl (1982) found that a number of intention-behaviour correlations were higher among state oriented individuals. These behaviours tended to be more highly routinised and socially determined behaviours such as brushing one's teeth. Kuhl (1982) attempts to explain this finding by suggesting that state oriented individuals may have a greater tendency to engage in externally controlled behaviours to compensate for their low self-regulatory capacities. Norman et al. (1997) explored this possibility by computing within-subjects intention-behaviour correlations for behaviours under attitudinal control (i.e., behaviours predominately predicted by attitudes) and normative control (i.e., behaviours predominately predicted by subjective norms). In line with predictions, state oriented individuals were more likely to act on their intentions for normatively controlled behaviours. Such findings demonstrate that personality and behaviour-specific factors affect cognition-behaviour relationships, implying that integrative models may have behaviour-specific implications for intervention development.

In conclusion, the literatures on personality traits and health-related behaviour, on the one hand, and cognitions and health-related behaviour, on the other, have developed in parallel with little cross-referencing. We would argue that personality and social cognitive influences on behaviour might be usefully integrated into a single account (see Bermudez, 1999; Evans, Dratt, Raines & Rosenberg, 1988, for similar views). In such an account personality dimensions are seen as distal predictors of behaviour, whose impact on behaviour may be mediated through more proximal determinants such as high-level goal specification, action control and self-regulation strategies and behaviour-specific cognition measures. Such integration could clarify the processes by which some widely applied personality measures predict behaviour (Bermudez, 1999) and simultaneously extend current motivational models of behavioural determinants. In addition, intervention designs which take account of dispositional differences could inform discussions concerning stability and change in personality and also clarify the findings of intervention evaluations by identifying groups who do and do not benefit from interventions (Fuhrmann & Kuhl, 1998). Future research could, for example, clarify whether the effects of high conscientiousness on health behaviour can be accounted for by TPB-like models or whether this trait represents a propensity for action which is not captured by cognition measures of motivation, perhaps through its effects on volitional processes. Such research could have important implications for interventions. For example, those low in conscientiousness might be seen as especially in need of motivational and self-regulation interventions.

CHANGING COGNITION TO PROMOTE BEHAVIOUR CHANGE: TOWARDS A PSYCHOLOGY OF INTERVENTION DESIGN

A number of chapters in this volume illustrate that models, such as the TPB, have a high level of 'practicality' (Brawley, 1993), in that they specify relationships between postulated cognitive determinants, provide reliable cognitive assessment tools, have predictive validity and indicate how cognitive change can lead to behavioural change. The range of cognitive models discussed by Abraham and Sheeran (in Chapter 1) can be used to design interventions and can help clarify why interventions are effective by identifying changing cognitions related to behaviour change. There have, however, been fewer interventions based on these models than might be expected. For example, van den Putte (1993) found only five studies employing the Theory of Reasoned Action/TPB as the basis of a behaviour change intervention. This may be due to a lack of clarity about how identified cognitive antecedents can be changed. In this section we highlight behaviour-related cognitions and discuss research findings suggesting how they may be applied to health promotion.

Knowledge. Knowing that particular behaviours promote or jeopardise health is, a priori, prerequisite to health-related behaviour change (Weinstein, 1988). Consequently, many health promotion interventions seek to inform people of the health risks and benefits of their actions. When such information seems relevant people are likely to attend to it. For example, reviewing patients' use of written information, Ley (1988) found that that on average, 72% of patients reported reading available leaflets and booklets. However, as McGuire (1972) pointed out, attention must be followed by comprehension, yielding and retention if it is to contribute to behaviour change. Comprehension is dependent on matching the presentation of information to the information processing skills of the audience. For example, written materials must be easy to read but Ley (1988) found that readability analysis of written materials available to patients in the UK suggested that approximately 70% of English-speaking adults would not be able to understand them. Such findings imply that health educational materials should be piloted to assess audience interest and comprehension.

Increasing 'knowledge' may mean different things in different health promotion contexts, depending on what kind of belief change is targeted. Cognitive models imply that some beliefs are more likely to lead to behaviour change than others and suggest that, for many target populations, it is not ignorance but a lack of motivation, action control resources and goal prioritisation that impede action. For example, a recent meta-analysis of correlates of reported condom use found weighted average correlations of 0.06 for knowledge, 0.32 for attitudes towards condom use, 0.43 for intentions to use condoms and 0.46 for having talked to one's partner about condom use (Sheeran, Abraham & Orbell, 1999). Such results suggest that campaigns which successfully increase knowledge may not promote behaviour change.

Perceived threat. Some interventions are designed to increase perceived threat by targeting beliefs concerning personal susceptibility to, and the severity of, illnesses. This is likely to be useful insofar as believing that one is invulnerable to a threat or that there are few negative consequences of an action maintains risk behaviour. For example, emphasising the threat of unhealthy behaviours has been found to have a significant effect on intentions in relation to alcohol use (Stainback & Rogers, 1983), dental flossing (Beck & Lund, 1981), dietary behaviour (Wurtele, 1988) and breast self-examination (Ripptoe & Rogers, 1987). Nevertheless, mere acknowledgement of threat may not constitute sufficient cognitive preparation for action. For example, Sheeran, Abraham and Orbell (1999) report non-significant average correlations of .06 and .02 between condom use and perceived susceptibility and perceived severity, respectively. Milne and Orbell (Chapter 3) found that perceived severity was significantly correlated with subsequent breast self-examination ($r = -.20$, $p < .05$) but perceived susceptibility was not. Quine, Rutter and Arnold (Chapter 4) found that perceived susceptibility was (just) significantly correlated with subsequent helmet wearing ($r = .17$, $p < .05$) and perceived severity was not. However, both Milne and Orbell and Quine et al. report that neither perceived susceptibility or severity were significant predictors of future behaviour in multivariate models. Thus, in populations where perceived susceptibility or severity is misleadingly low, interventions targeting these beliefs may be useful. However, behaviour change is only likely to follow when these interventions are supplemented with others targeting beliefs more closely associated with intention formation and action preparedness.

Fear. The findings reported above also have implications for interventions based on fear arousal. Presenting a health threat in a frightening manner may well make the threat more salient. However, since threat perception is not closely associated with action, this may only have minimal effects on behaviour change. For example, Sheeran, Abraham and Orbell (1999) report a non-significant correlation of .09 between reported worry or concern about HIV infection and condom use while Milne and Orbell found a non-significant correlation of .06 between reported fear and subsequent breast self examination. Unsurprisingly then, Rigby, Brown, Anagnostou, Ross and Rosser (1989) found no evidence that the Australian 'Grim Reaper' HIV/AIDS campaign, which depicted people as skittles in a bowling alley populated by giant grim reapers, had any impact on sexual behaviour. This does not mean that fear arousal has no persuasive effect. Leventhal (1970) and Sutton (1982) both concluded that the greater the fear aroused by communications the greater their impact on intention formation and behaviour. However, fear arousal is likely to have an impact on behaviour when it is included in interventions which have other cognitive effects, particularly those which prompt intention formation and action planning by clarifying the effectiveness of preventive action and explaining how to take such action (Leventhal, 1970). Thus it is difficult to separate the effects of fearful emotional responses to health promotion materials from their cognitive effects, that is, increasing perceptions of susceptibility, severity, response efficacy and self-efficacy as well as intention, and implementation intention, formation (through the provision of instructions). Further work is required to clarify what effects fear arousal may have when such effects are controlled (see Eagly & Chaiken, 1993 for a useful review).

Attitudes and normative beliefs. Models such as the TPB suggest that changing attitudes and norms in relation health-related actions is likely to be more effective in promoting behaviour change than increasing threat perception. According to the Fishbein and Ajzen model, attitudes are based on a variety of beliefs concerning the likely consequences of an action and evaluations of those consequences (Fishbein & Ajzen, 1975). Thus the first step towards applying the model is to establish which beliefs are relevant to the intention to undertake the recommended health behaviour (see Agnew, Chapter 5; Quine, Rutter & Arnold, Chapter 4). For example, if intenders, believe that a particular medication is very effective but non-intenders hold significantly weaker beliefs concerning effectiveness, then a campaign promoting medication effectiveness would be recommended. In this way a series of key beliefs underpinning intentions can be identified as intervention targets. Presenting a series of statements about a proposed health-related action which focuses on such key beliefs has the potential to change people's perception of the consequences of preventive action and, therefore, their attitudes and normative beliefs. For example, Parker, Stradling and Manstead (1996) found that a video showing how a young male driver might feel bad about himself as a result of being inconsiderate or dangerous as a result of speeding, resulted in more negative attitudes towards speeding. Similarly, they found that a video showing the driver's friends and partner disapproving of his speeding resulted in lower perceived social approval for speeding (compared to those who had not seen the video).

A series of other factors may affect the persuasiveness of such statements. The elaboration likelihood model (ELM) of persuasion (Petty & Cacioppo, 1986) proposes that the extent to which a message induces message-relevant thought will affect persuasion. When the arguments presented are strong such thought, or cognitive elaboration, will enhance persuasiveness but when weak arguments are presented then greater message-relevant thought may decrease persuasiveness. This 'central processing' of potentially persuasive messages involves assimilation and evaluation of presented arguments in relation to our established views and knowledge. This is most likely to occur when the message content is judged to be personally relevant and when there are few barriers to in-depth processing, for example, when the message is easy to understand and there is time to consider it, without distraction. When a message is not especially relevant to us or when it is difficult to process we may evaluate it in terms of more superficial features such as the attractiveness or expertise of the source or the number of arguments presented. Such 'peripheral processing' may also lead to persuasion in the sense that recipients are 'prepared to take the source's word for it' but such persuasion is less likely to be long term or to withstand future contradiction and so is less likely to affect subsequent behaviour. It is worth noting in this context, that Eagly and Chaiken (1993) suggest that fear arousal could discourage systematic processing and perhaps sensitise recipients to heuristic cues (such as the expertise of the message source). This could make poor arguments more persuasive but it could reduce the effectiveness of campaigns using strong arguments.

Thus health promotion should seek to present logical statements emphasising the positive outcomes of health-related behaviours in a manner which focuses on goals which are important to the intended audience. This may require clarification of the goal priorities served by health-related actions. For example, young people's alcohol consumption may be critically dependent on their perceptions of the importance of socialising (Oostveen, Knibbe & De Vries, 1996), rather than alcohol consumption per se. Messages need to attract attention and be easily understood and remembered. For example, Ley (1988) notes that simplification, categorisation of message components (e.g., 'this is what to do'), stressing important components, repetition and use of specific illustrations can enhance comprehension and retention of messages. Stressing positive outcomes relevant to the identity or self-concept of audience members is also likely to enhance persuasiveness. Messages from others with whom audience members identify, that is those categorised as belonging to the same group, may be more likely to prompt central processing so that strong messages from 'in-group' members may be most persuasive (Van Knippenberg, 1999).

Messages concerning the likelihood of positive or negative consequences of acting or not acting may be more or less effective if they are presented in terms of losses or gains. Prospect theory (Kahneman & Tversky, 1979) suggests that when people focus on gains they tend to avoid risks but when they focus on losses they tend to favour risk taking. Thus when a health preventive behaviour is regarded as risky it may be promoted most successfully by focusing on the potential losses of not acting than the potential gains of acting. However, if an action is not thought of as risky then it should be more successfully promoted by focusing attention on the gains of taking action. Thus preventive behaviours such as sunscreen use should be best promoted by emphasising the gains of action (Rothman, Salovey, Autone, Keough & Martin, 1993) because they are not thought to be risky in themselves. However, 'detection behaviours' (Banks et al., 1995) such as breast self-examination which involve the risk of worrying discoveries may best promoted by focusing on the potential losses on inaction (Meyerowitz & Chaiken, 1987). For example, Banks et al. (1995) found that messages focusing on loss appeared to promote mammography utilisation more effectively than messages focusing on gain. Loss focused messages included; 'failing to detect breast cancer early can cost you your life' and 'when you avoid getting a mammogram you are failing to take advantage of the best method for detecting breast cancer early'. Gain focused messages included;

'detecting breast cancer early can save your life', 'when you get a mammogram you are taking advantage of the best method for detecting breast cancer early'.

Inducing cognitive contradictions in recipients may also enhance persuasiveness. There is an extensive literature on the way in which perceived contradictions between our values or espoused beliefs and our behaviour can lead to attitude change. Such contradictions are thought to result in an unpleasant state that motivates attitude change (see e.g., Festinger, 1957; Greenwald & Ronis, 1978; Harmon-Jones, Brehm, Greenberg, Simon & Nelson, 1996). Thus persuading people to construct their own health protective messages and contrasting these with their own actions may be useful technique. For example, Stone, Aronson, Crain, Winslow and Fried (1994) found that when people who had been asked to construct persuasive safer sex messages were reminded of the circumstances in which they had failed to use condoms, they were more likely to buy condoms and to buy more condoms than those who had not been reminded of their own failures. This contrast is similar to the positive fantasy versus negative reality contrasts discussed by Gollwitzer and Oettingen (in Chapter 11) and both may work by arousing dissonance.

Perceived control. The constructs of perceived behavioural control and self-efficacy are closely related (Ajzen, 1998; Bandura, Chapter 13) and considerable effort has been devoted to designing interventions capable of increasing self-efficacy (see Bandura, 1997). As Bandura (1997) explains, there are four main sources of self-efficacy, each of which could be addressed in interventions. First, people can develop feelings of self-efficacy from personal mastery experience. For example, these could be generated by dividing a sequence of actions into sub-goals, so that the easiest are achieved before more difficult elements are attempted. Stock and Cervone (1990) report that sub-dividing a complex task into a series of sub-goals resulted in higher self-efficacy at task outset, heightened self-efficacy and satisfaction at the point of sub-task completion and greater overall goal persistence. Second, people may develop feelings of self-efficacy through observing other people succeed on a task (i.e. vicarious experience). This may be especially powerful if they perceive the model to be similar to themselves, in ability, attitudes or group membership. Note too that this means that observing failure amongst those perceived to have similar abilities can have adverse affects on self-efficacy and performance (e.g., Brown & Inouye, 1978). Third, people may gain in self-efficacy by being persuaded of their abilities. For example, Fisher and Johnston (1996) manipulated self-efficacy by inviting chronic pain patients to reflect on past experiences of high or low control and found that the manipulation altered levels of self-efficacy which, in turn, accounted for differential performance on a lifting task. Finally, one's own physiological and affective states may be used as a source of information, such that high levels of arousal or anxiety may indicate to the individual that he or she is not capable of performing a given action. As a result, relaxation techniques, reduced somatic monitoring and mood enhancing interventions may be employed to enhance feelings of self-efficacy (Bandura, 1997).

Each of these techniques have been used in intervention studies to enhance feelings of self-efficacy. For example, Maibach, Flora and Nass (1991) report the results of a year-long community health campaign to encourage the adoption of health behaviours. The campaign materials were all designed to reflect the main principles of Bandura's (1986) Social Cognitive Theory and used a variety of strategies including encouraging participants to set behaviour change goals, using community members who had successfully changed their behaviour as role models, using health experts to give advice about behaviour change and focusing on the skills needed to support behaviour change. The campaign was found to successfully increase feelings of self-efficacy which, in turn, were related to the adoption of new health behaviours. Interventions have also focused on more situation-specific feelings of self-efficacy. For example, Stevens and Hollis (1989) designed a smoking cessation programme based on research showing that situation-specific ratings of self-efficacy were predictive of the circumstances in which relapses occurred (Condiotte & Lichtenstein, 1981). In this study recently abstinent smokers identified potential relapse situations in which they perceived low levels of self-efficacy and then developed and rehearsed appropriate coping strategies over three weekly meetings. The intervention led to a greater abstinence rate at one year than both a discussion-only intervention and a no treatment control. Other studies which have attempted to improve behavioural skills to enhance feelings of self-efficacy have produced positive results in relation to alcohol use (Baer, Marlatt, Kivlahan, Fromme, Larimer & Williams, 1992) and dental hygiene (McCaul, Glasgow & O'Neil, 1992).

There is also some evidence that tailoring interventions to match fit people's existing control beliefs may lead to more effective interventions. Chambliss and Murray (1979a) devised a weight control programme in which participants were given placebo medication to help control their metabolism. After two weeks participants in one group were debriefed about the placebo medication and encouraged to attribute any weight loss to their own efforts over the previous two weeks. Participants in a second group were given further information about the efficacy of the medication and encouraged to attribute any weight loss to the medication. At two-week follow-up a significant interaction was found between the giving of information and participants' pre-program locus of control orientation, such that 'internals' lost more weight than 'externals' in the self-efficacy information group, while the opposite pattern of results was found for the drug information group. Similar results have been reported by Chambliss and Murray (1979b) in relation to smoking cessation and Quadrel and Lau (1989) found an interaction between health locus of control beliefs and the control orientation of a message to encourage breast self-examination. Women with strong internal health locus of control beliefs who received a message in a 'control' frame were more likely to perform breast self-examination at follow up but this effect was reversed if a neutral reminder was sent. Further evidence for a 'matching hypothesis' has been provided in relation to weight reduction (Wallston, Wallston, Kaplan & Maides, 1976) and smoking cessation (Best, 1975). Since locus of control is regarded as a relatively stable and global cognitive measure these findings further underline potential links between personality differences (e.g., action versus state orientation and conscientiousness and the cognitive control of action, see above).

Action control processes: intention formation and planning. Gollwitzer and Oettingen (Chapter 13) discuss how the formation of implementation intentions can make it more likely that intenders will act on their intentions. In this case simple rehearsal of when and where an intention will be enacted is enough to initiate action control processes that have a measurable impact on behaviour (see Gollwitzer, 1993; Orbell, Hodgkins & Sheeran, 1997). The effectiveness of these simple techniques to promote action planning raises questions about intention rehearsal. Is it possible, for example, to engender, or strengthen, intention formation by direct self-instruction? Does rehearsal of intentions such as, 'I intend to avoid eating biscuits and cake' result in their assimilation into current goal hierarchies? Such rehearsal could follow from focusing on discrepancies between positive fantasies relevant to health and negative reality. For example, as Gollwitzer and Oettingen note, an overweight person who considers her slim image of an ideal self and the difficulties of attaining this because of her current behaviour (e.g., impulse eating and a taste for high calorie foods) may formulate behaviour change goals. Do intentions based on an awareness of such discrepancies have different relations to attitudes and behaviour than intentions prompted by changes in outcome expectancies? It would be interesting to compare interventions using such rehearsal techniques with those targeting attitudinal change through persuasive communication (see above).

Self-regulation and behaviour change. Self-regulation processes refer to people's involvement in the management of their own cognitive change and behavioural regulation. For example, conscious consideration of the relative importance of potentially competing goals may lead to the reorganisation of goal hierarchies that may facilitate behaviour change. We have noted, for example, that young people's alcohol consumption may be regulated by the perceived importance of socialising (Oostveen et al., 1996) and Abraham, Sheeran, Norman, Conner, de Vries and Otten (1999) found that condom use was associated with the relative importance of protected intercourse versus having intercourse. Gollwitzer and Oettingen (Chapter 11) and Bagozzi and Edwards (Chapter 12) highlight the importance of goal hierarchies to health-related behaviour. Bagozzi and Edwards argue that, the regulation of body weight may be underpinned by linkages between this goal and personal reactions such as feeling happy because of social acceptance, feeling good because of looking good and elevated self-esteem, and enjoying life because one is feeling good. This may mean that linking health-related goals to widely-shared social values can promote goal hierarchy reorganisation that supports behaviour change. It would be interesting to explore whether changes of this kind underpin behaviour change prompted by advertising and health promotion campaigns.

In this context, it is interesting to return to Courneya et al.'s suggestion (in Chapter 8) that the 'processes of change' specified by the TTM may help us understand 'how' people change their behaviour. Prochaska and colleagues (Prochaska & DiClemente, 1986; Prochaska, Velicer, DiClemente & Fava, 1988) have identified ten change processes which, they argue, can partially explain progression from one TTM stage of change to another. These include; 'consciousness raising', i.e., increasing knowledge (e.g., 'I recall articles dealing with the problem of quitting smoking'), 'self liberation', i.e., commitment to act, or belief in the ability to act (e.g., 'I tell myself I can choose to smoke or not'), 'helping relationships', i.e., being trusting about problems with someone else (e.g., 'Special people in my life accept me the same whether I smoke or not'), 'stimulus control', i.e., avoiding stimuli which elicit problem behaviours (e.g., 'I remove things from my home which remind me of smoking'), 'counter-conditioning', i.e., substituting alternatives for problem behaviours (e.g., 'Instead of smoking I engage in some physical activity') and 'reinforcement management', i.e., being rewarded for making changes ('I can expect to be rewarded by others if I don't smoke').

Information seeking, for example, may be prerequisite to many of the cognitive changes discussed above. Becoming receptive to arguments that are inconsistent with one's current views and behaviours may be foundational to motivational change, including attitudinal change. Self-liberation appears to involve rehearsal of intentions and self-efficacy beliefs. This form of self-instruction is used in cognitive-behaviour therapy (e.g., Meichenbaum, 1977) and corresponds to techniques used to enhance self-efficacy (see above). Thus these particular 'change processes' refer to self-awareness of motivational changes. They are self-regulatory in the sense that they express a person's representation of internal motivational change. However, the changes they refer to correspond to change processes implied by decision-making models such as the TPB.

Seeking social support for behavioural change is likely to influence normative beliefs and could also affect self-efficacy, planning and the setting of goal priorities. Schwarzer (1992), for example, includes social support in his Health Action Process Approach as a situational factor that interacts with volitional processes such as action planning. Thus support seeking is a self-regulatory practice which has the potential to maintain and accelerate the individual cognitive changes involved in behavioural change. However, social support need not necessarily promote cognitive and behavioural change and only particular kinds of social support may do so. For example, Peirce, Frone, Russell and Cooper (1996) observed a buffering effect of tangible support (i.e., financial and resource support) on the relationship between financial stress and drinking alcohol to cope but no buffering effect for having a trusted advisor or someone to socialise with. Indeed it seems likely that being accepted or approved of (without change) could diminish motivation to change. Consequently, encouraging people to organise problem-specific social support may well enhance intervention effectiveness but this is likely to depend upon the supporter being motivated to bring about change in the supported person.

Stimulus control, counter-conditioning and reinforcement management are derived from an operant conditioning view of behaviour change and, as such, they pose an interesting challenge to cognitive models of motivation, action control and self-regulation. Stimulus control is a self-regulatory strategy involving acknowledgement of low situation-specific self-efficacy and automaticity in action control (see e.g., Abraham & Sheeran, Chapter 1; Bargh, 1990). Acknowledging that one has failed to control impulses and desires in particular situations highlights the need to establish action control processes to change behaviour in those contexts. These could involve the development of situation-specific self-efficacy and implementation intention formation (see Gollwitzer & Oettingen, Chapter 11). However, while such cognitive preparation is in progress avoidance of the specified situations may prevent lapses into now unwanted but previously established behaviour patterns. Counter-conditioning and reinforcement management involve manipulating the actual outcomes of action by taking time to reward oneself for intended action and removing rewards for behaviour which one is trying to change. From a cognitive perspective such action should alter outcome expectances and so change attitudes and strengthen intentions. It could also change goal prioritisation. It would be interesting to examine whether cognitive effects of this kind do, in fact, mediate the effects of such strategies on behaviour change.

Kuhl has also highlighted a set of self-regulatory processes which appear to support behaviour change. Fuhrmann and Kuhl (1998) found that those who scored more highly on measures attentional control (e.g., not attending to tempting stimuli or thoughts), impulse control (e.g., suppressing unwanted desires) motivational control (e.g., thinking of rewards and succeeding in self-regulatory goals) and decision-making control (e.g., making fast and stable decisions) were more likely to take advantage of opportunities to regulate their diet. These control strategies seemed to be especially important in the case of goals involving new behaviours (e.g., eat more of X) which were thought to be difficult and in the case of goals involving reducing previously established behaviour (e.g., eat less of X) which were thought to be easy. Further research could clarify the range of application of such strategies and explore how their effects are related to those of enhancing self-efficacy and planning.

Promotion of conscious consideration of, and intervention in, one's own cognitive regulation has been commonplace in the practice of cognitive-behaviour therapy (e.g., Meichenbaum, 1977). The challenge for cognitive theories is to link cognitive models of control with such self-regulatory intervention strategies. This may prove complex but it could generate more powerful intervention strategies which include; persuasion techniques targeting beliefs and attitudes (including threat perception and normative beliefs), various approaches to enhancing self-efficacy, instructions and rehearsal techniques designed to strengthen intention formation, implementation intention formation and planning, value-laden communications designed to prompt the reorganisation of goal hierarchies as well as self-regulatory techniques which support people in the conscious management of thought and action, while attempting to establish new behaviours. Further research could attempt to integrate these techniques and quantify their relative effects on behaviour change in various domains.

CONCLUDING COMMENTS ON FURTHER RESEARCH AND INTERVENTION DEVELOPMENT

The discussion above highlights the need to develop more theoretically integrated models of behaviour change. Such models should consider dispositional tendencies, motivational processes affecting intention formation, volitional processes affecting action regulation, goal hierarchies and self-regulatory strategies affecting cognition and action control. Although complex, such integrative models may be able to cast light on potential contradictory findings, e.g., those that suggest that a particular intervention is effective in some circumstances but not others or for some people but not others. Testing such theories requires controlled experimental work which allows attribution of effects to particular treatments and shows that such effects can be explained by predicted changes in mediating cognition.

The experimental examination of theory-derived psychological changes is important when evaluating interventions. Although the effectiveness of an intervention may be rigorously tested using a randomised control trial, this may not clarify why the intervention is effective. Thus, from a psychological perspective, it is important to test the effectiveness of intervention components to identify 'active ingredients'. For example, is an intervention effective because of its fearful presentation or because of its strong arguments promoting perceived susceptibility, severity and self-efficacy? Does it prompt intention formation or prompt intenders to act? Addressing such questions is likely to involve testing intervention components in sequential combinations or stages so as to establish what combination is responsible for observed effects on cognition and behaviour. It will also involve measuring disposition, cognitive, volitional and self-regulatory processes before and after interventions so that potential mediators of behaviour change can be identified. In this way a psychology of behaviour change and a science of health promotion can be managed in a co-ordinated manner.

A potential methodological problem may need to be addressed by such research; namely, the measurement of different types of change. Drawing upon research into change prompted by interventions used in organisational development (Golembiewski, Billingsley & Yeager, 1976), Norman and Parker (1996) note that different types of change may manifest themselves in measures of health-related cognition and behaviour. In particular, they note that as well as straightforward increases or decreases (alpha change) people may report change because they have recalibrated the dimension along which the construct is measured (beta change) or because they have re-conceptualised their reality and now think about themselves in different terms altogether (gamma change). In many cases psychologists may be concerned only with alpha change. However, it is important that beta and gamma changes are not confused with alpha change, especially when pre- and post- intervention scores are compared.

For example, an intervention might change people's view of control (e.g., through social comparison) so that they regard themselves as having relatively more control (because they see others as less in control) but, nevertheless, no more likely to perform a recommended action. This is a beta change which should not be confused with alpha changes in behaviour-specific self-efficacy. Such confusions can often be avoided by the use of precise measures of key constructs and Norman and Parker (1996) review some of the methods that are used to detect such changes.

This chapter, and much of this volume, has focused on the link between cognitive and behavioural change. This focus is appropriate to the development of a psychology of health-related behaviour change. However, any under-standing of health-related behaviour must be contextualised within an awareness of wider societal structures. For example, although we may be able to change attitudes towards a preventive action by using persuasive communication to alter outcome expectancies or by instructing people to change actual outcomes using self-regulating reward schedules, these attitudes may be more strongly influenced by consequences determined by social and political processes. For example, the consequences of buying cigarettes or healthy food may depend critically on pricing and taxation policies developed at corporate and government level. Similarly, reorganising goal hierarchies to prioritise health-related goals may be importantly facilitated by resources that give people control over their social environment. Thus understanding health inequalities depends upon a societal-level analysis (e.g., Alder et al., 1994; Wilkinson, 1996).

Social and political process will also determine investment in intervention development and evaluation. It is, therefore, important to demonstrate the benefits of such interventions to health care providers. For example, as well as contributing to the achievement of population-based health targets, psychological interventions can be cost effective because, for example, they may reduce demands for professional time and therapeutic drugs. Friedman, Sobel, Myers, Caudill and Benson (1995) show that behavioural interventions have resulted in substantial savings in US health services (e.g., in hypertension treatment, arthritis care and community services for the elderly). In some cases, such as post-surgical care, the cost offset may be ten times that spent on delivering psychological interventions. However, the development and evaluation of effective health-related behaviour change interventions may not generate profit and may, therefore, be dependent upon public and governmental support.

Similar processes are involved in the diffusion of effective interventions (such as the personalised, computer-based interventions described by Bandura in Chapter 13). Diffusion of interventions can be understood in terms of the social processes which determine innovation adoption, more generally. These have been studied in relation to industrial and farming innovations (e.g., Abraham & Hayward, 1985; Rogers, 1983) and more recently in relation to health promotion interventions (e.g., Paulussen, 1994). In line with previous research, Orlandi, Landers, Weston and Haley (1990), for example, argue that the diffusion process should involve a collaborative partnership between the group promoting a programme and its potential users, operating through what they call the 'linkage system'. This will involve tailoring interventions to the practicalities of the context in which they are to be implemented so that they are sustainable in routine practice and replicable across services (e.g., Wight & Abraham, in press). This, in turn, will require closer co-operation between service providers and those developing and testing interventions.

Thus, as Bandura reminds us (in Chapter 13) effective health promotion may depend upon developing 'collective self-efficacy' by raising public awareness of the implications of policy development and empowering people to become involved in political action which may influence corporate and political agendas. This highlights a community-development role for health psychologists. Public support may be essential to securing appropriate levels of investment in applying psychological theory to the development of behaviour change interventions and ensuring the growth of evidence-based health promotion.

REFERENCES

Abraham, C. & Hayward, G. (1985). Towards a more microscopic analysis of industrial innovation: From diffusion curves to technological integration through participative management. *Technovation, 3*, 3–17.

Abraham, C., Sheeran, P., Norman, N., Conner, P., de Vries, N., & Otten, W. (1999). When good intentions are not enough: Modeling post-intention cognitive correlates of condom use. *Journal of Applied Social Psychology*, 29, 2591–2612.

Ajzen, I. (1998). Models of human social behavior and their application to health psychology. *Psychology and Health, 13*, 735–739.

Ajzen, I. (1991). The theory of planned behavior. *Organizational Behavior and Human Decision Processes, 50*, 179–211.

Alder, N. E., Boyce, T., Chesney M. A., Cohen S., Folkman, S., Kahn, R. L. & Syme, S. L. (1994). Socio-economic status and health: The challenge of the gradient. *American Psychologist, 49*, 15–24.

Baer, J. S. Marlatt, G. A. Kivlahan, D. R., Fromme, K., Larimer, M. E., & Williams, E. (1992). An experimental test of three methods of alcohol risk reduction with young adults. *Journal of Consulting and Clinical Psychology, 60*, 974–979.

Bagozzi, R. P., Baumgartner, H., & Yi, Y. (1992). State versus action orientation and the theory of reasoned action: An application to coupon usage. *Journal of Consumer Research, 18*, 505–518.

Bagozzi, R. P. & Yi, Y. (1989). The degree of intention formation as a moderator of the attitude–behaviour relationship. *Social Psychology Quarterly, 52*, 266–279.

Banks, S. M., Salovey, P. Greener, S., Rothman, A. J., Moyer, A., Beauvais, J & Epel, E. (1995). The effects of message framing on mammography utilization. *Health Psychology, 14*, 178–184.

Bandura, A. (1997). *Self-efficacy: The Exercise of Control*. New York: Freeman.

Bandura, A. (1986). *Social Foundations of Thought and Action: A Cognitive Social Theory*. Englewood Cliffs, NJ: Prentice-Hall.

Bargh, J. A. (1990). Auto-motives: Preconscious determinants of thought and behaviour. In E. T. Higgins & R. M. Sorrentino (eds.) *Handbook of Motivation and Cognition: Foundations of Social Behavior*, (Vol. 2, pp. 93–130) New York: The Guildford Press.

Beck, K. H. & Lund, A. K. (1981). The effects of health threat, seriousness, and personal efficacy upon intentions and behavior. *Journal of Applied Social Psychology, 11*, 401–415.

Best, J. A. (1975). Tailoring smoking withdrawal procedures to personality and motivational differences. *Journal of Consulting and Clinical Psychology, 43*, 1–8.

Bermudez, J. (1999). Personality and health-protective behavior. *European Journal of Personality, 13*, 83–103.

Beswick, G. & Mann, L. (1994). State orientation and procastination. In J. Kuhl & J. Beckmann (eds.) *Volition and Personality: Action Versus State Orientation*. Seattle: Hogrefe & Huber Publishers.

Booth-Kewley, S. & Vickers, R. R. (1994). Associations between major domains of personality and health behavior. *Jorunal of Personality, 62*, 281–298.

Brawley, L. R. (1993). The practicality of using social psychological theories for exercise and health research and intervention. *Journal of Applied Sport Psychology, 5*, 99–115.

Brown, I. Jr. & Inouye, D. K. (1978). Learned helplessness through modeling: The role of perceived similarity in competence. *Journal of Personality and Psychology, 36*, 900–908.

Bryan, A. D., Aiken, L. S. & West, S. G. (1996). Increasing condom use: Evaluation of a theory-based intervention to prevent sexually transmitted diseases in young women. *Health Psychology, 15*, 371–382.

Budd, R. J. & Rollnick, S. (1996). The structure of the readiness to change questionnaire: A test of Prochaska and DiClemente's transtheoretical model. *British Journal of Health Psychology, 1*, 365–376.

Byrne, D. G., Byrne, A. E. & Reinhart, M. I. (1993). Psychosocial correlates of adolescent cigarette smoking: Personality or environment. *Australian Journal of Psychology, 45*, 87–95.

Canals, J., Bladé, J. & Domènech, E. (1997). Smoking and personality predictors in young Spanish people. *Personality and Individual Differences, 23*, 905–908.

Chambliss, C. A. & Murray, E. J. (1979a). Efficacy attribution, locus of control, and weight loss. *Cognitive Therapy and Research, 3*, 349–353.

Chambliss, C. A. & Murray, E. J. (1979b). Cognitive procedures for smoking reduction: Symptom attribution versus efficacy attribution. *Cognitive Therapy and Research, 3*, 91–95.

Cherry, N. & Kiernan, K. (1976). Personality scores and smoking behaviour: A longitudinal study. *British Journal of Preventive and Social Medicine, 30*, 123–131.

Condiotte, M. M. & Lichtenstein, E. (1981). Self-efficacy and relapse in smoking cessation programs. *Journal of Consulting and Clinical Psychology, 49*, 648–658.

Conner, M. & Abraham, C. (1999). Towards a more complete model of intention formation: The role of conscientiousness and its relationship to past behaviour. Manuscript under review.

Conner, M., Sheeran, P., Norman, P., & Armitage, C. (in press). Temporal stability as a moderator of relationships in the theory of planned behaviour. *British Journal of Social Psychology*.

Costa, P. T. & McCrae, R. R. (1994). Set like plaster? Evidence for the stability of adult personality. In T. F. Heatherton & J. L Weinberger (eds.) *Can Personality Change?* Washington, DC: American Psychological Association.

Eagly, A. H. & Chaiken, S. (1993). *The Psychology of Attitudes*. Orlando: Harcourt Brace, Jovanovich.

Eliot, T. S. (1974). *Collected poems 1909–1962 by T. S. Eliot*. London: Faber and Faber Ltd.

Evans, R. I., Dratt, L. M., Raines, B. E., & Rosenberg, S. S. (1988). Social influences on smoking initiation: Importance of distinguishing descriptive versus mediating process variables. *Journal of Applied Social Psychology, 18*, 925–943.

Festinger, L. (1957). *A Theory of Cognitive Dissonance*. Stanford: Stanford University Press.

Fishbein, M. & Ajzen, I. (1975). *Belief, Attitude, Intention and Behavior: An Introduction to Theory and Research*. Reading, MA: Addison-Wesley.

Fisher, J. D. & Fisher W. A. (1992). Changing AIDS risk behavior. *Psychological Bulletin, 111*, 455–474.

Fisher, K. & Johnston, M. (1996). Experimental manipulation of perceived control and its effect on disability. *Psychology and Health, 11*, 657–669.

Friedman, R., Sobel, D., Myers, P., Caudill, M. & Benson, H. (1995). Behavioral medicine, clinical health psychology and cost offset. *Health Psychology, 14*, 509–518.

Friedman, H. S., Tucker, J. S., Schwartz, J. E., Martin, L. R., Tomlinson-Keasay, C., Wingard, D. L., & Criqui, M. H. (1995). Childhood conscientiousness and longevity: Health behaviors and cause of death. *Journal of Personality and Social Psychology, 68*, 696–703.

Friedman, H. S., Tucker, J. S., Tomlinson-Keasay, C., Schwartz, J. E., Wingard, D. L., & Criqui, M. H. (1993). Does childhood personality predict longevity? *Journal of Personality and Social Psychology, 65*, 176–185.

Furnham, A. & Heaven, P. (1999). *Personality and Social Behaviour*. London: Arnold.

Fuhrmann, A. & Kuhl, J. (1998). Maintaining a healthy diet: Effects of personality and self-reward versus self-punishment on commitment to and enactment of self-chosen and assigned goals. *Psychology and Health, 13*, 651–686.

Godin, G. & Kok, G. (1996). The theory of planned behavior: A review of its applications to health-related behaviors. *American Journal of Health Promotion, 11*, 87–97.

Golembiewski, R. T., Billingsley, K. & Yeager, S. (1976). Measuring change and persistence in human affairs: Types of change generated by OD designs. *Journal of Applied Behavioural Science, 12*, 133–157.

Gollwitzer, P. M. (1993). Goal achievement: The role of intentions. *European Review of Social Psychology, 4*, 142–185.

Greenwald, A. G. & Ronis, D. L. (1978). Twenty years of dissonance: Case study of the evolution of a theory. *Psychological Review, 85*, 53–55.

Harlow, L. L., Prochaska, J. O., Redding, C. A., Rossi, J. S., Velicer, W. F., Snow, M. G., Schnell, D., Galvotti, C., O'Reilly, K., Rhodes, F. and the AIDS Community Demonstration Project Research Group (1999). Stages of condom use in a high HIV-risk sample. *Psychology and Health, 14*, 143–157.

Harmon-Jones, E., Brehm, J. W., Greenberg, J., Simon, L. & Nelson, D. E. (1996) Evidence that the production of aversive consequences is not necessary to create cognitive dissonance. *Journal of Personality and Social Psychology, 70*, 5–16.

Heafner, D. P. & Kirscht, J. P. (1970). Motivational and behavioural effects of modifying health beliefs. *Public Health Reports, 85*, 478–484.

Heather, N., Rollnick, S., Bell, A. & Richmond, R. (1996). Effects of brief counselling among male heavy drinkers identified on general hospital wards. *Drug and Alcohol Review, 15*, 29–38.

Heckhausen, H. (1991). *Motivation and Action*. Heidelberg: Springer.

John, O. P., Cheek, J. M., & Klohnen, E. C. (1996). On the nature of self-monitoring: Construct explication with Q-sort ratings. *Journal of Personality and Social Psychology, 71*, 763–776.

Kahneman, D. & Tversky, A. (1979). Prospect theory: An analysis of decision under risk. *Econometrica, 47*, 263–291.

Kalichman, S. C., Carey, M. P. & Johnson, B. T. (1996). Prevention of sexually transmitted HIV infection: A meta-analytic review of the behavioral outcome literature. *American Behavioural Medicine, 18*, 6–15.

Kendzierski, D. (1990). Decision making versus decision implementation: An action control approach to exercise adoption and adherence. *Journal of Applied Social Psychology, 20*, 27–45.

Kuhl, J. (1982). Handlungskontrolle als metakognitivier vermittler zwischen intention und handlen: Freizeitaktivitaeten bei hauptschuelern. *Zeitschrift für Entwicklungspsychologie und Paedagogische Psychologie, 14*, 141–148.

Kuhl, J. (1985). Volitional mediators of cognition-behavior consistency: Self-regulatory processes and action versus state orientation. In J. Kuhl & J. Beckman (eds.), *Action Control: From Cognition to Behavior* (pp. 101–128). New York: Springer.

Kuhl, J. (1992). A theory of self-regulation: Action versus state orientation, self-discrimination and some applications. *Applied Psychology; An International Review, 41*, 97–129.

Leventhal, H. (1970). Findings and theory in the study of fear communications. In L. Berkowitz (ed.) *Advances in Experimental Social Psychology, 5*, (pp. 119–186), San Diego: Academic Press.

Ley, P. (1988). *Communicating with Patients; Improving Communication, Satisfaction and Compliance*. London: Chapman and Hall.

Maibach, E., Flora, J. A., & Nass, C. (1991). Changes in self-efficacy and health behavior in response to a minimal community health campaign. *Health Communication, 3*, 1–15.

Marshall, G. N., Wortman, C. B., Vickers, R. R., Kusulas, J. W., & Hervig, L. K. (1994). The five-factor model of personality as a framework for personality-health research. *Journal of Personality and Social Psychology, 67*, 278–286.

Matthews, K. A. (1988). Coronary heart disease and type A behaviors: Update on and alternative to the Booth-Kewley and Friedman (1987) Quantitative Review. *Psychological Bulletin, 104*, 373–380.

McCaul, K. D., Glasgow, R. E., & O'Neill, H. K. (1992). The problem of creating habits: Establishing health-protective dental behaviors. *Health Psychology, 11*, 101–110.

McConnaughy, E. A., DiClemente, C. C., Prochaska, J. O. & Velicer, W. (1989). Stages of change in psychotherapy: A follow-up report. *Psychotherapy, 26*, 494–503.

McCrae, R. R. & Costa, P. T. Jr. (1987). Validation of the five-factor model of personality across instruments and observers. *Journal of Personality and Social Psychology, 54*, 81–90.

McCrae, R. R. & John, O. P. (1992). An introduction to the five-factor model and its applications. *Journal of Personality, 60, 175–215.*

McGuire, W. J. (1972) Attitude change: The information processing paradigm. In C. C. McClintok (ed.) *Experimental Social Psychology,* (pp. 108–141), New York: Holt, Rinehart & Winston.

Meichenbaum, D. (1977). *Cognitive Behaviour Modification: An Integrative Approach.* New York: Plenum Press.

Meyerowitz, B. E. & Chaiken, S. (1987). The effects of message framing on breast self-examination attitudes, intentions and behavior. *Journal of Personality and Social Psychology, 52*, 500–510.

Mutén, E. (1991). Self-reports, spouse ratings, and psychophysiological assessment in a behavioural medicine program: an application of the five factor model. *Journal of Personality Assessment, 57*, 449–464.

Norman, P. & Parker, S. (1996). The interpretation of change in verbal reports: Implications for health psychology. *Psychology and Health, 11*, 301–314.

Norman, P., Sheeran, P., & Orbell, S. (1997). Translating intentions into action: The moderating role of action control. *Proceedings of the British Psychological Society, 6*, 47. (B.P.S. Social Psychology Section Conference, Brighton).

Oakley, A., Fullerton, D., Holland, J., Arnold, S., France-Dawson, M., Kelley, P. & McGrellis. S. (1995). Sexual health education interventions for young people: A methodological review. *British Medical Journal, 310*, 158–162.

O'Brien, T. B. & Delongis, A. (1996). The interactional context of problem-, emotion-, and relationship-focused coping: The role of the big five personality factors. *Journal of Personality, 64*, 775–811.

Oostveen, T., Knibbe R. & De Vries, H. (1996). Social influences on young adults' alcohol consumption: Norms, modeling, pressure, socializing and conformity. *Addictive Behaviors, 21*, 187–197.

Orbell, S., Hodgkins, S., & Sheeran, P. (1997). Implementation intentions and the theory of planned behaviour. *Personality and Social Psychology Bulletin, 23*, 945–954.

Orlandi, M., Landers, C., Weston, R., & Haley, N. (1990). Diffusion of health promotion innovations. In K. Glanz, F. M. Lewis, & B. Rimer, (eds.) *Health Behavior and Health Education, 2nd ed.* San Francisco CA, Jossey-Bass, 288–313.

Parker, D., Stradling, S. G., & Manstead, A. S. R. (1996). Modifying beliefs and attitudes to exceeding the speed limit: An intervention study based on the theory of planned behaviour. *Journal of Applied Social Pychology, 26*, 1–19.

Paulussen, T. G. W. (1994). *Adoption and Implementation of AIDS Education in Dutch Secondary Schools.* Doctoral Thesis, Department of Health Education and Promotion, Maastricht University and Dutch Centre for Health Promotion and Health Education.

Petty R. E. & Cacioppo, J. T. (1986). The elaboration likelihood model of persuasion. In L. Berkowitz (ed.) *Advances in Experimental Social Psychology, 19*, 123–205, New York, Academic Press.

Pierce, R. F., Frone, M. R., Rusell, M. & Cooper, M. L. (1996). Financial stress, social support and alcohol involvement: A longitudinal test of the buffering hypothesis in a general population survey. *Health Psychology, 15*, 38–47.

Prochaska, J. O. & DiClemente, C. C. (1983). Stages and processes of self-change in smoking: Towards an integrative model of change. *Journal of Consulting and Clinical Psychology, 51*, 390–395.

Prochaska, J. O. & DiClemente, C. C. (1986). Towards a comprehensive model of change. In Miller, W. R. & Heather, N. (eds.) *Treating Addictive Behaviors: Processes of Change*. (pp. 3–27), New York: Plenum.

Prochaska, J. O., DiClemente, C. C. & Norcross, J. C. (1992). In search of how people change. *American Psychologist, 47*, 1102–1114.

Prochaska, J. O., DiClemente, C. C., Velicer, W. & Rossi, J. S. (1993). Standardized individualized interactive, and personalized self-help programs for smoking cessation. *Health Psychology, 12*, 399–405.

Prochaska, J. O., Velicer, W. F., DiClemente, C. C., & Fava, J. S. (1988). Measuring processes of change: Applications to the cessation of smoking. *Journal of Consulting and Clinical Psychology, 56*, 520–528.

Prochaska, J. O., Velicer, W. Guadagnoli, E., Rossi, J. S. & DiClemente, C.C. (1991). Patterns of change: Dynamic typology applied to smoking cessation. *Multivariate Behavioural Research, 26*, 83–107.

Quadrel, M. J. & Lau, R. R. (1989). Health promotion, health locus of control, and health behavior: Two field experiments. *Journal of Applied Social Psychology, 18*, 1497–1521.

Quine, L., Arnold, L., & Rutter, D. R. (1999). Development and evaluation of a theory based intervention to promote helmet use in school aged cyclists. Manuscript under review.

Rigby, K., Brown, M., Anagnostou, P., Ross, M. W. & Rosser, B. R. S. (1989). Shock tactics to counter AIDS: The Australian experience. *Psychology and Health, 3*, 145–159.

Rippetoe, P. A. & Rogers, R. W. (1987). Effects of components of protection motivation theory on adaptive and maladaptive coping with a health threat. *Journal of Personality and Social Psychology, 52*, 596–604.

Rogers, E. M. (1983). *Diffusion of Innovations*. New York: Free Press.

Rothman, A., Salovey, P., Autone, C., Keough, K. & Martin, C. (1993). The influence of message framing on health behaviour. *Journal of Experimental Social Psychology, 29*, 408–433.

Schwarzer, R. (1992). Self-efficacy in the adoption and maintenance of health behaviors: Theoretical approaches and a new model. In R. Schwarzer (ed.) *Self-Efficacy: Thought Control of Action*. (pp 217–243) Washington: Hemisphere.

Sheeran, P., Abraham, C., & Orbell, S. (1999). Psychosocial correlates of condom use: A meta-analysis. *Psychological Bulletin, 125*, 90–132.

Sheeran, P., Orbell, S. & Trafimow, D. (1999). Does temporal stability of behavioral intentions moderate intention-behavior and past behavior-future behavior relations? *Personality and Social Psychology Bulletin, 26*, 721–730.

Siegler, I. C., Feaganes, J. R., & Rimer, B. K. (1995). Predictors of adoption of mammography in women under age 50. *Health Psychology, 14*, 274–278.

Stainback, R. D. & Rogers, R. W. (1983). Identifying effective components of alcohol abuse prevention programs: Effects of fear appeals, message style and source expertise. *International Journal of Addictions, 18*, 393–405.

Stein, J. A., Newcomb, M. D., & Bentler, P. M. (1996). Initiation and maintenance of tobacco smoking: Changing personality correlates in adolescence and young adulthood. *Journal of Applied Social Psychology, 26,* 160–187.

Stevens, V. J. & Hollis, J. F. (1989). Preventing smoking relapse, using an individually tailored skills-training technique. *Journal of Consulting and Clinical Psychology, 57,* 420–424.

Stock, J. & Cervone, D. (1990). Proximal goal setting and self-regulatory processes. *Cognitive Therapy and Research , 14,* 483–498.

Stone, J., Aronson, E., Crain, A. L., Winslow, M. P.& Fried, C. B. (1994). Inducing hypocrisy as a means of encouraging young adults to use condoms. *Personality and Social Psychology Bulletin, 20,* 116–128.

Sutton, S. R. (1982). Fear arousing communications: A critical examination of theory and research. In J. R. Eiser (ed.) *Social Psychology and Behavioural Medicine,* (pp. 303–337) New York: Wiley.

Sutton, S. R. (1996). Can 'stages of change' provide guidance in the treatment of addictions? A critical examination of Prochaska and DiClemente's model. In G. Edwards and C. Dare (eds.) *Psychotherapy, Psychological Treatments and the Addictions.* (pp 189–205) Cambridge: Cambridge University Press.

Trafimow, F. & Finlay, K. (1996). The importance of subjective norms for a minority of people. *Personality and Social Psychology Bulletin, 22,* 820–828.

Tucker, L. A. (1984). Psychological differences between adolescent smoking intenders and nonintenders. *Journal of Psychology, 118,* 37–43.

Van den Putte, B. (1993). *On the Theory of Reasoned Action.* Unpublished doctoral dissertation, University of Amsterdam, The Netherlands.

Van Heck, G. L. (1997). Personality and physical health: Toward an ecological approach to health-related personality research. *European Journal of Personality, 11,* 415–443.

Van Knippenberg, D. (1999). Social identity and persuasion: reconsidering the role of group membership. In D. Abrams & M. A. Hogg (eds.) *Social Identity and Social Cognition,* (pp 315–331), Oxford: Blackwell.

Vingerhoets, A. J. .J. M., Croon, M., Jeninga, A. J., & Menges, L. J. (1990). Personality and health habits. *Psychology and Health, 4,* 333–342.

Wallston, B. S., Wallston, K. A., Kaplan, G. D., & Maides, S. A. (1976). Development and validation of the health locus of control (HLC) scale. *Journal of Consulting and Clinical Psychology, 44,* 580–585.

Watson, D. & Hubbard, B. (1996). Adaptational style and dispositional structure: Coping in the context of the five factor model. *Journal of Personality, 64,* 737–774.

Weinstein, N. D. (1988). The precaution adoption process. *Health Psychology, 7,* 355–386.

Weinstein, N. D., Lyon, J. E., Sandman, P. M. & Cuite, C. L. (1998). Experimental evidence for stages of health behavior change: The precaution adoption process applied to home radon testing. *Health Psychology, 17,* 445–453.

Weinstein, N. D., Rothman, A. J., & Sutton, S. R. (19998) Stage theories of health behavior: Conceptual and methodological Issues. *Health Psychology, 17,* 290–299.

Weinstein, N. D. & Sandman, P. M. (1992). A model of the precaution adoption process: Evidence from home radon testing. *Health Psychology, 11,* 170–180.

White, V., Hill, D. & Hopper, J. (1996). The outgoing, the rebellious and the anxious: Are adolescent personality dimensions related to the uptake of smoking? *Psychology and Health, 12,* 73–85.

Wight, D. & Abraham C. (in press). From psycho-social theory to sustainable classroom practice: Developing a research-based teacher-delivered sex education programme. *Health Education Research.*

Wilkinson, R. G. (1996). *Unhealthy Societies: The Afflictions of Inequality*. London: Routledge.

Wurtele, S. K. (1988). Increasing women's calcium intake: The role of health beliefs, intentions and health value. *Journal of Applied Social Psychology, 18*, 627–639.

Index

action identification theory, 18
anticipated affect, 8, 10, 17
anticipated regret, 75, 93
ASE model, 165–183
  alcohol use, 169
  dietary behaviour, 169
  exercise, 169
  smoking, 169–70, 171–7
attitude, 5, 8–12, 14–15, 27, 29–32,
  34, 37–46, 74–5, 77–8, 82–3,
  85–6, 88–90, 93, 101–10,
  115–33, 138–9, 166–7, 169,
  172–3, 175–6, 181, 191,
  194–202, 229, 263–8, 272–4,
  306, 308–9, 344
attitudinal control, 10, 12, 101–10,
  344, 351
attributions, 166, 248–9
automaticity, 14–16

behavioural beliefs, 27, 35, 39, 40–1,
  44–5, 77–8, 80, 83, 102,
  115–33, 166, 191, 274
behavioural willingness, 8, 11,
  137–56
  drink driving, 146–51
  sexual behaviour, 140
  smoking, 142–6
  substance abuse, 140

centrality, 279–80
cognitive behavioural therapy, 14–16
cognitive-social health information
  processing model, 69
collective efficacy, 328–32, 362
collective self, 106–8

conscientiousness, 349–50
control beliefs, 77–8, 80, 191
coping appraisal, 52–57, 60, 67
cues to action, 75–77, 80, 89, 171

decisional balance, 168, 190
Delancy programme, 325–6
depression, 242, 303–4
descriptive norms, 8, 10–11

elaboration likelihood model, 92,
  139, 354–5
energization theory, 243
extraversion, 344, 349–50

fear, 10, 53–4, 57, 59, 61–2, 64

goals, 16–18, 230–56, 261–93, 301,
  307–8, 343
guilt, 154–5

habit, 15–16, 66, 74, 171, 238–40
health action process approach, 207,
  346, 359
health behaviour goal model, 207
health belief model, 3–5, 73–93, 115,
  166, 229, 299, 301, 306, 343,
  350
  cycle helmet use, 9, 73–93
  road safety behaviour, 74
health locus of control, 77

implementation intentions, 14–16, 18,
  229–56, 261, 266, 346, 351,
  358–9
implemental mindsets, 233–4, 240–5

371